BOOKS PUBLISHED BY ALAN R. LISS, INC.
FOR THE NATIONAL FOUNDATION

GENETIC COUNSELING: FACTS, VALUES, AND NORMS

The National Foundation — March of Dimes
Birth Defects: Original Article Series, Volume XV, Number 2, 1979

GENETIC COUNSELING: FACTS, VALUES, AND NORMS

Editors:

Alexander M. Capron, LLB, Marc Lappé, PhD

Robert F. Murray, Jr., MD, MS, Tabitha M. Powledge, MS

Sumner B. Twiss, PhD, Daniel Bergsma, MD

Assistant Editor:

Sue Conde Green

ALAN R. LISS, INC., NEW YORK

To enhance medical communication in the birth defects field, The National
Foundation publishes the *Birth Defects Atlas and Compendium,* an *Original
Article Series, Syndrome Identification,* a *Reprint Series,* and provides a series
of films and related brochures.

Further information can be obtained from:

The National Foundation
Professional Education Division
1275 Mamaroneck Avenue
White Plains, New York 10605

Published by:

Alan R. Liss, Inc.
150 Fifth Avenue
New York, New York 10011

Library of Congress Cataloging in Publication Data
Main entry under title:

Genetic counseling.
    (Birth defects original article series; v. 15, no. 2)
    Includes bibliographic references and index.
    1. Genetic counseling.
    I. Capron, Alexander Morgan. II. National Foundation.
    III. Series.
    [DNLM: 1. Genetic counseling — Congresses. 2. Hereditary
    Diseases — Congresses. W1 BI966 v. 15 no. 2 / QZ50.3 G324 1978]
    RG626.B63 vol. 15, no. 2 [RB155] 616'.043'08s
    ISBN 0-8451-1025-X   [616'.042]   79-1736

Printed in the United States of America.

Contents

Contributors

Ray M. Antley, Director, Division of Medical Genetics, Methodist Hospital, Indianapolis, IN 46202 **[137]**

Sidney Callahan, 84 Summit Drive, Hastings-on-Hudson, NY 10706 **[217]**

Arthur Caplan, Associate for the Humanities, The Hastings Center, 360 Broadway, Hastings-on-Hudson, NY 10706 **[21]**

Alexander M. Capron, Associate Professor of Law, University of Pennsylvania Law School, Philadelphia, PA 19104 **[307]**

Kenneth Casebeer, The Law School, Box 248087, University of Miami, Coral Gables, FL 33124 **[279]**

James F. Childress, Professor of Christian Ethics, Kennedy Institute for the Study of Human Reproduction and Bioethics, Georgetown University, Washington, DC 20057 **[279]**

Arthur J. Culbert, Department of Community Medicine, Boston University School of Medicine, 80 East Concord Street, Boston, MA 02118 **[85]**

Jessica G. Davis, Director, Child Development and Genetics Program, North Shore University Hospital, 300 Community Drive, Manhasset, NY 11030 **[113]**

John Fletcher, President, Interfaith Metropolitan Theological Education, Inc., Washington, DC 20009 **[239]**

F. Clarke Fraser, Director, Department of Medical Genetics, The Montreal Children's Hospital, Montreal, Quebec, Canada H3H, 1P3 **[5]**

Y. Edward Hsia, Departments of Human Genetics and Pediatrics, Yale University School of Medicine, New Haven, CT 06510
Present Address: Departments of Genetics and Pediatrics, University of Hawaii Medical School, Honolulu, HI **[169]**

Richard T. Hull, Associate Professor of Philosophy, State University of New York at Buffalo, Buffalo, NY 14260 **[57]**

Seymour Kessler, Director, Genetic Counseling Option, Health and Medical Sciences Program, University of California, Berkeley, Berkeley, CA 94720 **[187]**

Marc Lappé, c/o Department of Health, Room 1253, 714 P Street, Sacramento, CA 95814 **[33]**

Carol Levine, Managing Editor, Hastings Center Report, The Hastings Center, Hastings-on-Hudson, NY 10706 **[123]**

Robert F. Murray, Jr., Professor of Pediatrics and Medicine, Howard University College of Medicine, Washington, DC 20059 **[71]**

Tabitha M. Powledge, Associate for Biosocial Studies, The Hastings Center, 360 Broadway, Hastings-on-Hudson, NY 10706 **[103]**

Philip Reilly, Fellow, Program in Law, Science and Medicine, Yale Law School, New Haven, CT 06520 **[291]**

Richard Roblin, Head, Molecular Biology of Tumor Cells Group, Basic Research Program, NCI-Frederick Cancer Research Center, Frederick, MD 21701 **[47]**

James R. Sorenson, Department of Socio-Medical Sciences, Boston University School of Medicine, 80 East Concord Street, Boston, MA 02118 **[85]**

Sumner B. Twiss, Associate Professor of Religious Studies, Brown University, Providence, RI 02912 **[201, 255]**

Preface

A clinical practice based on scientific and technologic capacities alone is not equipped to deal effectively with the social, economic, ethical, and legal issues engendered by modern medicine and biology. This is true of any medical specialty, but is particularly true of a specialty just coming into its own, as medical genetics is. The normative problems of genetic counseling seem especially exigent, partly because there is no public or even medical agreement about the idea of intervening in human genetics. What is clear, though, is that genetic counselors cannot by themselves resolve these problems.

Some hope for success may attach to a method that requires working at the junction of medicine, social science, philosophy, biology, public policy, and law. Thus, the Genetics Research Group of the Hastings Center, Institute of Society, Ethics and the Life Sciences, some time ago adopted the working assumption that critical and normative analysis of applied science and its implications — in this case, applied human genetics and the practice of genetic counseling — is best carried out by interdisciplinary inquiry.

This type of inquiry is characterized by two main features. First, it uses traditional modes of research appropriate to each of the disciplines represented. Second, it aims to achieve working rapport and a shared language among these disciplines. The first feature is necessary because valid normative inquiry requires accurate data on which to reflect — accurate biologic and medical data, and accurate sociologic and economic data. Moreover, if it is not to become merely esoteric, normative analysis requires the use of tested and well wrought techniques of argument from moral and social philosophy, law, and public policy. The second feature of interdisciplinary inquiry points to the unique advantages of intentionally crossing traditional disciplinary boundaries. Only through the shared and counterpoised reasoning of scientists and humanists, checking and rechecking their results by coming up against each other's points of view, can one escape from the preconceptions of each discipline and attain new (and valid) conceptual and normative advances.

In designing this volume and putting it together, the editors — with backgrounds in economics, law, experimental pathology, pediatric medicine, clinical genetics, evolutionary biology, philosophy, and religion — brought to bear several years of shared work on the moral and social problems of contemporary genetics, some of which work was also shared by many of the contributors. Thus there are, in this volume, some ideas and arguments that will be unfamiliar to those accustomed to the technical literature of genetic counseling, and others similarly novel for people trained exclusively in the humanities.

Birth Defects: Original Article Series, Volume XV, Number 2, **pages 1—3**
© **1979 The National Foundation**

Genetic counseling, in the form of "heredity counseling," was one of the earliest uses of human genetics in clinical medical practice. At first, such counseling was limited in scope. Until very recently counselors could only present clients with diagnoses of genetic defects after the birth of an affected child and with risk statements about future reproducti behavior based on Mendelian genetics or on knowledge of a few genetic diseases having identified modes of inheritance. In some cases, it was also possible to give empiric risk figures based on epidemiologic evidence. However, with rapid advances in knowledge about genetic diseases, and the advent of carrier detection and prenatal diagnosis, genetic counseling has become a more precise and extensively used clinical service.

The expansion of these counseling services has led to a significant effort by health professionals to establish operating principles for genetic counseling. Research and policy discussion has centered on the following sorts of questions: How can genetic counselors achieve a greater correlation between reproductive behavior and risk estimates? What are the appropriate professional qualifications and activities of the genetic counselor? What are the acceptable styles of counseling interaction?

But there are other questions, too, and they are often not addressed. A central unanswered question is: What is genetic counseling for? Counselors have taken many points of view on the aims of counseling, but often not explicitly, nor with critical analysis of those aims. Is counseling concerned solely with conveying accurate and value-neutral information? Is it intended to prevent suffering? Whose? The family's, the affected child's, even the counselor's? What is the family's obligation? What are standards of responsible parenthood, and how can they be achieved? What are some of the hidden transactions going on in a genetic counseling session? What are patients looking for besides obvious recurrence-risk information? What are counselors' obligations in this regard, and how able are they to fulfill them? Is there something about genetic counseling that makes it different from other kinds of counseling and different from other kinds of medicine, too? Should counselors pay attention to patient values, and, if so, how can counselors find out what they are?

The unanswered questions posed by the increase in genetic counseling are not limited to the problems for individuals, but extend to society as well. Is counseling done for the improvement of the human gene pool? Is such improvement technically possible? What is a "good" gene, anyway, if genetic functioning depends on context? Can a relatively esoteric specialty like medical genetics contribute to solving — or exacerbating — our problems of social justice? How much of our money should we, personally or as a society, be paying for medical genetics? What policy issues are engendered by the growth of medical genetics, and its consistent enshrinement in law? Should these questions be left to each counselor to answer for him- or herself, or are there norms of acceptable behavior which delimit "good counseling"? This book tries to address both the conventionally asked questions and these other ones, less obvious but no less important.

The book is composed of a series of critical inquiries into the conceptual problems and policy issues raised by current practices in genetic counseling. The Introduction sketches, both retrospectively and prospectively, the scientific and clinical contours of applied human genetics, thus setting the stage for subsequent exploration of the conceptual and normative dimensions of the practice of genetic counseling. In Part I, key concepts in medical genetics — genetic disease and genetic health — are analyzed in order to expose the deep evaluative presuppositions of genetic counseling. In Parts II and III, questions of moral and social policy concentrate on the following areas: dynamics and values of genetic counseling, individual rights and social obligations in medical genetics, legal protections for the counselor and client in genetic counseling.

Our hope is that something here will open a new window on the world of human genetics for each reader, bringing about a fresh examination of old ideas and perhaps even ideals. Our goal will have been accomplished if this book prompts you to say, "I never thought of it that way before."

The Editors

Introduction: The Development of Genetic Counseling

F. Clarke Fraser, MD

Twenty-five years ago, when a few lonely souls calling themselves medical geneticists were beginning to appear on the scene, most genetic counseling recognized as such was done by nonmedical geneticists, as a sideline to their main interests, research and teaching. Counseling was involved mainly with applying the Mendelian laws to a particular family situation. There was what seemed like quite a lot of information about the inheritance of human diseases in the literature, "enough to fill ten volumes," according to one author [1]. Yet much of it was misleading because of the tendency to choose strikingly familial cases for publication, failure to correct for ascertainment bias, overenthusiastic attempts to fit data to simple Mendelian patterns, and failure to appreciate the complexities involved in applying genetic principles to individual family problems [2]. There were a few textbooks on human genetics, and none that made reference to genetic counseling.

It is interesting to speculate on why physicians tended, in general, to ignore the practical applications of genetics to medicine, in spite of valiant efforts by a few pioneers to promote the teaching of genetics in medical school and its use in practice [3]. I suspect that disaffection with the eugenics movement was not the major cause of their indifference to genetics — physicians just were not aware of its relevance (see Chapter 1). For one thing, the diseases that showed simple Mendelian inheritance were all very rare, to the point of being esoteric, so that a physician might think that the chances of ever coming across one in practice were so slim it was not worth learning the rules. Also, the concept of "constitutional" diseases was well recognized and accepted — certain families are "predisposed" to certain diseases (the tacit assumption being that all family members inherited the predisposition). But this was contrary to the message of Mendelism,

Birth Defects: Original Article Series, Volume XV, Number 2, **pages 5–15**

namely that certain members of a family would inherit the disease and others would not. A related factor is, perhaps, the fact that physicians are used to making yes-or-no decisions and therefore find a probability prognosis dissatisfying.

A condition the relevance of which is not widely appreciated is "probability dysgnosia," a disorder frequently observed in medical students and graduates. Idiopathic in etiology, it results in marked abhorrence of the laws of probability. It appears not to be congenital; medical students who passed undergraduate courses in genetics without a qualm have become so severely affected that they blanch at the sight of a q^2. Results of treatment are generally poor, and the patient may complete his whole professional career suffering from the delusion that the laws of genetics are an impenetrable mystery.

Another reason why genetics did not appeal to physicians, in spite of its obvious significance, was the parlous state of specific knowledge about the genetics of particular diseases. Lectures on human genetics usually began with a series of apologies about why man was such a difficult subject for genetic research. This was supposed to account for the inadequacies and inaccuracies of our knowledge, whereas now it is probably true that, genetically, man is the *best* known eukaryote. Methods of documentation of large bodies of data and of bibliographic logistics were not well developed, and much of the available information consisted of reports of individual families. Suitable methods for the statistical analysis of human pedigree data were just being developed and were not widely applied. Paralytic poliomyelitis, for example, was made to fit a 1:4 segregation ratio by the simple approach of not excluding the proband, yet a physician dealing with the disease would know that it does not affect 1 in 4 of the patient's sibs. If a disease was shown to fit a Mendelian ratio in a few families, it was often tacitly assumed that this was so in all cases of the disease, without considering whether the series was representative. Polydactyly, for instance, was usually listed as showing autosomal dominant inheritance, whereas the observant pediatrician knows quite well that most cases are sporadic. The statement that "blue eyes are recessive" must have led to much unjustified recrimination in families that did not fit the laws. Genetic heterogeneity was recognized by some geneticists [4] but not generally taken into account by physicians, and the term itself was not coined until much later [2] . Thus, uncritical analysis of human data, and the blatant discrepancies that sometimes appeared between statements in the literature and observable fact, may have created some scepticism among physicians about the blessings of genetics. Perhaps this enhanced, and was enhanced by, the terminologic confusion of the time. "Hereditary" and "congenital" were often used synonymously. "Hereditary" was used for traits that showed vertical transmission (ie dominant), in contrast to "familial," for those that tended to occur in sibs. It was not generally recognized that a majority of cases of diseases determined by mutant genes are "sporadic" (ie the patient has no affected relatives). No wonder genetics had not been accepted as the guiding light of medicine, and was conspicuous only by its absence from most medical school curricula.

The first American genetic counseling center was probably the Eugenics Records office, founded by Davenport in 1915. In 1940 there was a Heredity Clinic at the University of Michigan and the Dight Institute of Human Genetics at the University of Minnesota. The term "genetic counseling" was introduced in about 1945 by Sheldon Reed, who did not like the eugenically tainted term "genetic hygiene" (personal communication). By 1955 it was possible to list 13 North American centers providing genetic counseling, 4 of them headed by MDs. Now the number of centers is in the hundreds, and probably those directors with medical training (some with genetic training as well) are in the majority.

In the 1950s a number of developments began to make genetic counseling more important to physicians, more interesting to ethicists, and more complicated for the genetic counselor. The control of nongenetic diseases (infectious, nutritional) was rapidly advancing, so attention began to focus more on the genetic ones. Accordingly, the number of diseases recognized as showing Mendelian inheritance began to increase rapidly. Empiric recurrence risk estimates became available for some of the commoner, familial, but not simple Mendelian diseases. Fogh-Andersen's [5] study on cleft lip and cleft palate was a trailblazer, and a series of such studies from Tage Kemp's Institute of Human Genetics in Copenhagen (the Opera ex Domo series [6]) contributed greatly to our knowledge of modes of inheritance and the risks of recurrence in various groups of relatives.

For a while there was a feeling that published lists of diseases and their recurrence risks were undesirable, as they would give those who used them, without appreciating their complexities and deficiencies, a false sense of security. Nevertheless, the rapidly growing body of knowledge, and the impossibility, for an individual counselor, of keeping up with the original literature, led to the acceptance of such lists, presumably on the grounds that a little knowledge is better than no knowledge, dangerous as it may be. One of the first of such lists [7] had about 170 entries, of which about 110 involved simple Mendelian inheritance. A current catalog, "Mendelian Inheritance in Man", lists over 2,000 Mendelian diseases [8]. Victor McKusick and The National Foundation must be credited with a major role in the promotion of medical genetics to the physician, by their collations of information [8–10] and the educational programs organized (the Bar Harbor course, the syndrome delineation conferences).

Another boost for medical genetics came with the dramatic advances in molecular and biochemical genetics, and particularly with the discovery that a biochemical defect resulting in mental deficiency (phenylketonuria) could be successfully treated and the mental retardation prevented. There were more or less successful treatments for other hereditary diseases (hemophilia, cretinism) but none had the dramatic impact of the treatment for PKU, where identifying the biochemical defect led to the rational development of a means of prevention. Continuing progress in biochemical genetics rapidly led to the identification of other inborn errors, development of methods of carrier detection, and the initiation of population screening programs for mutant genes [11].

The implementation of widespread, and often mandatory, screening programs was the first attempt to apply genetic knowledge on a societal basis since the notorious eugenics movement, and although there were unquestionable benefits, there were also unforeseen hazards. The complexities of the inborn errors — genetic heterogeneity in particular — had not been appreciated, and the necessity of adequate back-up facilities not anticipated. Screening was then extended to the clinically normal carriers of recessive mutant genes before the psychologic and social effects of discovering one is a carrier of a deleterious gene had been evaluated, and this has raised many problems [11] (see also Chapter 5). It was also screening that focused attention on the question of right to privacy and potential conflicts with the right to know. In short, the premature attempts to legislate screening programs provided us with another example of the problems evoked by trying to apply new knowledge before society is ready for it.

The third major event that contributed to the recognition of medical genetics, by the physician and the public, was the discovery of chromosomal diseases in 1959 [12, 13]. Until then the gene had been a hypothetic entity, known only by its manifestations, but now there were genetic disorders where one could actually see the cause under the microscope. The resulting increase in popularity of genetics among physicians was tremendous. In fact there was a phase when "genetic" became almost synonymous with "chromosomal," and Mendelian genetics tended to be ignored. Now perspective has been somewhat regained, but in the meantime the status of genetics in medicine had increased dramatically.

Finally, there was the advent of prenatal diagnosis of the chromosomal diseases and inborn errors of metabolism. This has become a practical approach only in the last few years [14], although amniocentesis for sex determination was reported more than 20 years ago [15]. Even more recently the multifactorial defects, represented by anencephaly/spina bifida, have become eligible for prenatal diagnosis [16]. Now improved methods of ultrasound and radiographic examination make it possible to detect major malformations, and amnioscopy has provided a means of obtaining fetal blood for the diagnosis of many of the hereditary anemias and, presumably, other hematologic disorders [17]. Biopsy of other tissues will probably be next.

The result of these advances has been to make the physician and the public progressively more aware of the practical applications of genetics in medicine, and this has led to a rapid increase in the demand for genetic health care services [18], including diagnosis (biochemical, cytogenetic, syndromologic), the prediction of recurrence risks and informing families about their medical and social implications (informative counseling, Chapter 11), providing support and making appropriate referrals for families who are working out their response to these implications (supportive counseling, Chapters 12 and 13), and follow-up of families where indicated. One would expect that the physician will become progressively better informed about genetics so that only the more complicated problems would need referral to a geneticist, but progress is slow. Genetics is still a very minor component of most medical school curricula, and what was taught in the first year has often been forgotten by graduation. Perhaps there should be a greater input into residency training programs, at which stage the need for it has become more obvious; this approach has been well received in our hospital, for instance.

What has been the effect of all this on the genetic counselor and on genetic counseling? The most obvious change is that the counselor's life has become infinitely more complicated. Patients with a tremendous variety of diseases and syndromes are now being referred for counseling, and the volume of relevant literature has expanded exponentially. In spite of a number of useful compendia [19], catalogs [8], atlases [20, 21] and various informational retrieval systems, the task of keeping up is overwhelming. The counselor must also keep up with progress in cytogenetics, and the bewildering array of deletion and mosaic syndromes now being recognized in ever-increasing numbers. A good counselor should also be familiar with the natural histories of the diseases about which he is counseling, so that he can inform his counselees about the implications of the recurrence risks he provides. He should also be skilled in interviewing, have some insight into the psychodynamics of the counseling process, and be aware of the moral and ethical implications of his counsel. In short, the genetic counselor, like the general practitioner, must be a jack-of-all-trades and may become master of almost none. One of the areas where most counselors are most deficient is knowledge of interviewing techniques and the psychodynamic interactions that go on during counseling (see Chapters 11 and 12).

The result of all this is that genetic counseling now requires a team. Optimally, the team operates in a major medical center, so that it can take advantage of modern laboratory facilities, diagnostic techniques, and expertise from a variety of disciplines, since genetic diseases affect all systems. Most, though not all, counselors feel that the informative counseling and supportive counseling is best done by an individual (though not necessarily the same one), since communication seems to work best on a one-to-one basis. The person who does the informative counseling need not be a physician (Chapter 7), but must rely on a physician in the team to take responsibility for any medical acts that may be involved. A growing practice is to have satellite centers in outlying areas around the genetics center that can provide regular clinics for the local population [22].

There is now increasing concern about quality control of genetic counseling. Undoubtedly medical genetics will eventually become a medical specialty, and genetic counselors, both medical and nonmedical, will need to be accredited by some official body (Chapter 19). The Canadian College of Medical Genetics has recently been incorporated as a professional body for this purpose [23]. It remains to be seen whether it will be recognized by other medical professional bodies and by state-supported health care programs. At least it is a positive step towards the goal of establishing genetic counseling as a bona fide health care service, and it is worth noting that provisions are made for recognizing genetic counselors without MDs, but with appropriate training in medical genetics centers.

The spectacular growth of genetics as a health care service has presented the counselor with a number of moral and ethical problems which, if not entirely new, are certainly more numerous and pressing than they were. Pressing, because the counselor who previously struggled with these problems in virtual solitude now benefits from (or at least is exposed to) the advice, exhortations, and sometimes remonstrances of a wide variety of experts in psychiatry, psychology, sociology, law, philosophy, theology, ethics, politics, and even molecular biology and physics. There is, incidentally, an interesting correlation between the degree of separation from the practice of medical genetics and the assurance with which views on its ethics are expressed.

Presented below are some of the questions that have troubled genetic counselors for a long time and have recently been attracting the attention of other experts as well.

1) *How directive should a counselor be?* Although it is practically a tenet of genetic counselors that one should never tell the counselee what to do, there is a wide range of opinions as to how far it is permissible to go in providing advice (a form of directiveness). Some counselors, particularly those medically trained, would not hesitate to state what ought to be done. Madge Macklin, for all her noteworthy contributions to the development of medical genetics, was dreadfully directive in her counseling [24]. Perhaps the fact that physicians are expected to provide explicitly directive advice in other areas influences them to do so in this one. Even some modern texts on counseling go so far as to suggest discouraging propagation when the risks are high [25]. At the other end of the spectrum are those who say that the counselor should simply provide the probability estimate required and let the family interpret this as they may. Many would agree with Milunsky [26] in trying to avoid the role of advisor, but providing all possible information that will aid the family to reach their decision. Yet it is almost impossible to avoid communicating by tone of voice, subtle changes of expression, choice of words, and even by what one does *not* say, some signals that are translated by the counselee(s) as directive. The counselor often is asked what he would do in the counselee's situation. Some would go so far as admitting what they *think* they would do in the same situation, hastening

to add that one never knows for sure what someone else would do, or even what one would do oneself in a situation not previously experienced. The latter group feels that if a counselee asks for advice by this indirect route he probably wants it, or even needs it. Some counselees will explicitly state that they have sought expert advice so that they could benefit by the counselor's wisdom and experience, and are disappointed if they do not receive guidance. Still, if the counselor feels that being directive is unethical, he should obviously try not to be. (Chapters 10–13 will extend this discussion.)

2) *Is abortion justifiable on genetic grounds?* To ask this question is to assume that abortion is justifiable on some grounds, a matter which has generated much debate. In the early days of counseling, obtaining a legal abortion was difficult. In cases where parents found that the risk and severity of a defect were so high that they wanted an abortion, the counselor could write a letter to the obstetrician in support of their request, which the obstetrician would then have to take before a hospital abortion committee. Depending on the attitude of the committee (which was often closely correlated with that of the Chief of Obstetrics), the request would be denied or approved. In any case, there were often difficulties and delays, sometimes with disastrous results [27]. This led to much soul-searching among counselors as to how high a risk, how severe a defect, and what family circumstances would justify terminating the pregnancy when the fetus might not even have the defect. The counselor might consider getting off the hook by being nondirective, in accepting what the parents considered to be the "right" decision, but in this case could not escape, since the obstetrician would want a letter stating that he, the counselor, considered that the indications justified the procedure.

The situation was exacerbated by the advent of prenatal diagnosis, which had the advantage (usually) of removing the probability element in the decision, since a definite diagnosis could be made. This probably increased the frequency of abortion for genetic reasons and attracted the attention of ethicists, lawyers, and other interested citizens to what was going on [26]. Fears were expressed that prenatal diagnosis with the expectation of possible abortion would diminish respect for life and lead to abortion being done for increasingly trivial reasons. The camel's nose argument appeared frequently — if you are not prepared to shovel, you should not let the camel get even his nose into your tent. That is, prenatal diagnosis should be stopped because it might have unfortunate social consequences. In my opinion, abortion for genetic reasons had little, if anything, to do with the recent, sudden, and dramatic change in public attitude towards induced abortion, and abortion for genetic reasons is such an unpleasant business for both mother, father, and obstetrician that it is not likely ever to be a trivial matter. I doubt, for instance, that many mothers will be willing to undergo abortion in the 16th week simply because the baby is of the unwanted sex, even though this reason seems to be becoming increasingly "permissible" [28]. But there are certainly some possible dangers. We should not deprive families of an opportunity to have healthy children, but we must be ready to protect them against negative social pressures that may develop as emphasis on the importance of not having defective children increases. (Chapters 14 and 15 elaborate on these questions.)

3) *Should genetic counseling be done if it is dysgenic?* Genetic counseling could be dysgenic (that is, tend to increase the frequency of deleterious genes) in certain circumstances. For instance, two carriers of a deleterious recessive gene ascertained in a screening program might find the 1 in 4 risk of a diseased child so formidable that they do not marry each other, but marry noncarriers instead. This would remove the opportunity for selection to act against the homozygote, and the gene frequency would slowly increase. Prenatal diagnosis and abortion of fetuses with autosomal recessive diseases would be dysgenic if there was reproductive compensation, since the subsequent child, if unaffected, would be more likely to be a heterozygote than a normal homozygote. Abortion of male fetuses when the mother is the carrier of an X-linked recessive deleterious gene would be dysgenic for similar reasons. However, the effects on gene frequency seem to be exceedingly small, even if applied on a large scale, and are generally considered to be insignificant relative to other factors influencing gene frequencies, such as our changing reproductive patterns [29].

4) *How does one protect both the welfare of the individual and of future generations when these are in conflict?* Two situations where such conflicts may arise are well known to genetic counselors. One concerns dominantly inherited diseases of variable age of onset, where it may be possible to identify carriers of the gene before the onset of overt disease. Huntington chorea is the best known example: a number of tests have been developed which, though none of them has proved reliable, have forced both potential gene carriers and counselors to face the question of whether it is better not to know. We have watched the members of a family faced with this decision sort themselves into those who would and those who would not want to take such a test and then, over a period of months, watched several members change sides. It is truly an agonizing decision. Knowing is a benefit to future generations if identified carriers refrain from having children, but knowing can be destructive to one who finds himself facing the prospect of inevitable mental and physical deterioration at some time in the future. If one decides not to take the test, the option remains, demanding an endless series of decisions. Should we then refrain from developing such a test? But this would withhold a potential benefit from those who would choose to know. It is a question that will have to be faced increasingly often as more tests are developed for more diseases of this kind. I do not believe that the solution lies in giving up our investigations, but we must be prepared to protect those who choose not to know from possible recriminations of a disapproving society.

A second kind of situation where conflict of interest is often met by counselors is that in which the need of an individual to know his family history conflicts with the right to privacy of one of his relatives. A piece of information about a relative vital to a person's genetic prognosis may reside in a hospital record which cannot be revealed without authorization which is not forthcoming. For example, a child whose grandmother has Huntington chorea is adopted, and comes for counseling when she wishes to marry. It is essential for her to know whether the mother (now 55) has the disease, but revealing her mother's identity is a breach of confidence, so how can she be traced? Does the right to privacy prevail over the right of an individual to know his genetic destiny? Sooner or later this question will have to be tested legally. Chapter 17 elaborates on this question.

5) *What nonmedical considerations should enter into decisions as to who gets screened for what?* The recent National Academy of Sciences report on screening [11] has discussed this question in some detail and only brief reference to some of the problems will be made here.

One concerns the advisability of screening for conditions that cannot be successfully treated, such as thalassemia or Duchenne muscular dystrophy. It can be argued that there is no point in identifying families at high risk of having children with serious genetic diseases unless the disease can be prevented by appropriate treatment or diagnosed prenatally and "prevented" by abortion. The anxieties and social stresses created by the testing may outweigh the (dubious) benefits, it is said. On the other hand, should one deny the knowledge that they are at risk to those who would prefer to know beforehand? For many conditions we simply do not have the necessary data and understanding to answer such questions. The question will arise with respect to an increasing number of diseases.

A related problem is the discovery of a genetic problem other than that being looked for. What does one do, for example, in a case where a (probably irrelevant) marker chromosome is found in two mentally retarded sibs; the rest of the family is karyotyped in an attempt to evaluate its significance; and the one "normal" brother, on whom all their hopes now rest, is found to have an XXY complement? The parents will resent the emotional stress thrust upon them by information that they did not seek, and which may alter adversely their attitudes toward the child. Yet it would be wrong to withhold the information, would it not?

Such problems will, no doubt, increase as the extent of, and potential for, screening increases. Perhaps accumulating knowledge and experience will provide some enlightenment. At least we may shun attempts to impose our value judgments on others through personal harassment and public pressure rather than the normally accepted methods of review, as in the unfortunate case of the XYY controversy [30].

We return again to the problem of prenatal screening and the question of how severe a defect justifies induced abortion. We are becoming able to detect disorders of increasingly benign effect, and if fetoscopy becomes practicable, the number will increase. Should a fetus be aborted who has an XXY karyotype? Cleft lip? Polydactyly? An XY karyotype when the parents wanted a girl? It would seem that being of the unwanted sex is already a valid justification in the eyes of some counselors [28]. Social considerations will become increasingly important. One father with a cleft lip suggested that prenatal sex determination should be done on his future children and the pregnancy aborted if the fetus was female, since the cosmetic defect would be far more severe for a girl, even though she would be less likely to be affected than a boy — a curious type of sex discrimination.

Social, economic, and even legal pressures may be brought increasingly to bear on families who do not avail themselves of the means to detect, and "prevent" individuals with genetic disorders (and nongenetic ones as well, for that matter). The increasing prevalence of socialized health care programs may hasten the process — for instance if a cost-benefit-minded Minister of Health decides to legislate economic penalties for those who choose to take, or ignore, a high risk of having a defective child. Where do we draw the line between the rights of the individual, of his relatives, of his future offspring, and of society? Although these are not specifically problems of genetic counseling, the counselor will see many of them at first hand, on an individual basis; he will be in a position to appreciate their complexities and to discern new ones as they begin to arise.

These and other ethical and moral problems will be discussed at length in the following chapters of this book. The present discussion has been designed to illustrate, with respect to genetic counseling, how scientific progress tends to outstrip society's knowledge of how to cope with the personal and social problems raised by the application of this progress. We hope that the rest of the book will help to reduce the gap.

REFERENCES

1. Gates GR: "Human Genetics." New York: Macmillan Co., 1946.
2. Fraser FC: Heredity counseling. The darker side. Eugen Quart 3:45–51, 1956.
3. Macklin MT: Medical genetics: A necessity in the up-to-date medical curriculum. J Hered 23(12), 1932.
4. Cockayne EA: "Inherited Abnormalities of the Skin and Its Appendages." London: Oxford University Press, 1933.
5. Fogh-Andersen P: "Inheritance of Harelip and Cleft Palate." Copenhagen: Arnold Busck, 1942.
6. Kemp T: Contributions from the University for Human Genetics, Copenhagen, vol 1–40, 1941–1958. Opera ex Domo Biol Hered Hum Univ Hafniensis, Copenhagen: E. Munksgaard, 40:3–15, 1958.
7. Fraser FC: Medical genetics in pediatrics. J Pediatr 44:85–103, 1954.
8. McKusick V: "Mendelian Inheritance in Man." 4th Ed. Baltimore: The Johns Hopkins Press, 1975.

9. McKusick VA: "Heritable Disorders of Connective Tissue." 4th Ed. St. Louis: CV Mosby, 1972.
10. Bergsma D (ed): The Clinical Delineation of Birth Defects Series. Parts I–XVI. White Plains: The National Foundation-March of Dimes, BD:OAS, 1969–1974.
11. Childs B: "Genetic Screening: Procedural Guidances and Recommendations." Washington: National Academy of Sciences, 1975.
12. Lejeune J, Gautier M, Turpin R: Etude des chromosomes somatiques de neuf enfants mongoliens. C R Acad Sci [D] (Paris) 248:1721–1722, 1959.
13. Ford CE, Jones KW, Miller OJ, Mittwoch U, Penrose LS, Ridler M, Shapiro A: The chromosomes in a patient showing both mongolism and the Klinefelter syndrome. Lancet 1:709–710, 1959.
14. Nadler HL: Antenatal detection of hereditary disorders. Pediatrics 42:912–918, 1968.
15. Sachs L, Serr DM, Danon M: Prenatal diagnosis of sex using cells from the amniotic fluid. Science 123:548, 1956.
16. Brock DJH, Sutcliffe RG: Alpha-fetoprotein in the antenatal diagnosis of anencephaly and spina bifida. Lancet 2:197–199, 1972.
17. Kaback M, Valenti C: "Intrauterine Fetal Visualization: A Multidisciplinary Approach." New York: American Elsevier, 1976.
18. Fraser FC: Genetics as a health care service. N Engl J Med 295:486–488, 1976.
19. Bergsma D (ed): "Birth Defects Atlas and Compendium." Baltimore: Williams & Wilkins for The National Foundation–March of Dimes, 1973.
20. Holmes LB, Moser HW, Halldorsen S, Mack C, Pant SS, Matzilevich B: "Mental Retardation. An Atlas of Diseases With Associated Physical Abnormalities." New York: Macmillan Co., 1972.
21. Smith DW: "Recognizable Patterns of Human Malformation." 2nd Ed. Philadelphia: WB Saunders, 1976.
22. Riccardi V: Health care and disease prevention through genetic counseling: A regional approach. Am J Public Health 66:268–272, 1976.
23. Miller JR: Canadian College of Medical Geneticists. Am J Hum Genet 28:312–314, 1976.
24. Macklin MT: The value of genetics in medicine. The Scalpel of Alpha Epsilon Delta, Feb. 1947.
25. Fuhrmann W, Vogel F: "Genetic Counselling." 2nd Ed. New York: Springer-Verlag, 1976.
26. Milunsky A (ed): "The Prevention of Genetic Disease and Mental Retardation." Philadelphia: WB Saunders, 1975, pp 64–89.
27. Fraser FC: Genetic counselling and the physician. Can Med Assoc J 99:927–934, 1968.
28. Fraser FC, Pressor C: Attitudes of counselors to prenatal sex-determination simply for choice of sex. In Lubs N, de la Cruz F (eds): "Genetic Counseling." New York: Raven Press, 1976.
29. Fraser GR, Mayo O: Genetic load in man. Humangenetik 23:83–110, 1974.
30. Hamerton JL: Human population cytogenetics: Dilemmas and problems. Am J Hum Genet 28:107–122, 1976.

I. Appraising the Legitimacy of Genetic Concepts: Introduction

Our understanding of the world and ourselves — and particularly of complex physical phenomena and the concepts through which we attempt to explain them — is conditioned by the language we use to describe the world and its inhabitants. Limitations in our means of communication are evident in scientific discussions, especially on the frontiers of knowledge where understanding is most hazy. These limitations become, if anything, only more pronounced as the topics being discussed move from the scientific realm to the medical and social. Thus, it is not surprising to discover that differences in terminology and concepts seem to lie behind much of the disputation and misunderstanding which have arisen in applied human genetics.

Mistaken concepts — such as the confusion of genes with the enzymes whose production they control — have often sent scientists off into blind alleys and have delayed the development of a field. More remarkable, however, are the instances in which accurate concepts also forestalled progress when they were misapplied or when their relationship to new subject matter was not perceived. Indeed, it is sometimes the very correctness of the misapplied concept that may explain its retarding effect; the simplicity and predictability of Mendelian genetics may thus actually have clouded geneticists' understanding of phenomena which defied such explanations. In the first chapter, Arthur Caplan analyzes the slow development of medical genetics and thereby helps to explain why genetic counseling has only recently come into its own as a legitimate specialty, backed up by sophisticated scientific understanding. He warns, moreover, that the conceptual blinders worn by human geneticists may cause further delays in the progress of their field. At the same time that we consider the slow acceptance of genetics into medicine, we may also wish to ponder, as subsequent chapters suggest, the effects on genetics as it becomes "medicalized," with consequences for the ways concepts will be used (in the doctor-patient relationship rather than in the scientific laboratory or textbook) and the new meaning that attaches to them (the difference connoted, for example, between a "*normal* fruit fly" and a "*normal* human baby").

Birth Defects: Original Article Series, Volume XV, Number 2, pages 17—19
© 1979 The National Foundation

Marc Lappé's essay expands on this point by demonstrating the complexity of the notion of "causation" in genetics. Needless to say, all branches of medicine face difficulties in explanation — in deciding "what is a cause of what" both for individual clinical cases and for entire areas of human functioning. But the very scientific rigor that is available for genetics, which can trace the roots of disease down to the cellular or even molecular level, invites narrow and oversimplified descriptions of causation. Lappé argues that it may thus be productive to compare the causal reasoning of geneticists with the mechanistic view that characterizes the physical sciences. Such a reductionistic analysis is inadequate to explain human genetics, as Lappé shows through case studies that display the problems posed for counselors by genetic heterogeneity, phenocopies, and the like. Especially in the case of diseases of late onset, it may make no sense to speak of "the genetic causes" of a disease or condition, as though they could be isolated from environmental causes and other factors dictated by human choice. Along with the many other difficulties that genetic counselors must face in diagnostic capabilities and personal knowledge, which are discussed later in this volume, Lappé's analysis suggests that geneticists may need to incorporate a recognition of uncertainties in causation into their thinking and counseling. Indeed, as with other medical and social phenomena, overcausation may prove to be the most accurate explanation for "genetic diseases."

The influence of specific terminology on our thinking is well illustrated by the very word "disease." Is a person with what is termed a disease different from other people in some categorical sense, or only as a statistical matter which would recognize all states as relative? Or even in the statistical view, may a person be so aberrant as to be substantively different? Some of these concepts may prove to be better explanations of certain conditions than of others; yet this may lead one to wonder whether the definition of a disease is dependent upon the physiologic tests presently available to medical science. Or may other factors — such as professional identification and social preference — not also play a crucial role in the way a person determines which conditions are "diseases" and which among these are "genetic"? These are among the topics addressed by Richard Roblin and Richard Hull in Chapters 3 and 4.

Genetic counseling is coming to be seen as a medical subspecialty, and to place the previous contributions into a pragmatic perspective, this section closes with a chapter by an author who is a physician — and an experienced genetic counselor as well. From a demonstration of the relative nature of "genetic health," which is so very much determined by time, place, and circumstances, Robert Murray argues that the concept is for the practitioner not only difficult to apply and perhaps meaningless but potentially extremely pernicious for patients and for society.

A common theme of all the chapters, then, is that terminology — and the world view it generates — are of critical importance to our approach to genetic counseling. Although the authors do not agree on the definitions themselves, they make clear the harm which can come from the inappropriate use of them. In genetic counseling, as in the rest of health care, the concepts which are used to explain patients' situations will set expectations about treatment and prevention which may be impossible to overcome despite the contrary wishes of the parties. The concepts circumscribe the questions that are asked and the solutions that are deemed responsive and hence responsible.

AMC

1. Genetic Counseling, Medical Genetics and Theoretical Genetics: An Historical Overview

Arthur Caplan, PhD

Although genetic counseling and medical genetics are relatively young disciplines, they abound with interesting theoretical and conceptual issues that can best be understood in light of a philosophic consideration of historical developments in genetics. Such understanding is invaluable for any scientist who is attempting to attain a sound comprehension of his chosen speciality, and it can also yield important practical consequences for the field's future development.

Perhaps the most intriguing problem in the history of clinical genetic counseling is understanding why this practice took so long to become an accepted part of medical science. This inquiry has traditionally been considered from the perspective of the more general issue of why human genetics took so long to become an independent subdiscipline within genetics. Since it seems reasonable to suppose that the existence of viable genetic counseling services is closely linked to the development of knowledge concerning human genetics, this essay will begin by examining the specific question of why medical genetics took so long to become a part of medicine.

In his Presidential Address to the American Society of Human Genetics in 1961, L.C. Dunn raised the problem of the slow development of a subdiscipline of human genetics in the form of a paradox [1]. "Why," Dunn wondered, "did human genetics develop so slowly?" when "by 1915 the general architecture of the hereditary material was known . . . or, even if we date the definitive elucidation of the physical basis of heredity as late as the publication of Morgan's "Theory of the Gene" in 1926 . . . the knowledge of heredity has been with us for thirty-five years" [2].

Dunn dismissed the stock excuse of many early geneticists that "we can't experiment with man, and his generation time is too long" [3], as being totally unsatisfactory since this excuse was no less valid in 1961 than it was thirty-five years earlier. Nonetheless, by 1961 a flourishing field of human genetics had

Birth Defects: Original Article Series, Volume XV, Number 2, pages 21—31
© 1979 The National Foundation

come into existence. Dunn noted that developments in human genetics were slow and plodding in other areas besides classic Morganian genetics. The basic principles of population genetics had been formulated by Hardy, Pearson, and the physician, Wilhelm Weinberg, in the first decade of this century, and the general theory of population genetics had been fully adumbrated by R.A. Fisher, Sewall Wright, and J.B.S. Haldane by 1930. Yet this theory had very little impact on human genetics and clinical medical practice for nearly thirty years. Archibald Garrod and William Bateson had discovered numerous connections between a variety of human ailments and genetically based metabolic disorders as early as 1908. Yet, in this case as well, human genetics did not incorporate the ideas of biochemical genetics and gene action into medical practice until the late 1940s. Not only was a science of human genetics slow to materialize, but even when it finally did arise shortly after World War II, it was slow to incorporate the nonclassic aspects of genetics: population genetics, biochemical genetics, cytogenetics, demography, and developmental genetics.

The slow development of human genetics may be analyzed from three vantage points: the development of the field of human genetics and clinical practice based upon Morgan's gene theory, the failure of a biochemical theory of human genetics to appear following Garrod's early investigations, and, the absence, even today, of a population genetic approach to human hereditary disorders despite the comprehensive efforts of Fisher, Haldane, and Wright in the 1920s and 30s. I shall try to show that while medical genetics and genetic counseling have been far from immune to the theoretical developments in biochemical genetics and population biology, a truly synthetic subdiscipline of human genetics, incorporating these areas of genetic concern, has not yet arisen to guide medical and clinical science.

I. GENETICS AND EUGENICS IN THE POST-MORGANIAN ERA

A good place to begin is by evaluating the answer offered by Dunn to the dilemma concerning why so much time passed before the findings of the classic Morgan school were extended from Drosophila to man. Dunn points to the abuses engendered by the eugenics movement and its culmination in the monstrous racial purity theories of the Nazi era as casting a dark shadow upon any sort of genetics research on human beings [4]. The aberrant social and racial concerns that fueled the eugenics movement so distorted the methods and findings of genetic science that any suggestion of extending classic Morganian genetics to include inheritance in humans and their medical complications was, Dunn argued, met with bitter scorn and critical revulsion.

The excesses of the eugenics movement in Europe and America, its effects upon immigration policies, segregation, and class structure have been extensively documented in a large body of scholarly books and articles [5]. Motivated, as the eugenicists were, by specific political, ethnic, or social concerns, most eugenicists took little time to sully their arguments for various social policies with actual biologic or genetic findings. Consequently, according to Dunn, the movement had little support or acceptance in the biologic community. As the preconceptions and biases of the eugenics movement and the notorious effects of its implementation in Germany became painfully evident to the scientific community and the general public, the power of the movement waned until, by the late 1940s, it was possible for geneticists to try and construct a valid empiric science of human genetics.

Although the eugenics movement, and the consequent racial madness of the Nazi period, did much to discredit the idea of a human genetics based upon classic principles of inheritance and gene transmission, other factors — biologic as well as sociopolitical — were at work in delaying the advent of human and medical genetics. For, while it may have been the case that the eugenics movement distorted and stunted the growth of a science of human genetics, it is also true that geneticists were not in a position to restrain the excesses of this movement on purely empiric or scientific grounds. A number of conceptual and methodologic obstacles within genetics proper had to be overcome in order to construct a valid science of human genetics and redress the excesses of the eugenics propagandists.

A. The "Extendability" Question — A False Lead

The most obvious methodologic difficulty facing the early geneticists was whether scientific findings concerning a particular species can be validly extended to another species. This "extendability" problem looms especially significant, since much of the work aimed at constructing a physical material base for Mendelian heredity was conducted on plants. Peas, beans, maize, and flowering plants of various species played a prominent role in the establishment of hereditary patterns and factorial explanations in the period following the rediscovery of Mendel's work. Yet, despite the obvious attractiveness of the thesis that geneticists were reluctant to extend or generalize their findings concerning plants to any animal species including man, this methodologic claim does not stand up to critical scrutiny. The fact remains that early pre-Morganian geneticists did a great deal of experimental work on a variety of animals, as well as plants, and the heritability studies of geneticists such as Correns, Cuenot, Bateson, Punnett, and others [6] convincingly demonstrated the universality of Mendelian patterns in the plant and animal kingdoms. Moreover, while the "extendability" problem may have given pause to early experimental work, it surely posed no problem for post-Morganian geneticists who could base all their heritability findings on Morgan's chromosomally-based physical theory of the gene. The definitive establishment by Morgan and his students; Sturtevant, Bridges, and Muller, in the early

1920s of the chromosomes as the material bearers of the Mendelian factors or particles, conclusively ended any serious suspicion that different systems of inheritance prevailed among different species.

B. The Mendelism-Darwinism Controversy

There is, however, one general theoretic issue, which arose prior to the formulation of a materially-based chromosomal theory of Mendelian heredity that, unlike the extendability question, did carry over into subsequent decades of genetic investigation. Mendelism, upon its rediscovery by Hugo de Vries, Correns, and Tschermak in 1900, was seized upon by many biologists as a viable alternative to Darwinian explanations of evolution [7]. William Bateson was an influential advocate of this theoretic view. He argued that there was little need to invoke principles of natural selection to explain organic evolution, when the processes involved in producing new variations and species could be understood on the basis of Mendelian segregation and recombination.

Bateson's Mendelian interpretation of evolution touched off a storm of critical reaction among neo-Darwinian theorists, foremost of whom were Karl Pearson and W.F.R. Weldon [8]. These scientists were known collectively as the biometricians since they made extensive use of the statistical techniques pioneered by Darwin's cousin, Francis Galton. They desperately tried to show that Mendelian segregation and inheritance patterns were incorrect, or, at any rate, superfluous, for understanding the variational base of Darwinian selection. Mendelian genetics was seen by the biometricians as a source of sudden, rapid change, analogous to the saltationist mutation theory advocated by the geneticist, Hugo de Vries. Sudden and rapid variation in phenotypes was totally incompatible with the slow and gradual picture of evolutionary change in organisms drawn by Darwin in his writings. Neither Bateson nor the biometricians understood that Mendelism and mutation provide the very variation in organisms requisite for Darwin's evolutionary theory.

Much of the subsequent research in genetics was directed toward a resolution of the Bateson/biometrician controversy that surrounded the birth of the subject. Morgan himself became interested in genetics as a consequence of his interest in Mendelism as an alternative theory to Darwinism. Despite his important work on the relationship between Mendelism and chromosomes, the real demonstration of the compatibility of Mendelian genetics and Darwinism was achieved by Morgan's student, H.J. Muller, through his work on radiation and mutations, and by the mathematical population geneticists, R.A. Fisher, Sewall Wright, and J.B.S. Haldane. Following in the mathematical footsteps of the biometricians, these men were able to show how, in principle, natural selection could act upon gradual slight variations, resulting from mutations and recombinations, to produce the vast panorama of organic diversity to be found in nature.

Since the synthesizing of Mendelian genetics and Darwinism was the task that occupied geneticists of all theoretic persuasions for much of the first half of the twentieth century, it is not surprising that a science of medical genetics failed to develop during this period. For although the requisite theoretical apparatus for constructing a science of human hereditary existed as early as 1925, genetics as a whole was struggling to become an integrated part of the dominant biologic theory of this century, Darwinian evolution. Genetics, in the form of population genetics, became the focal point of evolutionary inquiry and debate.

Moreover, despite the passionate and absorbing debate generated by theologians, human beings were assigned no special role within the context of evolution. Men, mice, flies, and maize simply became confirmational empiric tools for the theoreticians involved in formulating a coherent synthetic evolutionary theory. It was only when this theoretic work had been completed and confirmed by field naturalists, such as Theodosius Dobzhansky, Ernst Mayr, E.B. Ford, and Julian Huxley, that genetics could be diverted from its role as the lynchpin of evolutionary theory. While it may have been the case that the eugenics movement stunted scientific inquiry into the genetics of man, it is also true that the lack of empiric studies aimed at refuting the excesses of this movement, and the strange silence of the vast majority of genetic researchers concerning eugenics, can best be understood as the natural consequences of the attention of geneticists being focused on the controversy over Darwinian theory.

C. Polygenic Traits and Unit-Characters

Two other factors enter into the explanation of the failure of a science of human heredity to appear long after the Mendelian and chromosomal foundations of genetics were laid. The first is the prominent role played by discontinuous or unit-character traits in genetic studies of the early twentieth century. Before Morgan's work on chromosomes in Drosophila, geneticists, such as Bateson, W.E. Castle, and E.M. East, had debated the nature of the relationship existing between Mendelian factors or genes and continuous and discontinuous phenotypic variations in populations of organisms. Since it was easier to study transmission and inheritance by using features that were sharply distinguishable in a population, such as eye color, flower color or sex, geneticists concentrated their attention on these sharply discontinuous features in formulating their explanations of distribution and inheritance. Other traits, such as height, bristle number, weight, and kernel number seemed to be continuously distributed in populations of organisms. The heredity of such features did not admit of the simple unit-character or single factor analysis of discontinuous traits. For many years geneticists struggled to construct the necessary mathematical computations for deriving Mendelian ratios for every single character difference on the basis of a one-to-one correspondence with genes or factors. With the appearance in the mid-1920s of Morgan's chromosomal gene theory, it became evident that this "unit-character" hypothesis [9] was invalid; Morgan's thesis gained support, as the variations brought about by mutation, recombination, linkage, and position effects slowly came to light.

After the demise of the unit-character hypothesis the debate about continuous features shifted, in the 1920s and 30s, to the determination of polygenetic or multifactorial systems controlling such traits. Maize geneticists such as R.A. Emerson and M. Demerec advanced the hypothesis that every gene contained minute subunits or genomeres which could be unequally distributed in development and reproduction. The genomere hypothesis was opposed by H.J. Muller in a series of articles [10] in which he attempted to show, through studies of inheritance in mosaic fruit flies, induced by mutagenic agents, that the phenotypic variations observed from one generation to the next did not fit the distributions to be expected on the genomere view of genes. Eventually, Muller was able to show that continuous variations in organisms could be explained by multifactorial genetic assumptions without invoking the complex genomeres of the maize geneticists.

The theoretic debates concerning single gene, polygenetic, and multifactorial inheritance demonstrate the uncertainty that surrounded geneticists' attempts to understand continuous phenotypic variability. Since the vast bulk of human phenotypic traits are of the continuous sort, it would have been extremely unlikely that a science of human heritability or medical genetics would arise without the resolution of the unit-character, multifactorial, and genomere hypotheses of gene structure. In lieu of a theory of polygenetic or multifactorial Mendelian genetics, it was impossible to construct a valid science of human genetics regardless of the social or racial concerns of geneticists.

D. Germs, Genes, and Theories of Disease

Finally, medical science was not in a particularly receptive theoretic state for incorporating genetic analysis into its domain. Physicians and medical researchers in the 1920s and 30s were busily extending their new etiologic model of disease. Medical science had only recently come to replace the pneumatic and miasmatic disease theories of the late nineteenth century with Koch's germ theory of disease. Koch's postulates had focused medical attention on microbial sources of disease, infection, and abnormality. Consequently, physicians were simply not in a position to appreciate the etiologic model of genetically based abnormalities since they failed to conform to the basic methodologic paradigm employed at the time.

Furthermore, the miasma theory of disease had left a conceptual legacy, that of hereditary dispositions to abnormality and disease, in the guise of notions such as "hereditary degeneracy" and "diathesis" [11]. The idea of a general disposition or susceptibility to disease and mental and physical abnormality which could be acquired in a straightforward Lamarckian manner and transmitted in toto to future generations dominated medical views of human heredity well into the twentieth century. Medical science was hardly in a position to incorporate genetic research into its practices, given its preoccupation with the germ theory paradigm and its nineteenth-century conceptions of heredity.

Thus, conceptual problems in the field of genetics appear to have been crucial, along with the social and political factors that Dunn and others have traditionally expressed, in accounting for the curious delays in the development of human and clinical genetics. Physicians and geneticists were simply not in a position to add scientific credence to racial theories, correct the abuses of such views, or substitute a sound scientific approach to heredity in human beings.

II. THE FAILURE OF BIOCHEMICAL GENETICS TO BLOSSOM

If this argument concerning classic genetics is correct, it does not, however, explain why the specialty of biochemical human genetics failed to blossom into an area of medical concern. As early as 1908 a British physician, Archibald Garrod [12], had written and lectured extensively about what he referred to as the "inborn errors of metabolism." Garrod noted that the family distribution of such metabolic abnormalities was strongly suggestive of a hereditary base for these disorders. After consulting with William Bateson, Garrod realized that the distribution pattern of these disorders could be explained as a recessive Mendelian gene appearing as a consequence of inbreeding. Garrod wrote and lectured widely about the metabolic disorders he observed in his clinical practice and their relationship to the nascent science of genetics. However, as in the case of Morgan's classic heritability studies, little came of Garrod's work until the biochemical studies of George Beadle and E.L. Tatum reopened the science of human biochemical genetics in the 1940s. Indeed, it was only when contemporary medical geneticists such as Stanbury, Harris, and Hsia began to scour the historical references to locate the historical roots of their work that Garrod's research was rediscovered and appreciated.

A. The Gene/Enzyme Confusion

It would take a small monograph to explain properly the long neglect of Garrod's pioneering work on the genetic mechanisms of the metabolic disorders now so familiar to genetic counselors; nevertheless, it is possible to pinpoint two factors that greatly hindered the development of human biochemical genetics. Plant geneticists, such as Muriel Wheldale Onslow, carried out extensive research on the effects of gene action and metabolism in producing color pigments in flowers. A variety of flower colors result from differences and variations in the metabolic pathways leading to anthocyanin, the basic constituent of pigment cells in flowers. Animal geneticists, such as Sewall Wright and J.B.S. Haldane, carried out parallel studies on coat color pigments in mice produced by the action of certain genes involved in melanin production. Despite the existence of these studies, neither the plant nor animal workers were able to extend their studies to other organisms or to inborn errors of metabolism in humans. Both groups of geneticists realized that metabolism was in some sense associated with genetic factors, yet, both groups confused the control of enzymes and metabolism by genes with the notion that the genes themselves were enzymes [13]. This confusion greatly complicated the Mendelian analysis of metabolic variations and abnormalities. It was only when Beadle and Tatum succeeded in revitalizing Garrod's insight that factors or genes synthesized enzymes that the heritability of such units could be understood.

B. The Nuclein Misunderstanding

In addition to the gene/enzyme confusion, geneticists were hindered in their attempts to employ Garrod's findings by a basic biochemical confusion. Friedrich Miescher had, in the latter half of the nineteenth century, successfully pinpointed the nucleic acids as being key components of the chromosomal material. In 1895 E.B. Wilson [14] noted in his classic work, *The Cell in Development and Inheritance,* that "nuclein is in a chemical sense one formative centre of the cell, attracting to it the food-matters, entering into a loose combination with them, and giving them off to the extoplasm in an elaborated form." This conception of gene action sounds amazingly familiar to modern ears. However, physicians and geneticists were unable to utilize this understanding of the metabolic role of nuclein as a result of both a theoretical and an empiric error.

On the theoretical level, biochemical analysis of the nucleic acid materials seemed to indicate that these materials were far too simplistic and regular in their construction to synthesize the observable diversity of protein end-products found in every cell. The physical model of nucleic acids postulated by early twentieth century chemists depicted the nucleic acids as being composed of repetitive alternating sequences of purines and pyramidine nucleotides. This model restricted the amount of variability present in the nucleic acids and consequently diverted attention from the nucleic acids as a possible source of gene action.

On the empiric level, chemical analyses of chromosomal materials seemed to indicate that DNA constituted the central component material of chromosomes in animals while RNA constituted the bulk of the chromosomal material in plants. Thus, despite the fact that gene action was extensively studied in pigment formation in flowering plants by Onslow and others, these studies were not seen as indicative of genetic mechanisms in animals or humans. The unfortunate bifurcation by chemists of genetic materials in plants and animals and the simplistic model of nucleic acid structure current for most of the twentieth century effectively blocked the development of a science of human biochemical genetics and condemned Garrod's studies on metabolic disorders among humans to a long period of historical obscurity and neglect.

III. POPULATION GENETICS AND GENETIC EPIDEMIOLOGY: A CURRENT FAILURE

Having seen that a number of conceptual and methodological confusions contributed to the slow development of human genetics and, by extension, medical genetics and counseling services, it is tempting to inquire if similar sorts of confusions continue to prevent the incorporation of population genetics theory into human genetics. It is somewhat puzzling, given the extensive body of theoretical knowledge that has been developed concerning population genetics that a subdiscipline of genetic epidemiology does not constitute an important specialty within medical genetics. To a certain degree this situation can be understood when set in the context of current genetic counseling practice, which focuses on the individual and family as the key loci of medical concern. Still, it may seem surprising that the shift within genetic theory from an older, individually oriented conception of heredity to a population view of variation and inheritance has not been paralleled by a similar shift or broadening of perspective in the medical domain. But on close inspection, it appears that the incorporation of popular genetics theory into clinical genetics is hindered by a complex of factors.

Certainly the arcaneness of the mathematical models commonly employed by population geneticists, and their technical terminology, does not allow the theory to be easily assimilated into everyday genetics practice. But perhaps the most important factor forestalling such incorporation is the abstractness and idealization invoked in population genetic models of gene flow. In order to make the complex phenomena of gene transmission amenable to empiric and theoretical analysis, it has always been necessary for population geneticists to introduce simplifying assumptions and nonempiric conditional statements into their mathematical models. The complicated mating patterns, demographics, migration rates, mortality rates, and consanguinity affiliations found in interbreeding human populations have, until recently, simply been beyond the theoretical competence of the mathematical models commonly employed by population geneticists. Population geneticists often find that they simply do not have the theoretic apparatus at hand to deal with the particular conditions and restrictions obtaining in any real organic population [15]. It may be the case that, as better population genetic models are formulated, the "theoretical" aspects of population genetics will not prove to be such a stumbling block for practical empiric inquiry. Until this happens, however, it would seem that the rich body of theoretical data that has been accumulated concerning gene flow, drift, consanguinity, effective population size, and genetic load is doomed to remain inaccessible to practicing medical geneticists. The process of integrating this theory into medical genetics may, in fact, only begin when clinical geneticists and counselors succeed in accumulating the sort of empiric information necessary to properly flesh out and strengthen the mathematical models of the population geneticists.

IV. CONCLUSION

In suggesting reasons why human genetics took so long to become an independent discipline, this paper has attempted to provide a partial answer to the question why genetic counseling took so long to become a part of medical practice. Obviously, genetic counseling could not become a legitimate field of clinical practice until a science of human genetics had been established. However, as genetic counselors know only too well, the establishment of a clinical specialty, such as genetic counseling, does not necessarily follow as a logical consequence of the establishment of a scientific discipline such as human genetics. Conceptual difficulties, such as those that retarded the formulation of clinical sciences of genetic heritability, biochemical genetics, and population genetics, doubtless have their analogs in the history of genetic counseling. And to these must be added the special problems that arise in all clinical fields, with their norms of professional conduct and the nonscientific aspects of their educational format. One hopes that the analysis of human genetics presented here will permit and even stimulate a parallel inquiry into the recent history of genetic counseling. For the moment, it might be noted that, in comparison to the speed with which human genetics emerged, the progress of genetic counseling over the past fifteen years seems rapid indeed.

REFERENCES

1. Dunn LC: Cross currents in the history of human genetics. Am J Hum Genet 14:1–13, 1962. See also Childs B, Garrod A: Galton and clinical medicine. Yale J Biol Med 46: 297–313, 1973. Also Rosenberg CE: Factors in the development of genetics in the United States: some suggestions. J History Med Allied Sci 22:27–46, 1967.
2. Dunn LC: Cross currents in the history of human genetics. Am J Hum Genet 14:1, 1962.
3. Ibid, p 1.
4. Ibid, pp 7–9.

5. Haller M: "Eugenics." New Brunswick: Rutgers University Press, 1963. Ludmerer K: "Genetics and American Society." Baltimore: Johns Hopkins, 1972. Allen GE: Genetics, eugenics, and class struggle. Genetics 79:29–45, June, 1975.

6. Cf Dunn LC: "A Short History of Genetics." New York: McGraw-Hill, 1965.

7. Cf Carlson EA: "The Gene: A Critical History," chapters 2–6. Philadelphia: W.B. Saunders, 1966.

8. Provine WB: "Origins of Theoretical Population Biology," Chapter 2. Chicago: University of Chicago Press, 1971.

9. Ibid, pp 108–126.

10. Muller HJ: Variations due to change in the individual gene. Am Naturalist 56:32–50, 1922. Muller HJ: The measurement of gene mutation rate in drosophila: its high variability and its dependence upon temperature. Genetics 13:279–357, 1928.

11. Rosenberg CE: op cit, pp 28–37.

12. See Garrod's classic work: "Inborn Errors of Metabolism." Oxford: Oxford University Press, 1909, which was the published version of his 1908 Croonian lectures at Oxford.

13. Troland LT: Biological enigmas and the theory of enzyme action. Am Naturalist 51: 321–350, 1917. See also Allen G: "Life Science in the Twentieth Century." New York: John Wiley & Sons, Inc, 1975, pp 198–205.

14. Wilson EB: "The Cell in Development and Inheritance." New York: Macmillan, 1896, p 247.

15. See, for example, Cavalli-Sforza LL, Bodmer WF: "The Genetics of Human Populations." San Francisco: W.H. Freeman & Co, 1971, Chapters 8 and 9, and Lewontin RC: "The Genetic Basis of Evolutionary Change." New York: Columbia University Press, 1974.

2. Theories of Genetic Causation in Human Disease

Marc Lappé, PhD

THE PROBLEM

The presumption that we can achieve total knowledge of the biologic roots of human disease and through that, control over nature, is a modern phenomenon. It is part of the optimism of our age. In the last half century, we have turned increasingly to genetics for proof of the legitimacy of that conviction. Animal and plant breeders provided the earliest models. The genetic approach gave us a powerful model for controlling pathologic or desirable qualities in domesticated plants and animals. Animal husbandry was so convincing that even Charles Darwin came to believe that we ourselves should follow its example lest we continue "to breed our worst animals."

Genetic models of the expected outcomes of different crosses appeared to work so well in the past that it is understandable why we turn to them now in search for the roots of human attributes and disabilities. After genetics became a science, early calculations of hereditability demonstrated beautifully the extent to which we might expect "success" in breeding for hogback thickness, or egg number, or beef girth. Unfortunately, we find now that such calculations work much less well for the complex human phenomena which are under study in genetic counseling. Unless the limitations of the strictly genetic approach are learned concurrently with its strengths, it is likely that error, ignorance, and abuse will taint the emergence of genetic counseling as a scientific profession.

The central problem of the mid-20th century genetic counselor has been to determine the place of the genes in the origins of complex human characteristics — such as neural tube defects, cleft palate, diabetes, and congenital heart disease — in short, the major malformations and polygenic syndromes which make up the bulk of what we call birth defects. Of comparable importance in terms of genetic counseling is understanding the origin and incidence of the newly recognized genetic heterogeneity lying behind what had previously been regarded as simple, single-gene determined diseases.

Birth Defects: Original Article Series, Volume XV, Number 2, **pages 33—45**
© **1979 The National Foundation**

DEALING WITH GENETIC HETEROGENEITY

Phenylketonuria (PKU) has until recently been considered a classic example of a human metabolic disease determined by a single gene. The absence of a functional enzyme known as phenylalanine hydroxylase was thought to lead inevitably to a progressive buildup of the amnio acid phenylalanine in the blood. Researchers believed that the biochemic disturbances generated by this excess metabolite were responsible for the grave defects in both mental and physical development characteristic of PKU.

In the late 1950s the suggestion that a dietary restriction of phenylalanine could wholly or partially prevent this process evoked enthusiastic support. By the mid-1960s and prior to any systematic research, mass neonatal screening programs were begun in virtually every state with the intent of diagnosing PKU early enough to begin therapy before damage to the child had occurred. Within a few years, the screening had turned up some individuals with elevated phenylalanine levels who were genetically normal (benign hyperphenylalanemia), but this unexpected result was not immediately recognized.

Failure to acknowledge the complexity of this genetic disease led to unfortunate medical consequences. One classic example may suffice. A child in Maryland was diagnosed at birth as having PKU and was put on the special diet. Under ordinary circumstances, the restriction in circulating phenylalanine levels would have been more than sufficient to "cure" the child of any adverse effects of her genetic problem. Yet by the time the child was seven months old, she was mentally retarded [1]. On careful retesting, the child was not found to have classic PKU at all but a related metabolic defect which produced similar test results. In this instance, the deficiency was in an enzyme known as dihydropteridine reductase.

The lesson from such cases is that the genetic basic of even the most apparently straightforward human metabolic diseases is almost always complex. A consensus has emerged that most, if not all, human metabolic diseases might profitably be subjected to renewed scrutiny in light of the PKU example.

The new investigatory spirit has often led to surprising results. Some presumptively simple Mendelian-determined genetic diseases, like Tay-Sachs disease, have emerged as complex ones with greater or lesser heterogeneity, and others like cystic fibrosis have been found to generate extraordinarily diverse symptoms.

Cystic fibrosis was once thought to be a classic example of a unitary genetic disease, caused by a single autosomal recessive gene which leads to a disruption of the function of exocrine glands (those which discharge their products outside the organ instead of directly into the bloodstream). The pancreas, intestine, gallbladder, and lung are all affected. Until recently, it was assumed that any individual unfortunate enough to receive both genes for cystic fibrosis from his parents was doomed to death before the end of the teenage years. Indeed it is the most common lethal genetic disease of childhood among North American whites.

Now, all of these presumptions have to be reexamined in the light of a 1976 case report. The individual described had completed combat training at several special forces schools and ran eight miles a day. Only at the age of 30 had he sought medical attention because his formerly efficient breathing had become compromised; after running one-quarter of a mile, he found that he coughed spasmodically and brought up a large amount of sputum, a symptom not unlike that experienced by those of us who are amateur runners — and who run with a cold. Surprisingly, on examination he was found to have all the hallmarks of cystic fibrosis. His doctors described his previous adaptation as remarkable — a highly compensated genetic defect [2]. Certainly, he is an exception, but we now must realize that exceptions probably exist for virtually every "classic" genetic disease.

A geneticist may still believe that all that can be seen to be wrong with this man rests ultimately on disturbances at a genetic level. Virtually everything which makes up our biologic being is shaped and constrained in some way by genetic mechanisms. The range of our reactions to particular environmental opportunities or insults is almost certainly limited at some level by gene action. Yet, the actual net of events which interacts to "cause" a given perturbation in development, or generates a metabolic disease, is itself staggering in its complexity.

In spite of the growing appreciation of the complexity of genetic causation, attention seems repeatedly to swing from either a unilateral environmental viewpoint or towards a wholly genetic explanation. It is almost always a mistake to simplify models of gene-environment interaction by isolating the forces which eventually shape the whole. It would be unfortunate if the current generation of genetic counselors did not learn how often such an orientation generates a distorted view of the nature of the genetic processes that shape human beings.

PHENOTYPES AND GENOTYPES

The roots of a tendency to seek out either/or causal forces from the plethora of genetic and environmental factors can be traced to the origins of modern genetic thought. The ten years which followed the simultaneous rediscovery of Mendel's principles by Correns, von Tschermak, and de Vries in 1900 were marked by researchers who attempted to isolate genetic forces from environmental ones, in particular, Danish botanist Wilhelm Johannsen.

Johannsen studied the effects of different environmental and genetic backgrounds on the growth characteristics of the common French bean. He grew some of these plants in environmental conditions which were as nearly identical as possible, and others in widely different environments. Johannsen expected the bean seeds which he took from different plants to vary widely in genetic makeup, but those from any individual plant to be more similar, since they fertilized themselves.

Johannsen found that beans from widely separated sources indeed generated a range of plants, each with a range of different bean weights and shapes. But Johannsen noted that the bean plants derived from bean taken from even the most carefully inbred plants appeared to vary just as extensively. Moreover, the beans on such presumably genetically homogeneous plants varied depending on their position in the pod and the order of pod formation. Some beans appeared larger, some plumper, and others rounder than their brethren on the same genetically uniform plant. In spite of these external differences, when Johannsen planted beans which had grown on such a plant in as nearly identical environments as he could find, they produced a new generation of plants with beans which were almost precisely the same average size as those from their parents. More important, each line of bean plants which descended from the bean seeds of one plant bred true for generation after generation. The beans on each line consistently generated plants in which the average size of beans remained constant.

Johannsen concluded that the differences he originally observed in plant morphology and among beans on the same plant were due to forces outside the plant. These difference-generating forces, he presumed, were environmental in origin. The differences which he observed between various inbred plant lines he attributed to systematic, hereditary forces working inside the plants. Johannsen attributed these internal influences to "genetic" factors. The aggregate of internal sources of control over visible characteristics he termed the plant's *genotype*, a word he coined in 1909. The visible characters themselves, which fluctuated widely depending on environmental forces such as soil, sunlight and moisture, he termed the *phenotype* [3].

Johannsen's ideas encouraged a rigourous view of genetic causation which gave thinkers of his day a precise way of conceptualizing the relative roles of Nature and Nurture. The influence of his concepts is easily discerned in the writings of early geneticists. In this excerpt from an article written in 1924 [4], the dualistic view of causation is clearly discernible:

> Two sets of factors are involved in the development of an individual, and doubtless the same two factors are responsible for racial development, or evolution. One category of factors is intrinsic and seems to depend on the mechanisms that are involved in cell multiplication and differentiation: all such factors are here included under the term, "heredity." The other category of factors is extrinsic and seems to involve both environment and training: these factors are usually included together under the term "environment."

Many people still maintain the separate identities of these interacting components in spite of the fact that virtually every contemporary researcher rejects the notion that either genes or environments can independently determine any particular defect or behavior. Critical environmental events are often necessary to allow the expression of a given feature. For instance, a rat will not display its "genetically based propensity" for aggressive behavior unless its early postnatal environment permits a surge of testosterone, and then another set of environments releases the behavior when the rat becomes an adult. Environmental factors, in turn, cannot affect behavior or other characteristics except in interaction with the gene-directed biologic structure of the organism. And the action of any given gene is conditioned by other genes in the genetic repertory of the host.

Thus, neither the environmentalist nor the hereditarian view alone provides a useful model for explaining the complexity of forces which interact to cause the emergence of polygenically associated disease or disability. Certainly, all such phenomena are rooted in genetically directed biologic structures, many of which facilitate the very environmental interaction which leads to their appearance. But the issue is whether that interaction is adequately described by simple models of causation. If some higher biologic structures and functions are by their nature beyond simple reduction, then even a view which attempts to describe complex, polygenic features in terms of additive environment/gene interactions or covariance may still be potentially inadequate.

WHERE GENETIC CAUSATION DEFIES SIMPLE ANALYSIS

A common phenotypic variant called polydactyly, occurs in virtually all mammalian species including humans, where it is popularly presumed to be caused by a single dominant gene. Establishing the mechanism of genetic causation for this easily enumerated anatomic marker has proved elusive.

In 1934, famed population geneticist Sewall Wright [5] tested a wide variety of inbred strains of guinea pigs to plumb the genetic contribution to polydactyly. Wright found no clear-cut pattern of inheritance. It seemed as if the genes which allowed for multiple toes were radically affected by other genes in the organism. More interesting, the direct expression of these genes was further distorted by a wide variety of nutritional and environmental factors. Thus an animal with the requisite genetic complement for polydactyly might or might not express the variation, depending on the concerted influence of a cacophony of genes and environments threading in and out in a complex and seemingly indiscernable pattern.

Similar interacting forces often contribute to masking the actual "causes" of other mammalian birth defects. Often the pattern of defects commonly seen has defied analysis. For instance, genetically identical littermates in mothers exposed to a controlled amount of a teratogenic chemical like trypan blue or physical agents like x rays can show a complete range of responses — from death, to malformation, to seemingly unblemished survival [6].

To deal with this apparently insoluble indeterminacy, Wright postulated the existence of a critical threshold for the action of the genes. For Wright, "threshold" was a largely theoretical concept which described the conditions necessary for a gene to make its presence known. Genes with strong penetrance have low thresholds: their effects cut through all but the most resilient environmental counterinfluences. In contrast, genes with weak penetrance have very high thresholds and often become manifest only when environmental conditions are reduced or weakened.

One of the critical environments affecting gene expression in higher animals is the environment in which development itself occurs. For example, almost half of the newborns in a certain hybrid strain of mice develop cleft palate after their mothers are exposed to cortisone. If genetically identical mice gestate in the uterus of mothers that are resistant to cortisone's effects, little or no cleft palate occurs.* In like fashion, variations in number of vertebrae characteristic of one strain of mice only show up in embryos reared in mothers of their same genetic stock. On closer inspection, these and other genetically determined characteristics thus turn out to be heavily influenced by environmental forces.

To complicate matters, the relevant causative factors are often not only hard to identify, but their relative roles are not easily partitioned. Sometimes a whole array of contributing factors may be reviewed without producing a clear-cut picture. For instance, the authors of a collaborative study designed to isolate the effects of maternal weight, time of year, position in the uterus, fetal weight, and several other factors on congenital malformations were forced to conclude "that various non-genetic factors influence the response to teratogenic agents in not easily apprehensible ways" [8]. While other researchers have been more successful in isolating a few critical factors such as stress and diet, they are often still perplexed as to how they work in causing defects [9]. Since many of these factors are themselves subject to indeterminate influences, causation remains hidden.

A dramatic example of the intrinsic ambiguity of gene-environment interactions is found in mice with the mutation called "pallid." Affected animals have a double dose of a recessive gene and develop without the special stones (otoliths) in their middle ears necessary for proper balance in swimming. Supple-

*One simple procedure is to reverse the mating partners so that although the hybrid mice have the same genes, their uterine environment differs according to the parental phenotype. In Fraser's study A/Jax and C57BL mice were used, and the percentage of defects produced in each strain was 43% and 4%, respectively [7].

mental administration of manganese during pregnancy "overrides" the gene-related disability and allows normal development [10]. Similar supplementation, but with copper added to the maternal diet, greatly reduces the observable deleterious effects of a related gene called the "quaking."

Sometimes the presence or absence of a similar external agent can drive genetically based developmental programs awry, producing a mimic or pheno-copy of an entirely unrelated syndrome. The gross abnormalities produced by thalidomide provide a striking example. Thalidomide produces two broad classes of embryologic defects in humans, depending on the time of its ingestion in pregnancy. The first includes muscle paralysis, absence of ears, faulty develop-ment of the base of the spine and disordered kidney development; the second, a closed anus, a hernia, and a skeletal defect of the thumb. Both groups of anomalies occur in concert with the characteristic limb defects usually reported in the press. Parts of each of these syndromes are mimics of the effects of specific genetic mutations (at least seven in number), a fact which helped to delay recog-nition that an environmental trigger was operating in some but not all genetically prepared hosts [11, 12].

A new picture of human embryonic development has emerged from epi-sodes like this one. No longer is the embryo seen as a self-contained genetically programmed automaton, buffered and insulated against abuse from harmful agents in the outer world. Instead it is recognized as an extremely vulnerable entity whose essential functions are genetically fixed yet still broadly integrated to receive inputs from the outside world. The final expression of the genes, for good or ill is determined by a titration of these internal and external forces [13].

SOURCES OF VARIATION

An additional source of variability in genetic determination is the genetic background against which genes generate their products. Gene action is condi-tioned by the *other* genes carried by the organism. For instance, a gene known as "obese" in one strain of black mouse (C57B1/6) gives rise to a pleasantly plump animal with only mild evidence of diabetes. In an animal with a closely related genetic background (C57B1/Ks), the same gene produces a ravenous, grossly overweight animal with severe diabetes. Another gene known as "diabetes" is on a different chromosome, but can produce an effect indistinguishable from that of the "obese" gene when placed in the right genetic setting.

Similarly, diabetes in humans is thought by some researchers to be pri-marily genetically determined, with environmental factors affecting only the time of its appearance [14]. But the animal model would predict that other genes would be found which affect the expression of the diabetic phenotype. In fact, this is apparently the case. A team of researchers has recently put together data which shows that a person with the gene product known as HLA B7 has 14.5 times *less* chance of developing juvenile-onset diabetes mellitus as a brother or sister who lacks this gene [15].

Were these examples multiplied indefinitely, one might very well be content with a model of genetic determination.

But where human beings are concerned, a new factor involving gene-environment interactions must be added. Cultural forces are at least the equivalent to genetic ones in shaping human attributes. For instance, the extremely long period of intrauterine life and subsequent dependency are periods during which some of the most important interactions occur which shape the phenotype, morphological and behavioral, of the eventual adult. And it is here that the genetic counselor might otherwise fail to acknowledge critical, nongenetic contributions to syndromes, like Lesch—Nyhan, which are manifested by stereotypic behaviors.

Classical models of genetics only tacitly acknowledge that environments provide the critical challenges and conditions of development; in fact, according to two investigators, no adequate statistical models were available before 1973 to consider the complex circumstances of genotype-environment interactions in humans. Cavalli-Sforza and Feldman emphasize that simple models will not work in human beings where the phenotype is the result of a long and complex intrauterine experience and postnatal learning process. They conclude that "a purely 'cultural' inheritance" arises which "in the case of parent-offspring interaction is almost completely confounded with biological inheritance" [16].

Environmental factors overlayed on genetic variation can lead to widely fluctuating differences in the clinical manifestations of the symptoms associated with genetic disease, more so for dominantly inherited conditions, less so for recessive or sex-linked ones. Complex interactions can also confound the genetic analysis of complex phenomena which are of increasing interest to the genetic counselor. Some examples of this are discussed below.

BEHAVIOR DISORDERS WITH PRESUMPTIVE SINGLE-GENE CAUSATION: LESCH—NYHAN DISEASE

The behavior disorders which accompany Lesch—Nyhan disease, including compulsive head-banging and self-mutilation, have been considered by William Nyhan, codiscoverer of this disease entity, to be the direct result of a deficiency in an enzyme necessary for purine biosynthesis, hypoxanthine-guanine phosphoribosyl transferase (HGPRT). The gene determining this enzyme is recessive and sex-linked. Affected males are mentally retarded and suffer from an uncontrollable impulse to bite their fingers and lips beginning when they are about two years old. William Nyhan perceives these behaviors as an archetype of a pure genetic determination of behavior.

According to several researchers in this field, notably Dancis, Alpert, Anderson, and Herrmann, this pattern of self-mutilation may not be simply reflexive. They observed self-destructive activity in their two case studies more commonly when parents were present than when the children were left alone; the frequency of behavior varied in different environments; and the biting behavior responded to suggestion [17].

But was behavioral conditioning really biasing the expression of this gene? To Dancis and his co-workers, the observation that the therapist could produce biting behavior by threatening to leave the child alone provided a key to unlock the problem.

They tested the hypothesis that Lesch–Nyhan children are born with a far greater need for reinforcement than normal children. According to this theory, self-mutilation could occur because aversive control learning was grossly inadequate and failed to dampen even painful behavior. Dancis reasoned that Lesch–Nyhan children might respond to positive social reinforcement of their behavior.

Dancis tested the idea that these children would perform *any* physically feasible behavior that was sufficiently reinforced. The radical premise of their work was that children "try out" all behaviors on a random schedule. Lesch–Nyhan children simply get locked into a particularly bad pattern, not because they are genetically predisposed to bang their heads. By selectively reinforcing only noninjurious behavior, these researchers were able to suppress the self-destructive behavior of two boys.

One interpretation of this example (if verified) is that it demonstrates an elastic role for even the most powerfully disruptive genetic determinants. In this case, by failing to provide the necessary biochemical circuitry function, the enzymatic defect could be seen as opening a range of behaviors which would ordinarily be dampened by adaptive feedback mechanisms. By preventing the affected individuals from either selecting their environments, or being able to modulate their responses through learning, such a gene defect may be seen as *indirectly* creating the conditions for a child to have a high probability of self-destructive behavior.

Related studies on aggressive behavior reinforce this model of genetic causation.

BEHAVIOR DISORDERS WITH PRESUMPTIVE SEX-LINKED CAUSATION: AGGRESSIVITY

Behavior geneticists who have looked to the Y chromosome for the genes which "predispose" for aggression in animals have come up with extraordinarily perplexing data. Benson Ginsburg and his associates recently conducted follow-up studies of what had initially appeared to be the clear-cut association of specific

Y chromosomes and aggressive behavior in mice [18]. They discovered that genes on at least two other linkage groups not on the Y chromosome were involved in the expression of the behavioral trait [19]. Unfortunately, their previous work left the erroneous impression that a simple one-to-one correspondence between a given genetic background and expression of Y-linked aggressive behavior had been found, one that is still cited by researchers intent on simplifying the assumptions involved in explaining complex behavior in human beings.

The strong likelihood that significant genetic variation exists among human beings for comparable traits makes it highly unlikely that any simple genetic explanations of behavior will be forthcoming. Any behavioral or physiologic expression of any genetic makeup will almost certainly be mitigated by the *genetic* environment (ie the other genes the organism possesses) in addition to the effects of psychologic or social environments. These facts make it further unlikely that we will be able to predict the precise impact of an extra Y or X chromosome on any individual.

Social factors, in particular, profoundly influence the potential genetic influence on aggressiveness. A husband—wife team from Scandinavia demonstrated that four virtually independent mechanisms exist which can radically modify the aggressive behavior of experimental animals. Taking normally aggressive animals as their starting point, these two researchers proved that otherwise aggressive mice could be rendered nonaggressive by any of the following procedures: 1) selective breeding of nonaggressive littermates; 2) allowing an otherwise aggressive animal to be defeated in one or more fights; 3) handling it extensively in its early life; and 4) grouping it with similarly aggressive animals for long periods [20].

Other researchers have similarly shown that the early postnatal experience of the experimental animal exerts a profound and potentially overriding effect on its likelihood of exhibiting aggressive behavior. Undernutrition early in life heightens the tendency towards aggressiveness in some mouse strains [21]. Conversely, housing an otherwise predisposed male mouse with a rat will dampen its aggressive tendencies, as will drug treatments during the prepubertal period which prevent the normal surge of testosterone. All of these interventions suggest that complex events act in concert to "determine" the likelihood of a particular behavioral predilection.

BEHAVIORAL DISORDERS WITH PRESUMPTIVE POLYGENIC CAUSATION: ALCOHOLISM

Researchers who entertain the hypothesis that human alcoholism has a genetic basis frequently draw from several lines of animal research [22]. Often conflicting data from adoption studies in humans are by now commonplace. Nevertheless, variations in the rate and nature of the degradation of alcohol do occur among human groups with different patterns of alcohol abuse, suggesting a genetic component. For instance, persons of Asian origin clear alcohol more slowly from their blood than do Caucasians [23] . Such data have led a number of researchers to resurrect the hypothesis first introduced in 1947 that many of the factors which determine chronic alcoholism in humans have a genetic basis. But a closer look at the supporting evidence reveals the presence of potentially fatal confounding effects of gene-environment interactions.

In mice, for instance, the specific strain preference for alcohol solutions of different concentrations has traditionally been assumed to be under rigorous genetic control. The two critical test strains most often studied, C57BL/6 and DBA/2, have markedly disparate tendencies towards alcohol imbibition: the black strain exhibits a strong preference for alcohol solutions from 1—10% by volume, while the tan strain virtually avoids it altogether, even when dehydrated to the point of exhaustion.

Behavior geneticists working with alcohol-preferring strains like C57BL/6 had their first setback when it was found that the observable actions of the genes associated with alcohol preference differed depending on the *genetic background* of the animals involved [24] . Genes which appeared to "determine" alcohol preference in one strain would have virtually no effect when they were transposed to another strain. These differences have yet to be accounted for on a purely genetic basis.

A second and more serious obstacle to the pure genetic hypothesis of alcohol preference came in the early 1970s. In a classic experiment to determine the possible existence of social determinants of drinking behavior, two researchers placed young naive C57BL mice with adult nondrinking DBAs, and as a control, housed naive DBAs with C57BL adults who had already acquired their "drinking habits." In this carefully controlled experiment, both groups of naive mice "picked up" the behavioral characteristics of their older compatriots. The young black mice, who would otherwise be heavy drinkers, became virtually teetotalers when reared with nondrinking tans. The tans, in turn, became drinkers after seven weeks of mutual exposure. While neither strain assumed the total behavioral repertoire by cohabiting with opposite role models (neither ever drank as much or as little as the "pure" strain of origin), this experiment showed in a remarkable way the power of social factors in influencing behavior [25] . When analyzed in detail, it turns out that less than half of the observed differences in alcohol consumption among mouse strains can be attributed to genetic differences. Similarly, adoption studies which suggest closer relationships between the alcohol behavior of adoptive sons and their biological fathers, are likely to be flawed by uncontrolled social factors, such as the very fact of being adopted.

In mice, these experiments suggest that genetically similar mice housed together would come to interact in ways which allow the slight predilection of a *single* animal to spread through the remaining mice by behavioral mechanisms associated with socialization. A minimum genetic substratum for a particular characteristic would be all that is needed to allow the subsequent social amplification of its expression to bring this predisposition to the fore. Indeed, the phenomenon of social "pecking orders" in genetically identical mice has been confirmed for a wide spectrum of behaviors.

The existence of confounding effects of environment and gene interactions should give pause to the genetic counselor contemplating complex gene associated phenomena. The final outcome of any genetic system depends as much on the milieu in which it is acting as on the extrinsic forces with which it interacts. For people, the context of gene action includes the genetic background, the group in which it is being expressed, the cultural setting, and the prevailing environment. All of these components interact to dampen, reinforce, suppress or lift out the potential effects of the human genome [26].

Very few if any of the specific features of human ability or disability are thus likely to fall into a consistent, simple cause-and-effect relationship. Where human behavior is concerned, the genetic connection is likely to be even more tenuous. Rather than increasing the predictability of behavior or complex disease processes like diabetes, genetic underpinnings confound the possibility of knowing in advance what will happen. The true knots of interaction which characterize complex gene action and environmental forces skews all but the simplest systems into the realm of indeterminacy.

Indeterminancy in complex gene action almost necessarily arises from the fact that many, if not most, genes simply delineate a "reaction range" for an organism within a larger physiologic and behavioral reality. Physiology and psychology can interact to distort simple analogs of one gene-one enzyme. When human choices and not merely passive responses determine the reaction patterns, synergistic feedback loops become possible which can amplify any underlying genetic predilection for a given behavior or physiologic response. All of this means that the plasticity which we observe in human illness and well-being may indeed have a strong genetic base, but it is one which allows for almost infinite variations. And genetic counselors concerned with the human condition will do well to keep in mind the complexity which undergirds the expression of genes in people.

REFERENCES

1. Kaufman S, Holtzman NA, Milstein S et al: Phenylketonuria due to deficiency of dihydropteridine reductase. N Engl J Med 293:785–789, 1975.
2. Blanch RR, Mendoz EM: Fertility in a man with cystic fibrosis. JAMA 235:1364–1365, 1976.
3. Darlington CD: "Genetics and Man." New York: Shocken Books, 1969, pp 102–103. See also Johanssen's own summary from 1903. In Peters JA (ed): "Classic Papers in Genetics." Englewood Cliffs: Prentice Hall, 1959.

4. Cited in Newman HH: "Evolution, Genetics and Eugenics." New York: Greenwood Press, 1969, p 485.
5. Wright S: The results of crosses between inbred strains of guinea pigs differing in number of digits. Genetics 19:537–551, 1934.
6. Beck F, Lloyd JB: Embryological principles of teratogenesis. In Robson JM, Sullivan FM, Smith RL (eds): "Embryopathic Activity of Drugs." Boston: Little Brown & Co., 1965, pp 1–21.
7. Fraser FC: The use of teratogens in the analysis of abnormal developmental mechanisms. In "First International Conference on Congenital Malformations." Philadelphia: JP Lippincott, 1961, pp 179–186.
8. Kalter H: Some sources of non-genetic variability in steroid-induced cleft palate in the mouse. Teratology 13:1–10, 1976.
9. Barlow SM, McElhatton PR, Sullivan PM: The relation between material restraint and food, deprivation, plasma corticosterone, and induction of cleft palate in the offspring of mice. Teratology 12:97–104, 1975.
10. Erway L, Hurley LS, Fraser A: Neurological defects: Manganese in phenocopy and prevention of genetic abnormality of inner ear. Science 152:1766–1768, 1966.
11. Britain's Great Thalidomide Cover-up. Columbia Journalism Review, May 1975.
12. Lenz W: Phenocopies. J Med Genet 10:34–49, 1973.
13. Degenhardt KH, Kleinebrech J: Principles in teratology. In Raspe G (ed): "Advances in the Biosciences." New York: Pergamon Press, 1971, vol 6.
14. Rosenthal MR, Goldfine ID, Saperstein MD: Genetic origin of diabetes: Reevaluation of twin data. Lancet 2:250–251, 1976.
15. Van de Putte I et al: Segregation of HLA B7 in juvenile-onset diabetes mellitus. Lancet 2:251, 1976.
16. Cavalli-Sforza LL, Feldman MW: Cultural versus biological inheritance: Phenotype transmission from parents to children. Am J Hum Genet 25:618–637, 1973.
17. Anderson LT, Alpert M, Dancis J et al: An analysis of self-injury in Lesch–Nyhan disease. Summarized in Psychological Spectator 10:4, 1975.
18. Selmanoff MK, Jumonville JE, Maxson SC, Ginsberg BE: Evidence for a Y chromosomal contribution to an aggressive phenotype in inbred mice. Nature 253:529–530, 1975.
19. Selmanoff MK, Maxson SC, Ginsburg BE: Chromosomal determinants of intermale aggressive behavior in inbred mice. Behav Genet 6:53–69, 1976.
20. Lagerspetz KMJ, Lagerspetz KYH: Genetic determination of aggressive behavior. In Abeleen (op cit) pp 321–346.
21. Randt CT, Blizard DZ, Friedman E: Early life undernutrition and aggression in two mice strains. Dev Psychobiol 8:275–279, 1975.
22. Volume 197 of the Annals of the New York Academy of Sciences is devoted to "nature" and "nurture" questions about alcohol use.
23. Omenn G, Motulsky A: A biochemical and genetic approach to alcoholism. Ann NY Acad Sci 197:16–23, 1972.
24. Fuller JL: Measurement of alcohol preference in genetic experiments. Comparative and Physiological Psychology 57:85–88, 1965.
25. Randall CL, Lester D: Social modification of alcohol consumption for other complicating features of alcohol consumption in inbred mice. Science 189:149–151, 1975.
26. Hirsch J (ed): "Behavior Genetic Analysis." New York: McGraw-Hill, 1967, p 416.

3. Genetic Disease as Seen on a Continuum

Richard Roblin, PhD

   The definition of "genetic disease" and its diagnosis may be problematic, full of ambiguity, and a matter of argument for philosophers, but it is apparently not so for clinicians. There are now operational criteria for the diagnosis of several genetic diseases, and diagnosis of these genetic diseases consists of performing and interpreting particular biochemical or chromosomal tests. The results of these tests, especially when the tests are applied to a fetus in utero, lead to genetic counseling sessions with the prospective parents and, in some cases, to abortion of the fetus because it has a diagnosed genetic disease. For me, the fact that abortion decisions can hinge upon diagnosis of genetic diseases in utero makes complete presentation and comprehension of the information conveyed in genetic counseling a matter of considerable importance.

   In this chapter, I will sketch some operational criteria used to diagnose two representative genetic diseases, particularly as they illustrate varying degrees of certainty with which they establish the future occurrence of a given constellation of phenotypic characteristics — the genetic disease. My thesis is that biologic complexity and currently available operational criteria for diagnosis of genetic disease leave a margin of uncertainty regarding the future life-expectancy of those with the classic signs of a genetic disease. This margin of uncertainty creates both a dilemma and a temptation for those who bear the responsibility for genetic counseling. The dilemma is whether or not this margin of uncertainty ought to be conveyed in genetic counseling, and if so, how? The temptation is to simplify the situation for the prospective parents in genetic counseling, to gloss over the margin of uncertainty. I argue that to succumb to this temptation is to fall short of a standard of truth-telling which I believe ought to operate in the genetic counseling situation.

Birth Defects: Original Articles Series, Volume XV, Number 2, **pages 47—56**
© **1979 The National Foundation**

OPERATIONAL CRITERIA FOR DIAGNOSIS OF GENETIC DISEASES

Chromosome Analysis

In utero diagnosis of trisomy 21 (also called Down syndrome or mongolism) will be taken as an example of the manner in which chromosome analysis is used to detect genetic diseases. Desquamated fetal skin cells are isolated from the amniotic fluid obtained by amniocentesis; the cells are grown in, in vitro tissue culture; and the fixed and stained metaphase chromosomes are examined by microscopy. The normal human chromosome complement is 46 chromosomes, 22 pairs of autosomal chromosomes and 2 sex-determining chromosomes (XX for females and XY for males). Cells from individuals with trisomy 21 contain an extra copy of chromosome 21, 47 chromosomes in all.

Although the presence of an extra chromosome 21 is a discrete (present or absent) type of diagnostic characteristic, establishing the diagnosis of trisomy 21 is not always as simple as it might appear. In practice, when the number of chromosomes in a normal human cell are counted, the number 46 is not always obtained. Occasionally, a few chromosomes are lost from the spread-out field of chromosomes, and chromosome counts of less than 46 are obtained. Chromosome counts greater than 46 may also be obtained in normal cells, either because the same chromosome was counted twice, or because one or more chromosomes from an adjacent cell have become part of the group being counted. However, if a large majority of the cells show 46 chromosomes, the cells would be considered normal. Similarly, if most of the cells contain 47 chromosomes, and the extra chromosome can be shown to be No. 21 by special staining techniques, then trisomy 21 would be diagnosed. The probability of a correct determination of the chromosome number is a function of the number of separate metaphase cells whose chromosomes are counted. Counting a very large number of cells would maximize the probability of a correct determination, but counting chromosomes is a tedious process since it is still done manually in most laboratories. In practice, counting the chromosomes of about 30 metaphase cells has been recommended as being sufficient [1].

The existence of rare individuals who are mosaics, that is, those who actually contain cells with different numbers of chromosomes in their bodies, is an additional complication. For example, such an individual might have both cells with the normal 46 chromosome complement and cells with an extra copy of chromosome 21. In this case, chromosomal analysis of fetal cells might show approximately equal numbers of cells with 46 and 47 chromosomes, assuming that both types of cells survive equally well in the amniotic fluid and grow equally well in vitro. Differentiating mosaics from individuals with simple trisomy 21 is important because mosaics for trisomy 21 may not be as severely affected as individuals with simple trisomy 21. Milunsky has summarized this problem as follows [2]:

> Exclusion of true *mosaicism* could also prove extremely difficult to resolve. In line with the recommendations of Court-Brown et al. [ref. 1] for other tissues, it seems prudent in demonstrating the fetal karyotype to count at least 30 metaphases of the cultured amniotic fluid cells where possible. This approach, while not entirely excluding the possibility of mosaicism in the fetus, makes a potentially important error less likely. . . . It must be emphasized that counting an arbitrary number of cells is only a helpful guide and can never in itself disprove the existence of mosaicism.

The possibility that mycoplasma contamination of fetal cells prior to chromosome analysis may induce certain types of chromosome abnormalities in the cultured cells which are not originally present in the cells of the individual must also be considered. As Schneider et al [3] have concluded:

> Our results indicate that mycoplasma infection of cultured amniotic fluid cells leads to a significantly increased incidence of chromosomal alterations. Breaks and gaps induced by mycoplasma should not confuse prenatal chromosome diagnosis except, perhaps, in Bloom's syndrome or Fanconi's anemia. However, translocations and alterations of chromosome number could lead to false positive results. We therefore recommend that all amniotic fluid cultures which reveal chromosomal mosaicism, multiple or unusual translocations, or frequent breaks be examined for mycoplasma contamination. Parallel cultures of all amniotic fluid cells are also advised since, as in our case of chromosomal mosaicism, it may provide a source of uninfected cells. Biochemical as well as microbiological screening should be done since our study and previous studies indicate that mycoplasma contamination can be missed by microbiological testing alone.

The possibilities of mosaicism and of mycoplasma contamination generating chromosomal abnormalities in vitro, coupled with the technical aspects of chromosome counting and identification, combine to create a small margin of uncertainty regarding the diagnosis of genetic diseases due to chromsome abnormalities. Whether any of these factors were responsible for the few reported errors [4, 5] in prenatal diagnosis of chromosome disorders is unknown. While procedures such as the recommended mycoplasma testing can be instituted which will reduce this margin of uncertainty, such procedures increase the cost of each diagnostic test. Those who operate chromosome testing laboratories make implicit or explicit decisions balancing what they consider to be an acceptable margin of uncertainty against the practical necessity of keeping the cost of testing within reasonable limits. Since procedures for diagnosis of chromosomal disorders have not yet been standardized, considerable variation may exist between the practices of different laboratories.

Assuming that all the possible complicating technical factors in making a correct diagnosis of trisomy 21 in utero have been taken into consideration, in this disease there is also an added residual uncertainty regarding the predictability of the final outcome. Children with trisomy 21 exhibit a range of behavioral and intellectual deficits [6], not an invariable set of characteristics. In one rare instance, a child with Down syndrome proved to be capable of writing a book about his experiences [7]. To my knowledge, there is as yet no way to predict just how severely any given fetus with a diagnosis of trisomy 21 will be affected. Thus, a "correct" or "truthful" description of these facts would be some kind of probability statement. This statement would reflect the high probability that a fetus with an in utero diagnosis of trisomy 21 would exhibit subnormal intelligence and behavioral difficulties, but would also encompass the small margin of uncertainty in the correctness of the diagnosis and the degree of uncertainty in the predictability of the outcome. I will argue below why I think descriptive statements by genetic counselors to counselees should be more in this vein than absolutist statements which admit of no exceptions.

Biochemical Tests

In utero diagnosis of Tay-Sachs disease will serve as an example of the use of a biochemical test to detect a fetus with a genetic disease. Again, fetal cells obtained by amniocentesis are grown in vitro, and the amount of an enzyme known as hexosaminidase A contained in the fetal cell is measured [8]. Deficiency of the enzyme hexosaminidase A is thought to be reponsible for the abnormal accumulation of glycolipids in the brain, which characterizes Tay-Sachs disease. Hexosaminidase A cannot yet be measured directly, however. Advantage is taken of the observation that hexosaminidase A is more readily inactivated by heat than hexosaminidase B [9] to discriminate between these two enzyme activities. In practice, what one does is measure total hexosaminidase activity before and after heating, and express the fraction of the total activity lost upon heating as the "amount" of hexosaminidase A. For cultured amniotic cells from 16 normal controls, hexosaminidase A activity (as a percentage of the total) ranged from 62—79 [8]. For cultured amniotic cells from five fetuses in which the diagnosis of Tay-Sachs disease was subsequently confirmed, hexosaminidase A activity ranged from 1—12 [8].

The value obtained for the amount of hexosaminidase A activity is thus a quantitative, as opposed to a discrete (present or absent), type of biologic characteristic. That is, the value of hexosaminidase A activity is judged to be abnormally low (indicating deficiency and suggesting a diagnosis of Tay-Sachs disease) based upon comparison with a normal range. The number of normal control samples examined is thus of considerable importance in assessing the likelihood of the deficiency.

The data presented above, obtained from a paper published in 1971 [8], indicate that the control range for hexosaminidase A activity in cultured amniotic cells is sufficiently different from the low values obtained with Tay-Sachs homozygotes, so that the likelihood of an ambiguous test or mistaken diagnosis is small. However, only 5 Tay-Sachs cases were studied, and the size of the control group (16) was also small. Thus, it was possible that the full extent of variation in levels of hexosaminidase A activity in unaffected individuals had not yet been observed. Recent reports [10–12] of healthy individuals with apparent hexosaminidase A deficiency suggest that this is indeed the case.

There are several possible explanations for the existence of healthy individuals with no detectable hexosaminidase A activity. Navon et al [10] suggest that,

> [they] may have a sufficient amount of a variant isozyme of hexosaminidase A, which acts normally in vivo but is unable to cleave the synthetic substitute used . . . in vitro. [Alternatively] , at least two of the four exceptional [children] . . . must be heterozygous for the common mutant gene responsible for TSD [Tay-Sachs disease]. It is suggested that their other allele at that locus is a rare variant. It is postulated, therefore, that there are three alleles at this locus: T, the normal (dominant) one; t_1, the common mutant TSD allele; and t_2, the hypothesized rare variant. The six possible genotypes resulting from this system would probably produce five phenotypes: TT, clinically and biochemically normal; Tt_1, and Tt_2, indistinguishable from each other and clinically normal with reduced hexosaminidase A activity; t_1t_1, TSD with absence of hexosaminidase A; t_1t_2, the exceptional phenotype of the four sibs reported here; and t_2t_2, as yet unknown.

The existence of exceptional cases such as these again creates a small margin of uncertainty regarding the significance of the results of a biochemical test — in this case measurement of the hexosaminidase A activity. In the absence of any other tests, demonstration that an individual is deficient in hexosaminidase A activity no longer unambiguously establishes a diagnosis of Tay-Sachs disease. As Navon et al point out,

> As long as we are unable to distinguish between Tt_1, and Tt_2 individuals, the latter will be misclassified (for example, in population screening) as TSD heterozygotes and subject to whatever limitations this might impose. In marriages between them and genuine Tt_1 heterozygotes . . . t_1t_2 fetuses will be falsely diagnosed as having

TSD and therefore subjected to unnecessary abortion. The same may be the case in marriages of $t_1t_2 \times Tt_1$ individuals . . . half of whose hexosaminidase-deficient offspring could be non-TSD [eg, t_1t_2].

Fortunately, current circumstances under which genetic counseling for Tay-Sachs disease would be likely to take place partially mitigate this difficulty. Parents would be likely to seek genetic counseling either after already having had a child with Tay-Sachs disease, or after being identified as carriers in a heterozygote screening program. In both cases, the parents would have been tested and individuals who were t_1t_2 would have been identified as exceptional by virtue of their apparent lack of hexosaminidase A activity. The case that remains a problem, at the moment, for genetic counseling is the uncertainty whether individuals who are apparently heterozygous are Tt_2 as opposed to Tt_1.

Further research into the molecular basis of Tay-Sachs disease may eventually permit distinguishing individuals who are Tt_1 from those who are Tt_2. In the past several years, progress has been made toward detailed biochemical characterization of hexosaminidase A and determination of its molecular relationship to other hexosaminidase activities [13, 14]. Techniques for measuring hexosaminidase A activity using the glycolipid which accumulates in Tay-Sachs disease, rather than the currently used synthetic substrate, are being developed and the use of such techniques may increase the specificity of assaying hexosaminidase A activity. At present, the situation with Tay-Sachs disease illustrates a more general problem for genetic counseling: whether and how to translate this diagnostic uncertainty into terms understandable by those undergoing genetic counseling.

The situation of healthy individuals with apparent hexosaminidase A deficiency recapitulates the apparent genetic heterogeneity previously observed with elevated serum phenylalanine levels and phenylketonuria [15], and galactose-1-phosphate uridyl transferase deficiency and galactosemia [16]. Early in our experience with many recessive genetic disorders there appears to be a single mutant gene which, in the homozygous condition, leads to deficiency and associated genetic disease. As more and more individuals are examined, rare individuals with an apparent or real enzyme deficiency but no associated disease are detected. And the nature of the tests used to measure enzyme deficiency generally does not permit determination of the precise cause of the enzyme deficiency in different individuals.

OUGHT THE MARGIN OF UNCERTAINTY BE CONVEYED IN GENETIC COUNSELING?

As amply documented by other chapters in this book, the genetic counselor faces the problem of reducing a varied and complex set of facts and interpretations to a form comprehensible to those being counseled. The difficulties attending this process have been sufficiently described here and elsewhere so that one hesitates to add what may seem (to some) like unnecessary complications. Yet, it seems to me that there are significant practical and moral arguments in favor of including a discussion of the margin of uncertainty in genetic counseling.

The circumstances surrounding genetic counseling, with its possible decisions about fetal life and death, place a heavy stress on trust as an essential ingredient in the relationship between genetic counselor and counselee. By virtue of this trust placed in them, genetic counselors have a general obligation to convey the truth about their situation to those being counseled. Because difficult decisions with perhaps life-long consequences for those being counseled will be based upon what the counselor tells his counselees, a very high premium should be placed upon providing them with the truth. A description of the kinds of tests performed, the results obtained, the interpretation of those results, and any limits to the interpretation of those results (such as the margin of uncertainty) form the core of the truth which the counselor should convey.

Any margin of uncertainty which exists regarding the significance of tests to infer genotype is a significant piece of information for counselees, because different people may react to small degrees of uncertainty in different ways. It may be a significant fact for some counselees that the genetic counselor admits to a small degree of uncertainty regarding the future life-expectancy of a fetus with a third copy of chromosome 21, or a hexosaminidase A deficiency. In addition, as the principal or sole source of the information upon which the counselee acts, the genetic counselor should resist the temptation to simplify the situation by disregarding the exceptional cases.

In rare cases, discussion of the margin of uncertainty may protect the genetic counselor from the difficulties attending abortion of a nondiseased fetus which was diagnosed in utero as having a genetic disease. It is easy to imagine the detrimental effects of such events, even if infrequent, on the couple who were counseled, as well as on the counselor. However, to my knowledge, there is no current requirement that confirmatory diagnostic tests be done on fetuses aborted because of a genetic disease diagnosed in utero. Thus, the rare case of a nondiseased fetus aborted for genetic indications may never be detected. The temptation to ignore or cover up such a situation would be considerable.

Discussion of the margin of uncertainty with counselees encourages the genetic counselor to critically reexamine the primary data upon which his projections of fetal life-expectancy are based. In the course of so doing the counselor should consider the following questions: How many confirmed cases of the classic genetic disease have been reported? What is the frequency of the rare cases which mimic the classic genetic disease? What then can I infer to be the margin of uncertainty in my ability to predict that this particular fetus will be born with the genetic disease in question? Answering these questions will equip the genetic counselor with the raw materials for a discussion of the margin of uncertainty with those being counseled.

COUNTERVAILING ARGUMENTS

The complexity and unfamiliarity of the information to be conveyed in genetic counseling favors its simplification for presentation. In some discussions I have heard, genetic counselors have maintained the undesirability of attempting to give the counselee "a short course in genetics" during the counseling session. However, I believe what I have been describing is different from attempting to give counselees a complete understanding of genetics. Discussion of the margin of uncertainty provides not simply more facts but rather the counselor's best estimate of the probability with which the tests that have been done can predict the future. This is a far more relevant bit of information for evaluating the significance of the test results than many genetic facts would be.

It might also be objected that, while discussion of the margin of uncertainty might be desirable, it is impractical. This might be so for a variety of reasons — the difficulties inherent in reducing the margin of uncertainty to a single numerical probability, the difficulty counselees might have in comprehending such estimates, and the pressure of time. Although I have no practical experience in genetic counseling, none of these difficulties appears insurmountable to me. If there is no way to estimate the frequency of rare, variant genes (eg for hexosaminidase A) in the population, then would it be wrong to present counselees with the actual numbers? For example, the counselor might tell the prospective parents of a diagnosed, hexosaminidase A-deficient fetus, "There have been n cases of Tay-Sachs disease reported in the world medical literature, and x cases of rare variants of the gene for hexosaminidase A." The counselees could then make their own evaluation of the significance of these numbers for their particular case. I believe there is an important difference between presenting these facts and telling counselees, as fact, that their child will be born with Tay-Sachs disease.

It might be further objected that, by failing to *interpret* the primary data for counselees, the genetic counselor would be failing in one of the basic responsibilities to those being counseled. This view of the counselor's responsibility might be stated as follows:

My training has given me knowledge of the facts about genetic diseases and experience in evaluating the significance of these facts. Those whom I counsel start with much less knowledge and experience than I do. Part of my responsibility in genetic counseling is to impart some knowledge of the facts to those whom I counsel, but another part of my responsibility is to use my experience and judgment to help them evaluate the facts that I give them.

In part, the tension between this view and the one I have described could be resolved by separating facts and interpretation in time during the counseling session. If the counselor presented facts first and clearly indicated where the facts left off and interpretation began, then the two views are not very different. Counselors' attitudes toward this possibility will depend upon their conception of the dominant aspect of the counselor's role. Those who stress the role of the counselor as information-giver (see Chapter 11) may find it easier to separate facts and interpretation than those who stress the role of the counselor as moral advisor (see Chapter 13).

CONCLUSION

I have attempted to justify the view that giving counselees "the facts" about genetic disease ought to include a discussion of the margin of uncertainty of diagnosis and outcome by the genetic counselor. In part, I urge this course of action because it most closely approximates "the truth" about the counselee's situation. Because genetic counselors possess much greater knowledge about genetic disease than those whom they counsel, counselors should be particularly scrupulous about separating facts from inferences drawn from those facts. Simplifying the facts for the counselees by, for example, omitting discussion of rare variants, interposes the counselor's judgment of the significance of low probability events between the counselees and the facts. While many counselees may seek such judgments, others may not. Presenting the facts first would permit counselors to reserve their interpretations and judgments of significance until the counselees request them.

REFERENCES

1. Court-Brown WM, Harnden DC, Jacobs PA: Abnormalities of the sex chromosomes complement in man. London: Medical Council Special Report Series, 305:1, 1964.
2. Milunsky A: "The Prenatal Diagnosis of Hereditary Disorders." Springfield: Charles C Thomas, 1973, p 29.
3. Schneider EL, Stanbridge EJ, Epstein CJ, Golbus M, Abbo-Halbasch G, Rodgers G: Mycoplasma contamination of cultured amniotic fluid cells: Potential hazard to prenatal chromosomal diagnosis. Science 184:477–479, 1974.
4. Nadler H, Gerbie A: Present status of amniocentesis in intrauterine diagnosis of genetic defects. Obstet Gynecol 38:789–799, 1971.
5. Culliton BJ: Amniocentesis: HEW backs test for prenatal diagnosis of disease. Science 190:537–540, 1975.
6. Smith DW, Wilson AA: "The Child with Down's Syndrome: Causes, Characteristics and Acceptance." Philadelphia: WB Saunders, 1973.
7. Hunt N: "The World of Nigel Hunt, The Diary of a Mongoloid Youth." London: Darwen Finlayson, 1967.
8. O'Brien JS, Okada S, Fillerup DL, Veath L, Adornato B, Brenner PH, Leroy JG: Tay-Sachs disease: Prenatal diagnosis. Science 172:61–64, 1971.

9. O'Brien JS, Okada S, Chen A, et al: Tay-Sachs Disease: Detection by serum hexosaminidase assay. N Engl J Med 283:15−20, 1970.
10. Navon R, Padeh B, Adam A: Apparent deficiency of hexosaminidase A in healthy members of a family with Tay-Sachs disease. Am J Hum Genet 25:287−293, 1973.
11. Vidgoff J, Buist NRM, O'Brien JS: Absence of β-N-acetyl-D-hexosaminidase A activity in a healthy woman. Am J Hum Genet 25:372−381, 1973.
12. Dreyfus JC, Poenaru L, Svennerholm L: Absence of hexosaminidase A and B in a normal adult. N Engl J Med 292:61−63, 1975.
13. Beutler E, Kuhl W: Subunit structure of human hexosaminidase verified: Interconvertability of hexosaminidase isozymes. Nature 258:262−264, 1975.
14. Geiger B, Arnon R: Chemical characterization and subunit structure of human N-acetyl hexosaminidases A and B. Biochemistry 15:3484−3493, 1976.
15. Knox WE: Phenylketonuria. In Stanbury JB, Wyngaarden JB, Fredrickson DS (eds): "The Metabolic Basis of Inherited Disease." 3rd Ed. New York: McGraw-Hill, 1972, pp 285−290.
16. Segal S: Disorders of galactose metabolism. Ibid pp 185−186.

4. Why *"Genetic* Disease"?

Richard T. Hull, PhD

There are a few words and phrases which are continually employed in
genetic counseling, therapy, and research, but whose careful analysis has been
generally neglected. The more obvious of these (with the explicit valuational
component italicized) include expressions like *"mal*adaptive trait," "congenital
*mal*formation," *"defect," "deleterious* gene," and "inborn *error* of metabolism."
Even such terms as "genetic *ab*normality" and "chromosomal *aberration*," indicative of only a deviation from the normal range of variability, are, I suspect,
most frequently used in application to disvalued divergence.

Less obvious are the valuational components of the meaning of the important and constantly used expression "genetic disease," and they will be examined
in this paper. These components are in part etymologic, stemming from the
origins of the term "disease." But they also derive from two other sources: the
social and psychologic results of identifying a disease with only one of its causal
conditions, and the consequences of the selective focus on one particular range
of possible therapies, prevention, and research stemming from the decision to
call a disease "genetic." In the following sections, the sources of the valuational
aspects of the expression "genetic disease" will be traced to show the ways in
which they come into conflict in the genetic counseling situation.

ETYMOLOGY OF "GENETIC DISEASE": SOME SHIFTS IN MEANING

"Genetic"

There are two things to be said about the "genetic" component of the
term "genetic disease." The first can be stated in a couple of ways. Every nongenetic disease has a genetic component, describable in terms of the presence (or
absence) of one or more genetically determined traits. Susceptibility or resistance to infection by a given microorganism, injurability, and toxic reactability

Birth Defects: Original Article Series, Volume XV, Number 2, pages 57—69

are each in part a function of genetic endowment (although doubtless more frequently polygenic than monogenic in character). We may well suppose that individual resistance to, say, smallpox is a function of genetic endowment, yet we do not classify smallpox as a genetic disease. Why? Another way of putting the same point is this: every nongenetic disease has both genetic and nongenetic members of its set of nonredundant, jointly sufficient conditions. This raises the question of why and how some diseases come to be classified by appeal to their genetic component(s) and others by appeal to their nongenetic component(s). Whence our interest in only certain members of those sets of jointly sufficient conditions, and not others? I shall return to these points.

The second observation is this. Many so-called genetic diseases have known environmental components; the associated syndrome is manifested only in the presence of specific environmental factors or agents. For example, the hemolytic anemia associated with glucose-6-phosphate dehydrogenase (G6PD) deficiency is manifested only upon exposure to certain foods (such as *Vicia faba,* the common broad bean) or certain drugs (such as primaquine, used in treatment of malaria) [1]. Xeroderma pigmentosum skin cancer is triggered by sunlight and ultraviolet radiation, but otherwise its symptoms would not occur in persons homozygous for the recessive gene. Further, many genetic diseases involve the deficiency, or deficiency at a crucial stage of development, of some enzyme or hormone that plays a developmental or maintenance role. Insulin, whose absence produces the hereditary metabolic disease diabetes mellitus, can be artificially supplied, thereby allowing the patient to live a relatively normal life. Homozygotes for phenylketonuria (PKU) are unable to convert phenylalanine to tyrosine because of the lack of the liver enzyme phenylalanine hydroxylase [1]. So far, all individuals who have been discovered to excrete phenylpyruvic acid in their urine have shown some degree of mental retardation [2]. The amount secreted varies widely as a function of daily protein intake. The weight of evidence indicates that the presence of phenylalanine and its metabolites in large quantities hinders the laying down of myelin. Hence, a low phenylalanine diet, instigated at birth, allows more or less normal development of myelin to occur, thus avoiding or minimizing the associated mental deficiency. The diet may be relaxed after the first several years, since most myelin is laid down then and only maintenance of the sheaths is carried out thereafter. The point is that in these cases it is the absence of the enzyme which is "the cause" of the disease. The genetic abnormality of the enzyme is not necessarily itself sufficient for the disease, for the enzyme could (in principle) be supplied artificially, or the results of incomplete metabolism avoided by dietary control (just as the essential amnio acids and ascorbic acid must be acquired through diet in those species lacking the genetic basis for their natural production).

Even diseases such as sickle cell anemia, which seem under normal conditions to possess causally sufficient genetic antecedents, frequently are manifested through intermediate steps that are capable of reversal or interruption. Sodium cyanate has been used clinically in treatment of sickle cell anemia (although it is a suspected toxicant of the central nervous system), and a recent report indicates that dimethyl adipimidate may act on hemoglobin to increase its affinity for oxygen and restore the red blood cell membrane to normalcy without affecting red cell metabolism [3].

Finally, a number of genetic diseases that are thought to be due to a single (dominant or recessive) maladaptive allele may in fact involve the absence of some offsetting additional mutation. For example, several cases have been reported of healthy adults in families having Tay-Sachs or Sandhoff disease, in which the healthy adults appear to have a double dose of the associated lethal recessive gene [4, 6]. The evidence suggests that the effect is due to the presence of an offsetting mutation in the gene which both allows hydrolysis of the terminal N-acetyl-β-galactosamine of ganglioside G_{M2} (a natural substrate) and obscures any such activity within the artificial substrates usually employed in the routine diagnosis of such diseases [6]. Further, the second mutation may be undetectable in the way normal hexosaminidases A and B are, when it is coupled with a normal gene [5, 6]. So, if the presence of the second mutant is a sufficient condition for the nonoccurrence of Tay-Sachs or Sandhoff disease, its absence is as much a necessary condition for each of those diseases as is the commonly associated so-called lethal recessive in double dosage. What at first appears to be a classic case of the presence of a genetic factor homozygously fitting our definition of cause, so that we could without embarrassment identify it as *the* cause of the disease, turns out not to be so unequivocally.

This latter sort of case suggests a way to view even the most genetic of diseases in a nongenetic way. Our general understanding of such disorders indicates that in them the presence or absence of certain gene products in the internal biochemical environment of the body are the causes of those genetic diseases with no identifiable external environmental factor. But this raises the theoretic possibility of modifying the internal environment by means of introducing the essential product at its crucial point of interaction in some metabolic chain, or of suppressing the production, or otherwise offsetting the effect, of some gene product. Thus, strictly speaking, the presence or absence of the gene itself is not the cause of the disease, but rather the presence or absence of one or more chemicals which serve as partial determinants of the inner environment. To the extent that such products theoretically can be suppressed or supplemented by externally originating action, we may fairly characterize even the most "genetic" diseases as having nongenetic components.

These cases are tendered to suggest the possibility that no disease, or at most very few, has only genetic factors involved in its total set of individually necessary, jointly sufficient conditions. It is evident, then, that in most, if not all, cases of genetic disease, the application of the term "genetic" reflects a choice having been made to emphasize, among the causal factors, the genetic component and deemphasize the environmental one. There is some inductive reason to suppose that even the hard core of truly "genetic" diseases may shrink as our knowledge of euthenic engineering increases, enabling us to modify or control expression of the existing genetic information of individuals affected with diseases having genetic components, so as to result in a more desirable phenotype [7]. Hence, I am tempted to endorse the generalization that every genetic disease has nongenetic components, whether presently known and understood or not.

"Disease"

Conceptually, the notion of disease originates in the patient's complaints about bodily discomforts. A disease is identified, first and foremost, in terms of the dis-ease involved. In the subjective sense of the term, we speak of symptoms or abnormal feelings which the patient has. A disease is also identified in terms of abnormal states or conditions of the body which are publicly observable; these are sometimes also called symptoms, but here they will be referred to as signs. Some signs may be so obvious that they become part of the patient's complaint (eg rashes, paralyses); others may require more skilled observation to detect (eg dullness of some portion of the lungs under percussion).

Apart from physiologic knowledge of how an individual symptom or sign arises and may be made to recede, often little else is required for mere palliation. But the notion of disease has also come to involve, first, the idea of a syndrome, and, second, the idea of its cause. A syndrome is a set of *associated* symptoms and signs, associated both through their frequent joint occurrence and through the notion that they have a common cause. Frequently we are not satisfied with mere palliative measures; they must be constantly administered throughout the disease's natural course to suppress the occurrence of signs or symptoms, and they are often not fully successful. They involve conceiving of and treating symptoms individually, whereas we suspect that in most cases constellations of signs and symptoms can be thought of as manifestations of a common cause.

But it is overly simple to speak of "the cause" of a disease. One of the benefits of philosophers' investigations into the term is to show how idiosyncratic our use of "cause" can be. In its fullest sense, of course, the cause of something is the total set of its individually necessary and jointly sufficient conditions. In talking of the cause of a disease in more ordinary circumstances, however, this definition of cause is not employed, in large part because of the difficulty of satisfying its demand. Rather, "some one or more conditons within that set which were novel, unusual, or controllable" are usually cited in giving the cause [8]. Scriven [9] once described this common notion as follows: "A cause is a non-redundant member of a set of conditions jointly sufficient for the effect. . ., the choice between the several candidates that usually meet this requirement being based on considerations of context." What strikes us as novel, unusual, or controllable will be singled out as the cause, because our interests lie in uncommon, novel. or controllable phenomena.

Consider the following illustration, which is an example I recall from Scriven's lectures. A college co-ed has a premarital affair with a male student of whom her parents strongly disapprove and who has promised to marry her, and she conceives as a result. When he learns of it, her boyfriend jilts her. She comes from a conservative home and does not feel that she can turn to her parents for help and advice. Her roommate is studying hard for exams and rebuffs her attempts at soliciting a sympathetic ear. She becomes even further depressed over the reaction of the infirmary physician who confirms the pregnancy and lectures her on her loose ways but offers nothing but scorn at her tentative broaching of the subject of an abortion. She wanders out onto the San Francisco Bay Bridge and stands looking over the rail. A passing motorist yells, "Jump!" She climbs onto the rail; other motorists stop and watch her. She leaps off and drops into the waters of the bay. What was the cause of her death? Any of several of the conditions surrounding her could plausibly be pointed to as the cause (in the sense of "cause" which Scriven describes), in that we can point to a number of necessary conditions in the sequence of events which led up to her death. Such are events which, had they not happened or been prevented from happening, would have rendered the set of prior conditions insufficient to bring about the effect; depending on where our interests lie, we will cite some one or more of these as causes of her death. The coroner may list drowning as the cause; a policeman may list the cause as suicide by jumping off the bridge; various sociologists and psychologists with varying research interests may point to the seduction and abandonment, the coldness of the physician, the alienation from the parents, the preoccupation of the roommate, or even the jeers and passivity of the drivers on the bridge, as the event or events responsible for her death. The idea of cause as we most commonly employ it embodies the concept of human interest, in that it is in large part this which will determine which of several possible candidates for the cause of an event we will so identify.

The notion of a syndrome — a set of associated signs and symptoms thought to have a common cause — is not quite sufficient to capture the concept of disease as it is most commonly employed today. Indeed, there are some dramatic departures from the notion of disease as rooted in the patient's characteristic complaints together with associated signs. In its efforts to understand, control, and avoid disease, modern medicine has incorporated into the very identification of a disease the notion of the cause of the syndrome. This permits the individuation of similar syndromes with distinct causes into different diseases [10] . For example, the general classification of epilepsies along syndromic lines (petit mal, grand mal, temporal lobe) is augmented by classifications amounting to discrimination by cause; each type is further divided into ischemic, traumatic, and idiopathic. Thus, there are now three kinds of petit mal epilepsy; the symptoms are no longer definitive of the disease, but constitute manifestations of the disease; the disease is now identified with the underlying cause of the symptoms; and ischemic and traumatic grand mal epilepsy are spoken of as distinct diseases which manifest similar symptoms [11]. What has happened is that the root notion of disease — the syndrome — is replaced in its identification by the syndrome's cause. I shall return to this significant point.

Putting together the results of our inquiry, we see that the decision to call a disease "genetic" involves its identification with a nonredundant or individually necessary member of the set of conditions jointly sufficient for the associated syndrome, where there may be alternative necessary conditions with which it is not identified due to our relative lack of interest in them; further, the decision to call a disease "genetic" involves shifting the application of the term "disease" from the syndrome to "the cause" and the designation of the syndrome as a *manifestation* of the disease. It is this tendency to shift the application of the term "disease" to "the cause" that I shall attempt to disparage.

CRITERIA FOR APPLYING "GENETIC DISEASE": SOME VALUATIONAL DIMENSIONS

Sedgewick [12] and others [13] have defended the view that "illness and disease, health and treatment, . . . [are] social constructions. . . . All departments of nature below the level of mankind are exempt both from disease and from treatment — until man intervenes with his own human classifications of disease and treatment." Sedgewick suggests a set of criteria for something being a disease which I here modify so as to be necessary and sufficient for applying the term "genetic disease." For one to speak of something being a genetic disease, there must be reference made to: 1) a species in the welfare of whose members one takes an interest; 2) a state or item of behavior of some relatively small number of those members which deviates significantly from what is recognized as norms of appearance and behavior; 3) states or items of behavior which are disvalued; 4) only such states and items of behavior for which family history provides evidence of heritability, or for which our present scientific theories and technologies provide an identifiable genetic causal component; 5) only such states and items of behavior for which the present genetic technology and clinical practice hold promise of alleviation or avoidance (even if only by identification and nonreproduction of carriers); and 6) only such states and items of behavior for which alternative, nongenetic approaches to treatment or avoidance are disvalued. Several features of these criteria warrant specific comment.

First, it should be borne in mind that these criteria purport to describe the conditions that obtain when someone calls something a genetic disease. They are not intended to be prescriptive of how or when the term ought to be employed — all the more so, since it is one of the theses of this paper that the term ought to be eliminated. Second, note that it is a feature of this analysis that the term "genetic disease" has been relativized in a number of ways: to species of interest, to recognized norms, to individual and societal values, to current scientific theory, and to current and foreseeable technology. In turn, each of these is either value-laden or in some way determined by values. Given that pervasive interlacing of valuational considerations throughout every aspect of our operative criteria for "genetic disease" (and "genetic health," if its definition contains "the absence of genetic disease" as a necessary component [14]), we must conclude that the term is valuational both in its implications (eg that alternative typologies have been discounted) and its applications. A similar sort of analysis can be provided for the other terms mentioned at the start of this essay. Third, the criteria do not dictate what is to be called a disease; they only describe the conditions which are generally satisfied when one calls something a genetic disease. Specifically, either a syndrome or its cause could be labeled a genetic disease. I shall show how that choice of label may itself have important moral consequences.

The result of our various observations and analyses is that the causal classification of a disease (in the sense of a clinical syndrome) as genetic or otherwise (eg infectious, toxic, produced by a physical injury, etc) involves a decision to prefer one or a range of possible causal factors. But Sheldon [15] has observed that "the basis of the categorization of disease fundamentally determines what gets done about disease, even more than the organizational structures which develop to deal with it." If so, the decision to identify a disease as genetic may well determine a preference of a particular range of possible foci for therapy, prevention, and research. It thus becomes legitimate to ask, What are the moral dimensions of this decision? In short, why *genetic* disease?

USES OF "GENETIC DISEASE": SOME POLICY IMPLICATIONS

The positive benefits are by now obvious and familiar. They involve the furtherance of our knowledge of human development and variation as determined by the fundamental processes of human reproduction; the demythologizing of the occurrence of various kinds of disease (in particular, providing more cogent explanations of various disorders than their supposed visitation on persons as punishment for sin); the possibility of eradicating various kinds of disease by elimination of their genetic determinants from the gene pool; the possibility of improving the species and thus exerting control over evolutionary processes; and so forth. Rationales of these sorts generally hold up select long-term consequences in justification of the pursuit of genetic research, expressed in terms of the elimination of certain diseases, the advancement of knowledge, perhaps even the enhancement of desirable characteristics of the species, as likely future benefits.

But of course all such goals can be pursued whether we employ the typology "genetic disease" or not. Given that employing the term diagnostically does contribute in some way to a social and policy-making climate favorable to those goals, whether they provide adequate justification for such a use depends on whether there are significant negative considerations relevant to their employment. (I ignore, for present considerations, the question of whether even these goals may not have negative aspects.) The following considerations are divided into two classes: those which turn on the identification of *any* disease in causal terms, and those which involve the genetic typology [16].

Neville [17] has observed that ". . . short of a complete understanding of all the causes of a disease, decisions as to which to investigate are contingent upon the idiosyncracies of the clinicians and investigators, the state of their arts, and the policies channelling research and treatment funds." Few, if any, diseases are so well understood that we can justifiably identify the total cause and define the disease in terms of it. Yet, as Engel [18] notes, there is a profound tendency in humans to think in terms of substantive, unit causes. He cites two examples. The germ theory of disease, postulating as it does the existence of invisible, omnipresent entities which produce disease, had such a wide appeal that it became a dominant theme in medicine for some time, causing the earlier emphasis on homeostasis and other factors within the host to be relatively discounted. More recently, with the development of pathology and diagnostic techniques to detect functional and structural deviations, "the temptation has been to consider these findings the explanations for a disease rather than manifestations of the disease state. A disease, then, has substantive qualities, and the patient can be cured if the diseased ("bad") part is removed." To take the successes of surgical excision in treating disease as evidence for internal irregularities being the causes of the diseases is fallacious, since it ignores the role of other necessary conditions as well.

To build one causal factor into the very conception of a disease and thereby to prefer one causal hypothesis over others is to invite stagnation of research and treatment, and distortion of funding priorities. A case in point is that of the viral conception of the etiology of cancer, which has held sway in the funding of cancer research to the detriment of other approaches which have a higher likelihood of payoff in increased rates of cure [19].

Settling upon causal specifications discourages alternative conception of disease. For example, it has been recently observed [20] that "The success of Western science and related factors have produced a form of ethnocentrism, with biomedical diseases seen as the only real ones. This may have had the effect of rendering the search for new paradigms about disease partially illogical and inappropriate." The classic Western conception of disease focuses on its biologic import as specified in terms of disruption of normal functioning of biologic subsystems of the body. But an ethnomedical approach to disease would focus on "behavioral paradigms of disease . . . as devices for codifying and measuring a person's social functioning [where] . . . social behavior correlates of all kinds of interruptions in functioning are delineated regardless of the individual's culture. It is irrelevant (to an ethnomedical approach) whether outsiders judge that the alternations in behavior are caused by changes in sugar metabolism, toxic effects of an infectious or neoplastic disease, anxiety and depression, or, for that matter, the effects of preternatural influences. What is relevant, however, is the time-related changes in which the form of social functioning is altered or interfered with, and/or the changes in the way the person uses social symbols" [20]. A theory-neutral conception of disease in terms of symptoms and signs, while not independent of subjective factors, does permit the development of such alternative paradigms of disease as behavioral and biologic ones which selectively emphasize complementary aspects of the disease process. But to conceive and define a disease in terms of one causal aspect is to impose a priori the appearance of implausibility and confusion on other approaches.

Within the context of our own cultural institutions and practices in dealing with disease, some more specific negative consequences of the typology of "genetic disease" can be seen. Both Sheldon [15] and Engel [18] have emphasized the effect on therapeutic and preventive measures elected by the physician of the nomenclature employed in identifying a disease. "While our understanding of the processes involved is constantly changing, names are rarely changed, and they often continue to exert a weighty influence on the physician's concepts, at times blocking any approach contrary to what the name implies" [18]. In this way, identifying a disease with one range of necessary conditions (say, genetic) focuses attention on one range of treatment and/or prevention. This in turn may issue in perceptions of false or inappropriate dichotomies; for example, either one aborts a fetus identified through amniocentesis and karyotyping as having a genetic disease, or one produces an offspring with the disease. This dichotomy is false in cases where there exists an alternative way of avoiding the symptoms of the disease. For example, it is possible to diagnose G6PD deficiency prenatally. Avoidance of those foods and drugs that precipitate it is an alternative to both abortion and production of an offspring with the disease symptoms, but this alternative may be obscured by identifying the disease with the genetic antecedent. With genetic diseases for which prenatal diagnosis is not now possible, such as PKU, avoidance of production of an individual afflicted with the disease would be possible only if reproduction were denied altogether. But again this is a false dichotomy; in the case of PKU strict observance of a phenylalanine-free diet for six years avoids or greatly reduces the associated mental retardation [21]. Even in writers who appear not to fall prey to such false dichotomies, one finds evidence of a conceptual distinction between a disease and a set of symptoms as its manifestation that indicates that the disease has been identified with the cause. For example, in discussing the use of phenylalanine-free diets to avoid the mental retardation associated with PKU, Murray [22] writes: "The dream of the physician is, after all, the prevention of *the manifestation of disease* rather than its cure after it has been found" (italics mine). So it is the manifestation of the disease and not the disease itself that is prevented in the case of genetic diseases with manipulable components, and possession of the genetic component is a sufficient condition for possession of the disease, regardless of whether it is manifest. In this sort of conception, the genetic disease can be prevented only by preventing individuals who possess the genetic component.

The foregoing point is closely related to another one; namely, the stigmatization of persons who have genetic diseases. Not only have we come to use the term "carrier" for ones whose offspring may be at-risk for some genetic disease, thereby invoking folklore figures like Typhoid-Mary, but we also have long had practices based on the principle that those who are genetically diseased ought not to reproduce. By extension of the "carrier" metaphor, sterilization becomes a form of quarantine. We thus slide into social policies and attitudes which ought at the least to be squarely faced, independently debated, and adopted, if at all, both with the justification of a solid cost-benefit analysis and with full knowledge of the price paid in the currency of individual liberty and self-determination.

The identification of a disease with its genetic component, since it displaces the patient's complaint as the primary determinant of the occurrence of the disease, has other potential political and social consequences that raise grave concerns. One effect of separating disease from the diseased one's complaints is that the finding of disease can be made on the complaints, actual and anticipated, of others. The controversy surrounding the XYY syndrome serves as a case in point. An unproved low statistical association of criminality and the occurrence of an extra Y chromosome in males has been suggested. Walzer and Gerald of Harvard Medical School initiated a long-term study of newborn XYY males, in part to determine the degree of genetic (chromosomal) contribution to behavior problems. But they have been quoted [23] as holding that the XYY chromosome pattern "is a 'disease,' . . . and . . . children who have it are entitled to medical treatment just as they would be for any other disease" — this, despite their admission that while "some XYY children are 'hard to handle', others are 'perfectly fine'." The associated syndrome seems to have at best only an indirect relation to the complaints of XYY individuals; rather it is the complaints of parents, teachers, and those who have been victimized by XYY criminals that constitute a large part of the syndrome. And, XYY individuals are all classified as diseased, irrespective of whether they are 'hard to handle" or 'perfectly fine," because they possess the genetic basis for the disease. It appears evident that there is an enormous environmental component in the determinants of the anti-social behavior of those who are hard to handle; how does calling the XYY in-

dividual diseased on the basis of his chromosomal pattern enhance our understanding of why the behavioral syndrome occurs? Given that the incidence of
the correlation is low, it looks as though the identification of the disease with
the genetic component only serves to direct attention to a relatively unimportant component of the total cause. And, so directed, we are led to the utterly
useless stigmatization that all XYY individuals are incurably diseased [24].

Finally, let me cite the case of some research that is in progress into the
genetic components of cancer, and point to two possible ways of handling the
outcome. It has long been known that susceptibility to bronchial carcinoma in
cigarette smokers is varied; the occurrence of lung cancer in individuals who have
a similar history of rate and duration of smoking is markedly dissimilar (a fact
which has bolstered the claims of cigarette manufacturers that it has not been
proved that smoking causes cancer). In recent years, the National Institutes of
Health have supported research into the basis for such variability. Recent reports
indicate that the variability centers about low, intermediate, and high inducible
aryl hydrocarbon hydroxylase activities, with susceptibility to bronchogenic carcinoma being associated with the higher levels of activity; these levels of activity
are in turn thought "to result from two alleles at a single locus with the three
(levels of activity) representing homozygous low and high alleles and the intermediate heterozygote" [25]. This and other research has prompted one researcher for Hoffman-LaRoche Pharmaceuticals to observe: "The studies in the
journal by Kellerman and his associates suggest that the measurement of BP
(benzopyrene)-metabolizing enzymes in human lymphocytes may allow us to
detect members of the population who are uniquely sensitive, or who are resistant to carcinogens in cigarette smoke, and further studies along these lines are
to be encouraged" [26].

As I view it, the question is not whether such research ought to be continued, but what is to be done with its results. Will it, for example, prompt concern for those individuals who are carcinogenically sensitive to cigarette smoke
and reinforce legislation to protect them from unintentional exposure to tobacco
smoke by restricting the sale and private use of tobacco cigarettes to individuals
known to be resistant? Or, will the results of these researches be used to identify
bronchial cancer as a manifestation of a genetic disease, thereby rendering the
individual responsible for avoiding the noxious substance? Depending on what is
done with the knowledge resulting from the research, what many regard as a
matter calling for regulation in the public interest may become a matter involving only prudential considerations for individuals having a genetic disease —
despite the fact that bronchial carcinoma is a condition resulting from the interaction of genetic and environmental factors. In light of the valuational components of the criteria listed earlier for the use of "genetic disease," the socialization of the anticipated results of this and similar research should be highly
instructive.

In sum, I maintain that the disbenefits for the typology "genetic disease" far outweigh any benefits that accrue to research and therapy from the use of the term. If, nonetheless, it is viewed as desirable to have some indication of a disease's etiology encapsulated, if not in its identification at least in some systematic form of reference, it may be valuable to discriminate between different types of the same disease (specified in terms of an associated syndrome or family of syndromes) in terms of differential causal analyses. But, lest we repeat there the sins outlined above and once again fall into the grip of the simplistic equation of "one disease, one unit cause," we would do well to develop some sort of characterization of the whole cause of a disease in terms of a density function which would give some specification of the relative contributions made by genetic and various types of environmental factors. In that way, we could perhaps preserve the virtues of the present system of classification while avoiding the nomenclature of "*genetic* disease."

Little of the foregoing may seem relevant to the task of the genetic counselor. In a sense, I have attacked the very foundations of that profession, and I do not want to be misunderstood. I hold that genetic counseling is an important resource to an individual who is in jeopardy, or whose prospective progeny are in jeopardy, of contracting a disease about whose genetic component considerable is known. Indisputably, there are diseases for the avoidance of which manipulation at the genetic level offers the only hope. Let the genetic counselor go so far; but, more importantly, let the genetic counselor live up to the charge not to impose values on clients, by becoming aware of the danger of unwittingly influencing decisions by employing unnecessary terminology with hidden valuational components.

REFERENCES

1. King R: "A Dictionary of Genetics." 2nd Ed. New York: Oxford University Press, 1974.
2. Slater E, Cowie V: "The Genetics of Mental Disorders." London: Oxford University Press, 1971.
3. Lubin B et al: Proceedings of the National Academy of Sciences. Sci News 107(9): 136, 1975.
4. Navon R, Padeh B, Adam A: Apparent deficiency of hexosaminidase A in healthy members of a family with Tay-Sachs disease. Am J Hum Genet 25:287–293, 1973.
5. Vigdoff J, Buist N, O'Brien J: Absence of β-N-acetyl-D-hexosaminidase A activity in a healthy woman. Am J Hum Genet 25:372–381, 1973.
6. Dreyfus J-C, Poenaru L, Svennerholm L: Absence of hexosaminidase A and B in a normal adult. N Engl J Med 292:61–63, 1975.
7. Lederberg J: Biological future of man. In Wostenholme G (ed): "Man and His Future." Boston: Little, Brown & Co, 1963.
8. Taylor R: Causation. In Edwards P (ed): "The Encyclopedia of Philosophy." New York: Macmillan and Free Press, 1967, vol 1.

9. Scriven M: Explanations, predictions and laws. In Feigl H, Maxwell G (eds): "Minnesota Studies in the Philosophy of Science." Minneapolis: University of Minnesota Press, 1962, vol 3.

10. Whitbeck C: The relations between the concepts *syndrome* and *disease* in contemporary medicine. In Baker R, Lowinger P (eds): "The Psychosurgery of John Doe." (Unpublished manuscript)

11. Pincus J, Tucker G: "Behavioral Neurology." New York: Oxford University Press, 1974.

12. Sedgewick P: Illness – Mental and Otherwise. Hastings Cent Stud 1(3):19–40, 1973.

13. Dubos R: "The Mirage of Health." New York: Harper & Row, 1971.

14. Lappé M: Genetic knowledge and the concept of health. Hastings Cent Rep 3(4):103, 1973.

15. Sheldon A: Toward a general theory of disease and medical care. Sci Med Man 1:237–262, 1973.

16. Lappé M: Reflections on the cost of doing science. Ann NY Acad Sci 265:102–111, 1976.

17. Neville R: Gene therapy and the ethics of genetic therapeutics. Ann NY Acad Sci 264:153–161, 1976.

18. Engel G: A unified concept of health and disease. Perspect Biol Med 3:459–485, 1960.

19. Kopkind A: The politics of cancer. The Real Paper, March 31, 1976.

20. Faberga H Jr: The need for an ethnomedical science. Science 189:969–975, 1975.

21. Erbe R: Therapy in genetic disease. N Engl J Med 291:1028–1029, 1974.

22. Murray R: Screening: A practitioner's view. In Hilton B et al (eds): "Ethical Issues in Human Genetics." New York: Plenum Press, 1973.

23. Culliton B: Patients' rights: Harvard in site of battle over X and Y chromosomes. Science 186:715–717, 1974.

24. Borganokar D, Shah S: The XYY chromosome male – Myth or syndrome? Prog Med Genet 10:135–222, 1974.

25. Kellerman G, Shaw C, Luyten-Kellerman M: Aryl hydrocarbon hydroxylase inducibility and bronchogenic carcinoma. N Engl J Med 289:934–937, 1973.

26. Conney A: Carcinogen metabolism and human cancer. N Engl J Med 289:971–973, 1973.

5. Genetic Health: A Dangerous, Probably Erroneous, and Perhaps Meaningless Concept*

Robert F. Murray, Jr, MD, MS

DEFINITIONS OF HEALTH

Health is commonly defined as a state of complete physical, mental, and social well-being of mind and body [1]. But health can be defined, in a pragmatic sense, as the absence of detectable disease, and disease can, in turn, be viewed as a disturbance or abnormality in the function of mind, or body, or both. Mechanic [2] states that the concept of disease refers to some abnormal functioning which has undesirable consequences because it produces personal discomfort or adversely affects the individual's future health status.

A myriad of biologic, biochemical, and physiologic processes go on in an effort to maintain a state of equilibrium or homeostasis of the mind-body complex with its internal and external environment essential for the organism's survival. When internal and external homeostasis exist and the human organism is functioning with reasonable efficiency, it can be described, in an operational sense, as healthy. The physician usually describes a patient as healthy when there appears to be no sign of disease, manifest either as symptoms (eg pain or other types of discomfort), or disturbance in function.

There are now many examples of disturbances in the biochemistry and/or physiology at the cellular level which can be identified long before the function of the organism is disturbed in any clinically detectable way. Examples of such disorders include Gaucher disease, type II hyperbetalipoproteinemia, and alpha$_1$-antitrypsin deficiency. Does the presence of a disturbed metabolism without disturbed mind-body functions mean the individual has a disease? Is a person unhealthy merely because the potential for disease exists?

If one adheres to the strictest possible definition of disease including any disturbance in mental or physical function, temporary or prolonged, actual or

*Partially supported by MCH project grant No. 414 and NIH grant HL 15160.

potential, one would also have to consider as diseased, persons who are significantly overweight, people with mild viral illnesses (either respiratory or gastrointestinal), persons with allergies, and even persons who are judged to have excessive drives and desires. People with physiologic or biochemical differences associated with the future development of illness would also have to be labeled as unhealthy.

Another way of looking at health is in relationship to human "entropy" or so-called "natural aging." Loosely stated, entropy refers to the tendency toward degradation of all matter and energy in the universe to an ultimate state of inert uniformity [3]. Stated another way, all energy-containing systems are running down (ie working to resist the tendency to lose energy), and, therefore, all living organisms from the time that they function independently are in the process of running down to eventual death or termination. All life can be conceived, in one sense, as a struggle against the effects of entropy. But it is a losing struggle. Even though essentially all cells of the body renew themselves on a regular basis, tissue and organ degeneration occur at fairly predictable rates in most people. And although everyone experiences a gradual loss of efficiency, function, and well-being as they get older, elderly persons are often called "healthy" even though they show degenerative changes in their tissues or organs at the expected chronologic age. If they feel good and function well within predicted limits, physicians say they are in good health. According to the strictest definition of health, aging is a disease. But if human entropy is accepted as an immutable law of the biologic universe, statements about the health of an individual can only be made relative to other members of the population of the same age.

According to the strictest definition of disease, everyone has a disease at some time or other, and all suffer from a disease called aging that begins at birth. No one is truly healthy. Health is only an ideal physiologic state which the body struggles to achieve but rarely does. The concept can be used, but only in relative terms and then only really by defining the context in which it is being used. If these are the limits of the general concept of health, what then can be said of genetic health?

THE VARIOUS CONTEXTS OF GENETIC HEALTH

According to current theory, all chemical and physiologic functions in the body are under the control of one or more genes. Inherited variation or mutations in these genes are sometimes responsible for disturbed or frankly abnormal function of certain essential processes so that homeostasis is upset and a "diseased" physiologic state is said to exist. In this situation, the relative state of health (or disease) is directly and primarily determined by variant (often abnormal) genes (called Mendelian genes or single mutant genes of large effect) which have, with rare exceptions, been inherited from one or both parents. The individual carrying genes that cause disease now or that will cause disease in the future can be said to have a genetically determined disturbance of his or her health.

Abnormalities in body function are also produced by foreign organisms like bacteria or viruses or toxic materials, such as alcohol or certain other drugs, that disturb or disrupt cellular processes. There is evidence that whether or not an individual becomes ill from exposure to certain of these foreign agents is likely to be a consequence of inherited factors. These genetic factors may also determine what kinds of microbes the immune system of a given person may be able to combat successfully. In some cases of inherited immune deficiency disease, even harmless bacteria become dangerous [4]. Inherited variation in enzyme function, such as glucose-6-phosphate dehydrogenase (G6PD) deficiency, may prevent one person from detoxifying a chemical or drug while another person without the variant enzyme handles it with no difficulty. This is an example of a pharmacogenetic disorder, an inherited variation in ability to detoxify or metabolize drugs [5]. In other words, genes affect health (disturb homeostasis) not only when they directly disrupt smoothly operating body functions, but also when they interfere with the body's ability to destroy or inhibit the spread of potentially lethal microbial invaders. They significantly influence the neutralizing of chemical agents that might cause harm and may also play a role in causing the side effects that can come from taking a wide variety of drugs.

Considered in the broadest sense, then, it can be said that virtually all disease is to a greater or lesser extent genetic in its etiology. It is the degree to which the genetic material contributes to the etiology of the particular abnormality that leads geneticists to label some diseases as "genetic" and others not. Or, stated more precisely, it is the extent to which we are able to recognize a clear genetic component in the manifestation of the disease that leads us to call that condition "genetic."

The expression of the information encoded in genes is always to some extent influenced by the environment(s) in which it operates. These consist of the microenvironment of the cell and tissues and the macroenvironment of the blood stream, and the rest of the body organs, as well as the environment external to the organism. Changes at any one or all of these levels can profoundly influence the range of expression of a gene or genes. An example of this is seen when the nutritional environment of an infant homozygous for a mutant gene that determines phenylketonuria (PKU) is altered by drastically lowering the level of phenylalanine in the diet. The degree of mental retardation that would almost always occur if this change were not made is thereby averted. Variation in other genes in the genetic makeup of the individual, the so-called "genetic environment," also influences the degree to which a disease that is produced by a variant or mutant gene is expressed and, in some cases, whether it will be expressed at all [6].

THE BENEFITS OF "BAD" GENES

Genes that can produce disease under one circumstance can also promote health in others. The child homozygous for the mutant gene that codes for an abnormal beta polypeptide chain in hemoglobin S will suffer in varying degrees from chronic hemolytic anemia and recurrent attacks of pain leading to organ damage and eventual death. If a child only carries one such gene, he or she will usually enjoy good health and have an increased chance of surviving in an environment where falciparum malaria is endemic. This parasitic disease, transmitted by mosquitos, kills primarily in childhood. There is much evidence showing that carrying this gene, which may produce ill health or disease under some conditions, confers protection against the lethal disease under other conditions [7]. Therefore genes that can cause disease can also prevent disease depending on the circumstances. G6PD deficiency, an X-linked red cell enzyme defect like the sickle cell gene, geographically follows the distribution of falciparum malaria. It is responsible for self-limited hemolytic anemia that occurs if certain oxidative drugs (eg primaquine) are administered to a male who carries the gene for this condition. But it, too, presumably confers on these males resistance to the lethal effects of falciparum malaria [8].

Carrying a single gene in heterozygous form for several variant or abnormal hemoglobins or for thalassemia (where the mutant gene causes a reduced rate of hemoglobin synthesis) is primarily beneficial in a malarial environment, but is potentially more harmful in a nonmalarial environment, because of the risk of having a child homozygous for the genes that determine a particular hemoglobin disease. It is clear, then, that the genes causing hemoglobinopathies and G6PD deficiency can promote health and be responsible for disease, but always in a relative sense, since even in the malarial environment the risk of the diseased child also exists. Clearly the environment, both external and internal, is a vital key to the relationship of a variant gene to health or disease.

GENETIC DISEASE AND THE ENVIRONMENT

Most human traits are controlled by multiple genes (involving two or more loci) modified by the internal and external environment. They are called polygenic or multifactorial traits. In many, if not most, cases, it appears that the environment may play the major role in whether or not there is clinical disease, and how severe it is.

Gout is an abnormality of uric acid metabolism in which there are recurrent acute episodes of arthritis with progressive joint damage associated with an elevated serum uric acid. It appears to be particularly common in males ranging from a frequency of 0.3—8.0% of males affected in different populations [9] . Gouty arthritis, for instance, is more frequent in Philippino males than in males of non-Philippino background [10] .

Long before any episodes of acute arthritis occur, an increase in serum uric acid can often be detected. Its pattern of occurrence in families is consistent with its inheritance as a multifactorial trait [11] . A male at risk to have gout who lives in a harsh rural environment of the Philippines on a diet low in purine-containing foods (purines are the metabolic precursors of uric acid) and high in carbohydrates is unlikely to have clinical gout. He is also not likely to have an increased level of serum uric acid [10] . When the same person moves to a more industrial environment, adopts a diet which is relatively rich in purines, and lives under much less physically rigorous conditions, there is a much higher probability that an elevated serum uric acid level will appear, and he may even develop overt gout. Evidence for this effect of environment was seen during World Wars I and II, when a decrease in the frequency of gout occurred when purine rich foods were in short supply in the Philippines. But the frequency returned to previous levels when the shortage was relieved. Gout has also become much more common in the Japanese population with the increase in protein consumption in the population in the past two decades [9] . It appears that the environment plays a primary role in determining whether or not variant genes produce gout. There is, on the other hand, evidence for a positive correlation between uric acid levels, drive, achievement, and leadership in one study [12] and drive and range of activities in another study. If these important human qualities are promoted by elevated uric acid levels and they are considered to enhance adaptive behavior, then genes responsible for gout are apparently both unhealthy and healthy (if we can agree that high achievement is consistent with health).

WHAT IS GENETIC HEALTH?

What then is meant by genetic health? Does one mean that the state of genetic health is that condition in which there are no genes in the total genetic makeup of a given individual that will produce or predispose to disease? Or does one mean that the individual in question has no disorder significantly related to genetic factors that will disturb the individual's internal or external equilibrium with the environment for a significant period of time, or lead to premature death?

There is a very limited context in which one can discuss genetic disease or genetic health and that is from the perspective of the individual carrying a gene(s) that drastically disturbs the body's equilibrium with its internal and external environment causing organ or tissue damage, or that accelerates the process of human aging. Examples of this context occur in 1) individuals heterozygous for or who carry a mutant gene of large effect determining a disease process inherited as an autosomal dominant, X-linked dominant, or (in males) an inherited X-linked recessive character or 2) individuals homozygous for a mutant gene of large effect inherited as an autosomal recessive trait and which produces serious disease, disturbing function and/or well-being. Examples of genetically determining conditions which are harmful and *also* beneficial have already been given. It is clear that it is not just the quality of the gene product but also its quantity that may determine its relationship to health or disease. It is related to the status of the individual person heterozygous for mutant genes which in double dose will determine a serious or even lethal disease. Those persons who have coined the concept of genetic health most likely have this situation in mind.

ARE CARRIERS OF MUTANT GENES GENETICALLY UNHEALTHY?

Is an individual who is heterozygous for a gene which when present in homozygous state determines sickle cell anemia or cystic fibrosis, or who is a female carrier (heterozygous) for the X-linked gene determining Duchenne muscular dystrophy genetically unhealthy? If one considers that they are, then everyone is, in a strict sense, genetically unhealthy. This is because on the average, everyone is heterozygous not only for one but probably for 3–5 gene mutations which, if they occurred in homozygous state would produce a lethal disease – intrauterine death or sterility [13]. This estimate does not include genes which are semilethals, which in the homozygous state produce disease which may shorten the life-span or significantly compromise the individual's ability to function. One can also add to this the 2–20% of eggs or sperm in each individual that carry a newly mutant gene detrimental to varying degrees [14]. If genetic health consists of not harboring potentially harmful genes in one's genetic makeup, no one is genetically healthy. Indeed, one can really only consider genetic health a measure of the relative frequency with which one carries genes and/or expresses disease that has a significant genetic component. One would also have to consider the potential severity of the expressed gene: whether it would be lethal at or before birth, produce sterility, cause disease leading to early death in childhood or young adulthood, or produce chronic debilitating disease.

In order to examine an individual's "genetic health" in this way, it would be necessary to be able to look at the composition of the individual's entire genome. As a minimum, one would have to examine a representative fraction of the genome to make some estimate of an individual's relative genetic health because it cannot be done in any absolute sense. A conservative estimate sets the number of gene loci in man at 100,000 [15]. Our current knowledge of the human genome, based on the number of gene loci listed in McKusick's catalog, is slightly less than 2% [15]. This objective knowledge of the genome is not only rather small, but may very well not be truly representative. A great deal has been learned about the composition of the human genome in the past 20 years, but many more loci need to be identified, understood, and characterized before one can say with any real confidence that the composition and function of the human genome is understood. The ability to detect the heterozygote is confined to an even smaller fraction of the total human genome. Since the composition of human genes and the ability to detect the carrier status of mutant human genes are so inadequate, it makes little sense to attempt to determine what the state of genetic health of the genome of a particular person might be even if there were agreement on what the characteristics of a "healthy" gene are.

REPRODUCTIVE GENETIC HEALTH

Differential reproduction is one of the areas in which the adaptive or mal-adaptive functions of genes are especially important. In the context of reproduction, genetic health may be a more meaningful and acceptable concept. The presence or absence of disease in the offspring is still the major method of identifying parents who are carriers of disease-causing or potentially disease-causing genes. In this sense, it is a mating *couple* that might be classified as genetically unhealthy. *Individuals* might be classified as genetically unhealthy only when they possess an X-linked or autosomal dominant trait in which the affected child need receive only one mutant gene from a parent in order for the conditon to be fully expressed. Since virtually everyone is heterozygous for several mutant genes which in homozygous state produce disease, there is a significant probability that every mating couple is at risk for producing children with genetically determined disease, depending on the potential combination or combinations of genes resulting from their genomes. Even if a couple is at a 1 in 4 risk to produce an affected child because both members are gene carriers of the same recessive gene, there is a 3 in 4 chance that each offspring of the couple will *not* be affected with that particular condition. So a large fraction of the time parents classified as genetically unhealthy by this reproductive criterion will not have diseased offspring. On the other hand, if a particular couple that produces or has the potential to produce a child with a genetically determined disease is classified as genetically unhealthy, then it follows that every single couple is potentially genetically unhealthy because of the small possibility that one or more new mutations may occur.

POPULATION GENETIC HEALTH

If a couple cannot be strictly classified as genetically unhealthy, then perhaps, it is the population that should be called genetically healthy or unhealthy. By examining the frequency of individuals at different ages with genetically determined disorders in populations in the same or similar environments one could determine whether the carrier frequency for mutant genes of various kinds was significantly more frequent in one population than another. As long as it was clear that there were not significant differences in the frequency of inbreeding in the populations compared and that environmental factors were not playing a significant role, one might surmise that when the frequency of disease-causing genes was increased in one population over that in another population, its genetic health was poorer (or its genetic *un*health was greater) than in that other population. However, keep in mind that there is evidence that the heterozygous state of some disease-producing genes confers increased resistance to certain environmental hazards. It might be that while one population has an increased genetic disease frequency because of an increased proportion of disease-causing genes, through increased heterogeneity in its gene pool it may have an increased adaptive capacity to resist potential environmental hazards [16]. Good genetic health of a population measured as a very low level of detectable genetic disease, may actually indicate reduced adaptive capacity, since part of the genetic resiliency of a population is thought by some to be related to its ability to respond to unforeseen environmental hazards.

Even if we agree that there are certain circumstances under which we might define an individual, or a couple, or even a population, as genetically unhealthy, can it be considered an ethically acceptable concept? If we know only a small fraction of the human genome and a small fraction of the mutant genes that produce disease in individuals is it *just* that a particular segment of the population be branded as genetically unauthorized because they happen to have, by chance, genes that we can characterize? It seems unjust, especially when the members of that particular group of individuals do not take part in determining what the definition of good or bad genetic health may be, and when that definition is so inexact. People get their genes by accident. If one receives "unhealthy" genes by accident, not only might there be undeserved suffering, but other ethical values such as freedom and well-being are likely to be seriously abridged.

There is the possibility that in our haste to eliminate persons considered genetically unhealthy or genes considered unhealthy from the population at large, potentially unhealthy *or* adaptive genes may be inadvertently, or through ignorance, removed from the population. In this sense, the concept of genetic health is dangerous. Within the complexity of the genetic makeup of an individual are not just genes which determine disease, but also genes that may bring benefits, such as improved intellectual capacity, or genes that may be beneficial to individuals who carry them or to the population at large. Unless there is some idea of what some of these are so that they can be preserved, particularly in a rapidly changing environment, human adaptability may be seriously harmed.

SUMMARY

At least three dimensions define the state of health. These are time, place, and person. In this context, as a measure of the dimension "person," genetic health may in special cases have meaning. But the utility of this concept is limited.

The concept of genetic health, like the concept of health in general, is relative and often nebulous. It must be defined according to specific conditions of time, place, and person. The concept is in a way erroneous because a gene in and of itself is neither healthy nor unhealthy. The benefit or harm of a particular gene is most likely to be a function of the internal and external environment in which it operates and its interaction with many of the other genes that are present. The concept is dangerous because there is so much we do not know about the human genetic makeup and the functions that so-called mutant genes play in human adaptability. Furthermore, to attempt to act on this concept would very likely be unethical, in my judgment, because many people who carry so-called genetically unhealthy genes would not be included or identified, and accidental recipients of unhealthy genes would bear a painful burden that would cause suffering and infringe on other values as well. The term is, in a sense, meaningless because one cannot be certain that a gene which appears to produce ill health may not be associated with, or linked to, genes that are at the same time providing some benefit to that individual, or other individuals in the family, or to the population at large.

For scientific and ethical reasons, it seems unwise for genetic counselors to invoke the concept of genetic health in trying consciously to improve the gene pool of future generations by discouraging reproduction in known carriers of disease-producing genes. Even if counselors are successful in doing this, they may merely eliminate genetic heterogeneity that has probably been responsible for the evolutionary success of the human species in coping with the hostile environment of the planet earth, not to mention the possibility of producing other, as yet unknown, side effects.

REFERENCES

1. Agnew LRC et al: "Dorland's Illustrated Medical Dictionary." 24th Ed. Philadelphia: WB Saunders, 1965.

2. Mechanic D: "Medical Sociology: A Selective View." New York/London: The Free Press/Collier-Macmillan, 1968.
3. In Gove PB et al (eds): "Webster's Seventh New Collegiate Dictionary." Springfield: G and C Merriman, 1972.
4. Bergsma D, Good RA (eds): "Immunologic Deficiency Diseases in Man." New York: The National Foundation–March of Dimes, BD:OAS IV(1), 1968.
5. Kalow W: "Pharmacogenetics. Heredity and the Response to Drugs." Philadelphia: WB Saunders, 1962.
6. King RC: "A Dictionary of Genetics." London: Oxford, 1968.
7. Allison AC: Protection afforded by sickle cell trait against subtertian malarial infection. Br Med J 1:290–294, 1954.
8. Motulsky AG: Hereditary red cell traits and malaria. Am J Trop Med Hyg 13:147–155, 1964.
9. Wyngaarden JB: Gout and other disorders of uric acid metabolism. In Wintrobe MM et al (eds): "Principles of Internal Medicine." 7th Ed. New York: McGraw-Hill, 1974, pp 607–617.
10. Blumberg BS: Heredity of gout and hyperuricemia. Arthritis Rheum 8:627–647, 1965.
11. Hauge M, Harvald B: Heredity in gout and hyperuricemia. Acta Med Scand 152:247–257, 1955.
12. Brooks GW, Mueller E: Serum urate concentrations among university professors: Relation to drive, achievement and leadership. JAMA 195:415–418, 1966.
13. Muller HJ: Our load of mutations. Am J Hum Genet 2:111–176, 1950.
14. Hartl DL: "Mutation in Our Uncertain Heritage – Genetics & Human Diversity." Philadelphia: JB Lippincott, 1977, pp 275–295.
15. McKusick VA: "Mendelian Inheritance in Man." 4th Ed. Baltimore: Johns Hopkins University Press, 1975.
16. Dobzhansky T: Man and natural selection. Am Sci 49:285–299, 1961.

II. Genetic Counseling in Psychological and Social Perspective: Introduction

The agonies surrounding the birth of a defective child and the vexing question, "Could it happen again?" are recurrent nightmares of the human condition. In ancient China, a malformed newborn was considered a "Green Misfortune," symbolic of a chance departure from the orderliness of creation. Other societies considered congenital malformations much more ominous omens or punishments visited on a whole people for collective misdeeds. The societal response to defect probably reached its nadir of rationality in the Middle Ages when, as Diderot reported in his Encyclopedia, the malformed were considered to be affronts to the perfection of creation. Diderot's contemporaries cleverly resolved the matter by assigning the cause of such defects to an imperfect fusion of two otherwise perfect eggs. Animal monstrosities or sex-reversed hens were deemed a sufficient outrage to the order of God's universe to be brought to courts of law for disposition. Pigs and cocks were actually burned at the stake in 16th century France, just one manifestation of the irrational fear which accompanied the birth of defective newborns.

The emergence of genetic counseling as a formal profession can be seen as an attempt to demystify the irrational and cope with crises which have been an eternal part of the human condition. Unlike past societies, however, our contemporary social structures insure that genetic defects are experienced individually, within the privacy — and isolation — of the family unit. Without the collective social supports of the past, the crises surrounding the birth of a defective child are potentially more frightening, and perhaps fraught with even more social opprobrium than when everyone shared the burden of accidents of birth.

The configuration of genetic counseling suggests that a profession may be as pleiomorphic in its manifestations and as heterogeneous in its origins as the most complex polygenic trait. As James Sorenson and Arthur Culbert show, what began as the special province of the human geneticist or pediatrician has become populated by a plethora of specialists — and nonspecialists — often with quite different social and value perspectives. Tabitha Powledge concentrates on

Birth Defects: Original Article Series, Volume XV, Number 2, pages 81–83
© 1979 The National Foundation

one of these emerging groups — the counselor who is not a doctor — and identifies the recognition (and nonrecognition) of the roles which such persons can
usefully play in the counseling process.

As the chapters in this section demonstrate, the proper roles of the counselors and responses of the families who experience these ultimate confronta-
tions with fate are still uncertain. Counselors are idiosyncratic in their approaches
and attitudes toward what constitutes "good counseling." The often disparate
perspectives of counselors and their clients are explored by Jessica Davis and
Carol Levine, respectively. The social and psychological responses to defect constitute a shifting sand of fear and ambiguity as science uncovers specific causes
for some malformation syndromes and leaves others as indeterminate as they
were a thousand years ago. Where certainty is possible, specific recurrence risks
coupled with amniocentesis virtually eliminate the irrational source of fear. But,
as the chapter by Levine demonstrates, such measures still leave a residuum of
anxiety and doubt. Where counselors can only assemble empiric estimates of risk,
these fears may be exacerbated, leading to exaggeration of the guilt, denial and
depression which can accompany the birth of a genetically handicapped child.

Up until the past few years, parental doubts and anxieties were met by a
firm, directive approach from counselors, which rested on great assurance in the
biomedical community about the right courses to follow, and perhaps also a
wide stripe of paternalism. Today, the growth in concern by patients and others
about their rights and autonomy renders most counselors shy about acknowledg-
ing how large a part they can play in the decisions supposedly made by counselees. Thus, even when speaking of the "counselor as decision-maker," most
counselors would now probably not want to acknowledge a role broader than
that of "facilitator" described by Ray Antley. Nevertheless, as can be seen between the lines of Antley's paper — and in the other descriptions, such as those
of Seymour Kessler and Sumner Twiss — the counselor's influence can be a profound one, even when unacknowledged.

Edward Hsia presents a divergent view, drawing from his own counseling
experience to advocate a predominantly indirect role of the counselor as an information giver rather than a decision maker. Sumner Twiss examines some of
the normative questions of counselors' functions, and suggests that the counselor
might best be seen as a moral advisor to clients faced with life and death decisions
about newly born, or as yet unborn, children.

Whether the counselor is described as an active party to the counseling
process, or merely as a facilitator of it, he or she nonetheless is privy to the most
personal, and often heartrending, events which we experience. Without exception, observers of the counseling process concur that psychodynamic forces of
the most powerful sort come into play, often with devastating effect. Permitting
a client to express his or her anger or resentment, and balancing these potentially

destructive emotions within the context of a spousal relationship, require the most adept and perceptive psychological skills. Kessler identifies such skills and advocates the psychotherapeutic function of the counselor as uppermost in the delivery of genetic counseling care. According to this perspective, lifting depression, lessening denial and ultimately affording avenues for acceptable futures are among the key functions of the counselor.

How society responds to its burden of genetically affected individuals is not readily controlled or shaped by individual genetic counselors and other concerned professionals. Perhaps, then, this section points to an unfinished task — partially taken up in the next section and partially left with the reader — to identify the social relationships and institutions which will surround genetic counseling to give support to the families afflicted by genetic disease or disability and to validate the critical importance of the roles of the genetic counselor in ameliorating the social and psychological sequelae of events still outside of human control.

ML

6. Professional Orientations to Contemporary Genetic Counseling*

James R. Sorenson, PhD and Arthur J. Culbert, MS

A group of medical and genetic professionals [1] recently defined genetic counseling as:

> . . . a communication process which deals with the human problems associated with the occurrence, or the risk of occurrence of a genetic disorder in a family. This process involves an attempt by one or more appropriately trained persons to help the individual or the family to: (1) comprehend the medical facts, including the diagnosis, the probable course of the disorder and the available management; (2) appreciate the way heredity contributes to the disorder and the risk of recurrence in specified relatives; (3) understand the options for dealing with the risk of recurrence; (4) choose the course of action which seems appropriate to them in view of their risk and their family goals and act in accordance with that decision; and (5) make the best possible adjustment to the disorder in an affected family member and/or to the risk of recurrence of that disorder.

This definition, published in the "American Journal of Human Genetics" (AJHG), suggests that genetic counseling, at least as viewed by this group, has three elements: a) provision of medical and genetic information (components 1 and 2), b) exploration of reproductive-parenting options for individuals or couples in counseling (component 3), and c) assistance in helping counselees†

*Data from a survey supported by the Russell Sage Foundation. Paper prepared for Genetics Group, Institute for Society, Ethics, and the Life Sciences; Hasting-on-Hudson, New York. Citation or quotation only with written consent of the senior author.

†The authors are aware that people seeking genetic counseling are referred to in a variety of ways by counselors, eg clients, consultees, patients, counselees, even "our mutants." For the purpose of this paper, we use the label "counselees."

Birth Defects: Original Article Series, Volume XV, Number 2, pages 85—102
© 1979 The National Foundation

select a course of action and adjust to that action (components 4 and 5). This definition places a heavy burden on the counseling process, presumably giving as much emphasis to the word "counseling" as to the word "genetic." (In the absence of any commentary in the AJHG article to the effect that some components are more important than others, we assume each component to be of equal importance.) This dual emphasis, in turn, suggests that a variety of skills are required of and various tasks face the genetic counselor, including not simply counselee education but some discussion of counselee family attitudes and goals.

While this definition is only one of several, it does seem to include elements that have been suggested, with differential emphasis, in most other published definitions [2]. In fact, it seems that most counselors proffering a definition of counseling always include counselee education, in terms of genetic and medical information. Major variability in definitions of counseling seems to occur in terms of professional opinions about discussing family and personal (psychosocial) topics with counselees. While it is at variance with the AJHG definition, some counselors advocate a near single focus on medical–genetic knowledge transmission [3], while others endorse counseling approaches with varying degrees of involvement of psychosocial topics [4].

While much literature on genetic counseling has been published, to a large extent it reflects the views of those professionals in counseling who publish. We have little information on how most counselors view their activity. In addition, much of the published literature provides a limited view of the orientation with which a counselor may approach counselees. This is so because much of the published literature does not go into the specifics of the counseling process but remains aimed at a normative, as opposed to a descriptive, analysis of various counseling orientations.

In order to provide a more general view of genetic counseling this article will: (1) provide an empiric description of how nearly 400 professionals are oriented to their genetic counseling, (2) present an empiric assessment as to how various orientations are related to attitudes about the process of counseling, and (3) discuss what the different counseling orientations identified in this chapter may mean for counselees utilizing such services.

THE STUDY

The data to be reported here were gathered as part of a national survey and interview study of professionals in genetic counseling. The data-collection phase spanned the period from January 1973 through April 1975.

Full details of the sampling procedure, questionnaire, and interview protocols, as well as data analysis procedure, are being presented elsewhere [5]. For purposes of this paper it is adequate to comment briefly on population ascertainment and response bias.

At the present time genetic counselors do not constitute a distinct group of professionals with specific training or licensing. Genetic counseling is practiced by private physicians, professors of biology, and biomedical researchers, among others. Because of the relative newness of the area, it is probably the case that most medically or genetically complex counseling cases are referred to a specialized genetics clinic. More routine cases may be handled by private physicians, but the general lack of training of most physicians in medical genetics, and the very low frequency with which cases present in private practice, probably induces general practitioners to make use of available genetics clinics when problems arise. In fact, one study of practicing physicians in Massachusetts suggests this may be the case [6]. More widespread genetic counseling, especially for routine cases, may become more common as physicians become increasingly acquainted with genetics in their formal education and training. For the present, however, genetic counseling is probably obtained most often by referral to a specialist in a genetic counseling clinic.

For the purpose of this research we studied the specialists in genetic counseling clinics. These professionals provide the bulk of counseling today and certainly are highly visible to and very instrumental in defining the nature and scope of genetic counseling for physicians in general. To identify such professionals we employed two methods. First, we wrote to the directors of all genetic counseling clinics listed in the 1971 "International Directory of Genetic Services" [7]. We asked these directors to supply us with a list of the professionals in their center involved on a regular or part-time basis in actually seeing people in genetic counseling. We also asked for the names of professionals, not based at the clinic, known to be providing counseling on a regular basis. Second, we wrote to all 50 state departments of public health, soliciting the names of institutions and individuals known to be providing genetic counseling in each state.

These procedures resulted in the identification of 741 individuals as providing genetic counseling. Upon direct contact, 80 of these reported that they did not counsel at all, while an additional 17 reported such infrequent counseling as to make their experience too limited from which to generalize. This resulted in a target population for our survey of 661 individuals. Of these, 509 (79%) returned questionnaires, of which 496 (77%) were usable. Of the remaining 135 (21%) who did not return a questionnaire, 79 (12%) agreed by phone to participate but did not; 37 (6%) were virtually unreachable; and 19 (3%) refused to participate. A comparison of the 496 respondents with the total target population of 661 in terms of geographical distribution, organizational setting, and departmental placement revealed no significant differences. Thus, to the extent that the original target population was a fairly complete enumeration of professionals providing secondary and tertiary levels of genetic counseling in this country, the data gathered by this survey is representative of those counselors recognized in the medical, voluntary health, as well as public health communities

as having expertise in genetic counseling. They represent as a group one significant component of what organized American medicine has to offer in its battle
against birth defects and genetic disease.

WHO PROVIDES GENETIC COUNSELING

Of the 496 professionals providing counseling who returned questionnaires,
the majority held the MD degree, while smaller percents (Table 1) held the PhD
or the MD and the PhD in combination. Only a small percent had neither degree.

The historical legacy of genetic counseling in this country is reflected in
Table 1. Genetic counseling began largely as the province of self-proclaimed experts in social reform [8]. Subsequent to the demise of the eugenics movement,
counseling became largely limited to academic settings [9]. In the late 1950s
and especially into the 1960s, applied human genetics became increasingly associated with the medical world, especially through medical research [9]. There is
still a close connection of clinical genetics to research as reflected in the 19% of
contemporary expert genetic counselors who hold the PhD degree alone, or in
combination with the MD.

The fact that counselors can be broken down into three general groups
(MDs, PhDs, and MD/PhDs) does not provide an adequate description of the
variety of professionals in counseling. Accordingly, Table 2 presents information
on the professional background of counselors, and Table 3 arrays areas of professional interest. As shown in Table 2, the majority of MDs that are involved in
counseling report pediatrics or internal medicine as their specialty. In fact, about
77% of those that claim one of these areas are board certified in it. MD/PhDs
reflect similar medical backgrounds, coming primarily from pediatrics and
medicine. However, only 37% of this group is board certified in these specialties.

As can be seen in Table 2, as one would expect, PhDs come predominantly
from genetics, general biology, and zoology. The academic background of the
MD/PhDs reflects a similar professional origin.

The professional background of a counselor does not, of course, necessarily
reflect one's interests. To ascertain an impression of counselors' interests we
asked them to indicate current professional interests. Table 3 presents the proportion of each of the three groups indicating various areas.

While a number of generalizations are suggested by Table 3, two are of
particular interest. First, the professionals in genetic counseling today are more
research than clinically oriented. Eighty-nine percent of the MD/PhDs, 85% of
the PhDs, and 57% of the MDs are primarily interested in one or another form of
research. Twenty-seven percent of the MDs and 5% of the MD/PhDs are primarily
interested in practicing medicine, and, perhaps most significantly, only 11% of
the MDs, 6% of the MD/PhDs, and 13% of the PhDs are primarily interested in
providing genetic counseling.

Table 1. Degrees Held By Respondents

Degree	Percent	N
MD only	72	357
PhD only	11	54
MD/PhD	8	40
RN only	2	12
Other	7	33
Total	100	496

Table 2. Specialty Areas of MD, PhD, and MD/PhD Counselors

MD only			PhD only		
Area	Percent	N	Area	Percent	N
Pediatrics	64	225	Genetics	61	33
Medicine	16	58	Biology (Gen.)	11	6
Ob/Gyn	5	17	Zoology	11	6
Pathology	5	16	Psychology	7	4
Other	11	41	Other	9	5
Total	101[b]	357	Total	99[b]	54

MD/PhD					
Area	Percent	N	Area	Percent	N
Pediatrics	55	21	Genetics	44	16
Medicine	24	9	Biology (Gen.)	31	11
Other	21	8	Other	25	9
Total	100	38[a]	Total	100	36[a]

[a] Number less than original (Table 1) due to nonresponses

[b] Rounding error

The latter observation has to be interpreted carefully. The fact that relatively few counselors are interested in counseling as their primary professional activity does not mean that they have no interest in it. Nevertheless, it is the case that expert genetic counseling is today practiced mostly by physician—investigators or research scientists. To some extent, most of the counselors in this study can be considered accidental practitioners with respect to genetic counseling. That is, they provide counseling for a host of reasons, including the fact that it provides them with a research setting in which to operate. Also, many realize that if they do not provide genetic counseling, there is a chance that it will not be done or will be provided by someone with less adequate medical/genetic preparation.

Table 3. Current General Areas of Primary Professional Interest of MD, PhD, and MD/PhD Counselors

Areas	Percent		
	MD	MD/PhD	PhD
Basic research	13	26	34
Clinical research	40	63	32
Behavioral research	1	0	17
Research on clinical practice	3	0	2
Practicing medicine	27	5	0
Genetic counseling	11	6	13
Other	5	0	2
Total	100	100	100
N	327*	35*	47*

*Numbers not equal to original because of nonresponse

ORIENTATION TO GENETIC COUNSELING

Above we noted that published counselors express a variety of opinions on the role of psychosocial discussion in genetic counseling. While all are concerned with presenting genetic and medical facts (information provision), some think it important, in addition, to raise and discuss with counselees such topics as counselee religious beliefs, attitudes toward contraception, and/or the counselee's economic situation, in general what we may call psychosocial issues. Others consider raising such issues to be beyond their professional obligations. How, in fact, do most counselors in our study view the role of information provision and psychosocial discussion in genetic counseling?

In approaching this topic in our national survey, counselors were asked to indicate which of three activities they considered to be a primary, secondary, or tertiary task, and which they considered not to be a professional task. The specific tasks listed were: 1) the establishment and delivery of an accurate diagnosis and valid recurrence risk estimate; 2) the establishment of counselee comprehension of the genetic mechanisms involved in his problem and its etiology; and 3) an examination of the counselee's personal attitudes toward his situation and his personal perspective on his problem.

To some extent, each of these tasks can be seen as an indicator of a more general orientation to genetic counseling. For example, the first task can be seen as an orientation emphasizing knowledge provision, be it specific knowledge about a particular disease or explanation of how a particular recurrence risk has been determined. Such an orientation is suggested in the first two components of the AJHG definition of genetic counseling offered at the beginning of this chapter.

The second task can be seen as one reflective of a concern with assuring counselee comprehension of the genetic etiology of a specific medical problem.

Finally, the third task can be seen as reflecting a desire to explore with counselees their personal views, providing a psychosocial context into which the medical and genetic facts may be placed. Components 3–5 of the AJHG definition can be seen as part of this orientation.

For the purposes of this discussion we will focus only on the comparative emphasis which counselors give to the first (information provision) and third (psychosocial discussion) tasks as orientations to their counseling, since they correspond reasonably well to elements of the AJHG definition.*

For the 447 MDs and/or PhDs, who assessed the first task we find that 394 (88%) consider information provision a primary obligation and 51 (11%) consider it a secondary or lesser obligation. Only two (< 1%) said it was not a professional obligation. Turning to the 443 MDs and/or PhDs who assessed the other task — psychosocial discussion in counseling — we find that 99 (22%) con-

---

* Respondents were asked to assess the three tasks — disease-risk information provision, client comprehension, and psychosocial discussions — as professional obligations in counseling. They could assess each task as a primary, secondary, tertiary, or nonprofessional obligation. Question wording suggested, and most respondents did rank the tasks. Since our main focus in this paper, as well as in the AJHG definition, is on the first and third tasks, we have decided to focus exclusively on respondent comparative assessment of these two tasks.

By focusing on only two of the three items assessed, one might ask whether or not this procedure may violate the spirit in which the question was asked. Our focus on two of the three items does not violate the spirit of the question. This is so because most respondents ranked the tasks in a hierarchy. Logically it makes no difference for our analysis in what sequence the respondent ordered these three tasks, since, as will be seen below, we are interested in the relative positioning of disease-risk information provision and psychologic discussion. Our analysis preserves whatever ranking the respondents gave to these tasks. Also, in the analysis to follow, we rely upon this single question and ranking of each of the two tasks to analyze variation in counseling orientations. This may raise questions about placing so much weight on only two statements as valid and reliable indicators of what are obviously complex counseling orientations. Our defense of this procedure is twofold. First, we appeal to the face validity of the question and the described tasks themselves. They do seem to be relatively clear statements reflective of disease-risk information provision and psychosocial discussion orientations. Second, on an empiric level, there is statistical support for the validity of these statements as acceptable indicators of each orientation. For example, 72% of counselors holding psychosocial discussion as a primary obligation consider it very important to discuss with the counselees their attitudes about the disease. Only 26% of those with no interest in psychosocial discussion want to discuss such attitudes with counselees. We would expect such a strong association if our single indicator of psychosocial interest is valid and reliable. In a similar fashion, our single item indicator assessing an information provision orientation correlates with independent criteria. For example, whereas 73% of those counselors holding information provision as a primary obligation consider the recurrence risk estimate as a very important reproductive decision factor, only about half of those who feel a lesser obligation to focus on information provision endorse the recurrence risk as such an important decision factor. Again, we would expect such an association if our indicator of an information provision orientation is valid and reliable.

sider this a primary obligation while 324 (73%) view it as a secondary or lesser professional obligation. Twenty, or about 5%, of the counselors said that discussion of psychosocial issues with counselees is not a professional obligation.

These data suggest that generally counselors are more disposed to putting information provision above psychosocial discussion, but counselors are far from wanting to exclude the latter from the counseling process altogether.

A second way of examining the data is to classify counselors into groups based on their responses to disease-risk information provision and psychosocial discussion as professional obligations. Table 4 shows the number and percent of MD and/or PhD counselors who endorse various counseling orientations combining different levels of commitment to information provision and psychosocial discussion.

Table 4 shows that the largest number of counselors (39%) endorse a counseling strategy placing disease-risk information provision as a primary obligation and psychosocial discussion as a secondary one. The second largest group (36%) consider disease-risk information provision as a primary obligation and psychosocial discussion as a tertiary one. Nineteen percent view both disease-risk information provision and psychosocial discussion as primary obligations, while 6% see psychosocial discussion as a primary obligation and disease-risk information provision as secondary or tertiary ones. It would appear from this assessment that about 19% of contemporary counselors give approximately the same relative emphasis to knowledge provision and to psychosocial discussion implied in the AJHG definition.

COUNSELING ORIENTATIONS, GOALS, AND PROFESSIONAL OBLIGATIONS

The four orientations to genetic counseling suggested in Table 4 reflect very general views on the role of the professional in counseling. It is likely that the particular orientation adopted by a counselor will be related to the topics he feels willing to discuss during counseling, as well as the goals he holds for his counseling. To some extent the former constitutes the elements or components of what we may call an agenda with which a counselor approaches his counseling task.* His goals constitute the raison d'etre or justification for why he approaches counseling as he does.

In this section we would like to examine briefly how the counseling orientations identified above relate to more specific counseling topics, as well as counseling goals.

---

* We realize that a counselor's approach to his counseling will vary from case to case, to some extent. However, we feel that this variation will take place about a set of ideas or attitudes that the counselor holds about what he is doing. These basic reference points are what we mean when we talk about a counselor's "agenda."

Table 4. Percent of Counselors Giving Varying Degrees of Emphasis To Information Provision and Psychosocial Discussion in Counseling*

	Obligation orientation			
	Psychosocial discussion — primary; information provision — secondary or teritary	Psychosocial discussion and information provision — both primary	Information provision — primary; psychosocial discussion — secondary	Information provision — primary; psychosocial discussion — tertiary
Percent	6	19	39	36
Number	23	75	157	144

	Disease-Risk Information Provision			
	Primary	Secondary	Tertiary	Not an obligation
Primary	A 75	B 21	C 1	D 1
Secondary	E 157	F 2	G 7	H 0
Tertiary	I 144	J 13	K 0	L 1
Not an obligation	M 15	N 4	O 1	P 0

For the purposes of this paper, we have opted to discuss only cells A, E, and I separately, and cells B and C combined as one. We are excluding cells D, F, G, H, J, K, L, M, N, O, and P because cell N's are too small for reliable analysis. This procedure leaves us with a total of 399 counselors for our analysis.

* Respondent assessments of both disease-risk information provision and psychosocial discussion were coded into four categories: 1) primary professional obligation, 2) secondary professional obligation, 3) tertiary professional obligation, and 4) not a professional obligation. Cross classifying these responses provides a 16-cell table as indicated below.

As part of our national survey we asked counselors to indicate whether or not they felt certain issues should be discussed in counseling, and if so, who has an obligation to raise the issues, the counselor or the counselees. Table 5 lists 11 issues presented to counselors, as well as the percent of counselors representing each of the orientations identified above who feel a professional obligation to raise the specific issues during the counseling session.

The specific issues presented in Table 5 are far from an exhaustive listing of topics that may be covered in counseling. Taken together, however, they represent a variety of types of issues that may or may not be discussed. For example, some of the topics, such as a counselee's financial situation and the effects of a defective child on the family, focus on a counselee as a member of a family and the consequences on a family of having children with a genetic problem. Other topics, such as consideration of the social stigma associated with various disorders as well as the possible societal economic burden of a sick child, are issues which place the counselee's problems in an extra familial or social perspective. Finally, some issues, such as the last four, focus specifically on counselee reproductive attitudes and behavior. Thus taken together these 11 topics provide for a variety of types of issues that might arise during any counseling session.

Table 5 contains some interesting data. First, disregarding the orientations we have identified, it can be see that, on only 5 of the 11 items, do 50% or more of all counselors feel a professional obligation to raise and discuss the specific topic with counselees. On the average, counselors want to discuss the familial impact of defective children, alternative forms of parenthood, and notification of extended family members who may be at-risk to be carriers of a deleterious gene. Smaller majorities want to discuss patient contraception and a family's financial situation. On three items, only a minority feels a professional obligation to raise and discuss the specific issue. Sterlization, a couple's sex life, and the possible societal economic burden of a defective child are not popular topics for discussion by counselors in this study. Nor, for that matter, are discussion of a couple's religious views or the social stigma that may be associated with a particular disorder. These data suggest, among other things, that in general counselors are more likely to want to discuss those topics that keep genetic counseling defined as a medical-familial consultation. They are not as interested in the social (social burden/stigma) nor even private-personal aspects (religious beliefs) of the problem counselees may bring to counseling.

A second observation suggested by the data in Table 5 is that there is substantial variability in counselor opinion about his obligations to discuss many of these items. Some insight into these differences may be gained by examining the four counseling orientations identified earlier, and their relationships to the topics listed.

In some respects, counselors who hold psychosocial discussion and disease-risk information as both primary professional obligations have the most complex of the four orientations identified, while those who hold information provision primary and psychosocial discussion tertiary have the least. While it may be reasonable to draw some limits on the requisite disease-risk information to be provided in a particular situation, it would seem to be much more difficult to do so for possible psychosocial topics, which may require extensive discussion and coverage of many issues. Not surprisingly, when we compare these two counseling orientations in Table 5, we see that 50% or more of the counselors with the dual orientation want to discuss 8 of the 11 items, while among those with a basically information provision orientation, 50% or more want to discuss 5 of the

11 items, suggesting a somewhat less complex counseling agenda. More importantly, the range of the eight issues that a majority of dual-oriented counselors express an interest in runs the gamut of topics listed in Table 5, including reproductive, personal, familial, and societal topics. On the other hand, the five issues in which a majority of essentially information provision oriented counselors express an interest in focus on only reproductive and familial topics.

Genetic counseling as a form of medical consultation revolves about the discussion with patients of certain topics, which almost all professionals feel are necessary. Variability in approaches to counseling, consequently, should be seen less in opinions about discussing such core issues, but more, perhaps, in opinions about the appropriateness of other topics for counseling. A perusal of Table 5 suggests what may be some core issues, and what may be topics of more variable interest to counselors, depending on their general philosophic orientations to counseling.

Three of the 11 topics listed in Table 5 receive high endorsement by counselors of all four orientations. These are discussion of: 1) the effects of affected children on the family; 2) alternative forms of parenthood; and 3) notification of extended family members at-risk to be carriers or have a disease. There is some difference among counselors with the four orientations in terms of the percents endorsing these as topics of professional responsibility in counseling. For example, the topic receiving the most endorsement by the most psychosocially oriented counselors is discussion with counselees of alternative forms of parenthood. Among counselors of the three other orientations, the item receiving the most endorsement is discussion of the family effects of an abnormal child. Generally, however, all counselors, regardless of orientation, view these as topics requiring discussion.

The major differences among the four orientations in Table 5 appear to arise for two sets of issues: a group of personal-social topics — items A, B, D, and E; and a group of reproductive topics — items H, I, J, and K. We will discuss each set separately.

The group of items making up reproductive issues reveals some interesting differences among the four orientations, and in particular strong differences between the most (column 1) and the least (column 4) psychosocially oriented counselors.

As can be seen in Table 5, for all reproductive issues, a larger percent of psychosocially oriented counselors view them as necessary topics for discussion than do the least psychosocially oriented counselors. In general, the trend is quite consistent, in that as there is a lessening in the psychosocial orientations of a counselor (as we move from left to right columns), there is a lessening in the percent of counselors who feel a professional obligation to raise and discuss such topics.

Of the four reproductive items, the ones that display the largest differences between the most and the least psychosocially oriented counselors are items H, discussion of limitation of family size because of risked abnormal offspring, and item K, discussion of the counselee's sex life. The remaining two, discussion of contraception and sterilization, show lesser, though largely consistent variation across orientations. To some extent item H, limitation of family size, can be seen as one of the central issues confronting most counselees.* Based in part on the information provided by the counselor, most counselees will be making a decision about reproduction. As we can see in Table 5, almost three-fifths of the most psychosocially oriented counselors want to raise and discuss this issue with counselees, whereas slightly less than two-fifths of the least psychosocially oriented counselors are so disposed. In some measure, contraception, sterilization, and the counselee's sex life may be viewed as practical adjuncts affecting the extent to which a counselee may be able to act effectively on reproductive decisions, be it to continue or cease reproduction. Hence we would expect, as we find in Table 5, that these items relate to counseling orientation in a fashion similar to item H.

The other sets of items that show significant variation among counseling orientations are items A, B, D, and E. This is a mixed set, and each item requires separate discussion, to some extent.

As can be seen in Table 5, as counselor psychosocial orientation lessens, there is a gradual, then a dramatic, drop in counselor interest in discussing counselee religious views. In terms of a counselor's interest in a counselee's financial situation, we see a shift in professional interest that is carried through for items D and E as well. For these three topics, the greatest interest is shown by counselors who hold both psychosocial discussion and information provision as primary professional obligations, while fewer counselors of the other three orientations, including those committed primarily to psychosocial discussion, report as much interest.

In attempting to summarize the data presented in Table 5 it will be helpful to use the notion of a counseling agenda, introduced above, as a way of viewing how counselors of different orientations approach their counseling. The agenda of the most psychosocially oriented counselors is one, we think, that places primacy on the expectations, values, and personal beliefs of the counselees. Compared to the agendas of the other counseling orientations, these counselors are more interested in exploring the private beliefs (eg religion), personal circumstances (eg sex life, contraceptive practices), and counselees' parenting expectations or desires (eg limitations of family size) than counselors with different orientations. Such discussion permits these counselors some insight into their counselees, and some appreciation of what counselees would like out of life. In

---

* This position is premised on the assumption that most people who seek counseling have not totally ruled out the possibility of reproduction, or they would not be seeking counseling. An increasing number of cases in counseling involve prenatal diagnosis and the decision to continue or terminate a pregnancy. Many of the issues raised in Table 5 nevertheless are applicable to this case.

Table 5. Percent of Counselors With Different Orientations Expressing a Professional Obligation to Raise and Discuss a Variety of Issues with Counselees*

Issues	Obligation			
	Psychosocial discussion primary, information provision secondary or tertiary	Psychosocial discussion and information provision primary	Information provision primary, psychosocial discussion secondary	Information provision primary, psychosocial discussion tertiary
A Counselee's religious views	57	55	39	30
B Financial capacity	50	68	60	51
C Family effects	76	97	92	85
D Social stigma	36	54	39	35
E Social economic burden	23	32	16	24
F Alternative forms of parenthood	86	76	81	78
G Extended family members	77	75	77	83
H Limited family size	57	56	52	39
I Contraceptives	71	64	68	63
J Sterilization	48	43	43	38
K Sex life	48	41	32	30
Maximum N per single item	23	75	157	144

* Since the response rate for this study equaled 77% of the target population and, as assessed by several indicators, was nonbiased, tests of statistical significance provide no additional information to that provided by noting percentage differences. Any differences suggested by data in Tables 5 and 6 are, for all practical purposes, real population differences. The substantive signifcance of percentage differences are discussed in the body of the paper.

an interesting fashion, counselors with this agenda, compared to others, are not as interested in discussing such topics as a family's financial situation or the social stigma associated with a particular abnormality. These latter issues may be seen as suggesting that what is primary in making a decision about reproduction are the consequences of having an abnormal child, and secondary are the values and parenting expectations of the counselees. In short, the most psychosocially oriented counselors seem to want to focus very much on the prior beliefs and expectations counselees bring to the counseling session as basic elements for discussion. On the other hand those counselors with less, but some psychosocial interest seem to prefer to discuss more so the consequences of, or the qualifications for, reproduction as basic discussion elements.

COUNSELING GOALS

Perhaps more insight into the counseling orientations identified in this study can be gained by looking at the goals counselors hold. Table 6 reports on counselor orientation and goals.

As part of the national survey, counselors were asked to indicate how important it was to them that their counseling achieve a variety of outcomes. In almost all cases if the counselor were to attempt to achieve these counseling goals, he would be required to control not only the knowledge and attitudes of his counselees, but their behavior as well. This is obviously not possible. Nevertheless, one may look at endorsement of various counseling goals as reflective of basic counseling strategies that underlie the way in which a counselor approaches his obligations and tasks. As such, by examining the endorsement of these various goals, we may better understand and gain some insight into the counseling orientations identified above.

Table 6 lists the seven goals counselors were asked to endorse in this study. Also reported are the percent of counselors of each of the orientations identified above who consider acknowledgment of the goals as important or very important for their counseling. The seven goals listed, while reflecting a diversity of possible outcomes, do not exhaust the possible goals that counselors may hold. The list does retain, however, commonly held goals, such as disease prevention and reduction of counselee anxiety, as well as some less commonly held goals, such as improvement of general population health and vigor, and reduction in the number of carriers of deleterious genes in the population.

As can be seen in Table 6, there is general agreement among almost all counselors, regardless of their relative emphasis on patient education and psychosocial discussion, that some goals are highly desirable, while others are much less so. For example, a large majority of counselors of all types endorse the goals of lessening counselee anxiety/guilt (B), advancing an understanding of genetics in disease (E), and increasing counselee happiness (F). On all other items, however, a rather marked difference emerges between the most psychosocially oriented counselors, and counselors of the three other orientations, which, with some variation, appear to be quite similar in terms of goals.

An examination of Table 6 suggests that the most striking difference between the most psychosocially oriented counselors and all the rest is that the former are, in general, much less "prevention" oriented. This difference appears for both prevention of somatic abnormality (item A) as well as genotype abnormality (items C and G).

Table 6. Percent of Counselors With Different Orientations Endorsing Various Counseling Outcomes (Goals) As Important or Very Important

Counseling outcomes	Obligation Orientation			
	Psychosocial discussion primary, information provision secondary or tertiary	Psychosocial discussion and information provision primary	Information provision primary, psychosocial discussion secondary	Information provision primary, psychosocial discussion tertiary
A Disease prevention	48	77	88	87
B Lessening counselee anxiety/guilt	100	97	97	98
C Preventing deleterious genes	13	32	31	30
D Improving population vigor	13	39	25	26
E Advancing understanding	74	81	87	80
F Counselee happiness	87	81	87	80
G Reducing carriers of deleterious genes	13	34	21	20
Maximum N per single item	23	75	157	144

It would appear from this limited analysis that the agendas of the most and lesser psychosocially oriented counselors are quite different in terms of their prevention orientations. To some extent this difference fits with the conclusion we came to in discussing the data presented in Table 5. To the extent that the most psychosocially oriented counselors approach counseling wanting to use counselee values and expectations to shape their counseling, we would not expect them to view their counseling goal as that of disease prevention or reduction in the number of carriers of deleterious genes in the population. To do the latter would entail giving limited attention to the values and expectations of the counselees, even though these at times may coincide with prevention goals. The most psychosocially oriented counselors, we think, want to let counselees define the end point of counseling, and for counselees to do this the genetic counselor can not adopt a view of genetic counseling as preventive medicine. For psychosocially oriented counselors, if counselees want prevention, then counseling can be oriented to it. But, the thrust of counseling must be shaped by the values and expectations of the counselees, more so than by the genetic expect as preventer of somatic disease or genetic abnormality.

DISCUSSION

The data presented above suggest to us two basically different orientations among the counselors in this study. The first and most common orientation is one in which genetic counseling is viewed largely as preventive medicine. Many of the things that a counselor with this orientation wants to discuss with counselees focus on the consequences of reproducing and having an abnormal child; that is, failure to achieve disease prevention. We see the clinical logic of such counselors based on two premises: 1) prevent the birth of abnormal children; and 2) assess the reasonableness of reproducing in any given situation in light of the possible/probable consequences of having an affected child. To a large extent the more than 30 published evaluations of the efficacy of genetic counseling to date have adopted these premises [10]. To assess the success of genetic counseling these studies have focused primarily on counselee reproductive attitudes and behavior subsequent to counseling as a function of: 1) the magnitude of the recurrence risk; and 2) the severity of the disease or disorder, in light of the efficacy of available therapy.

The logic of this prevention approach enables one to see the reproductive decisions of counselees as more or less "rational," and to assess the success of genetic counseling in a similar vein. From the view of such an orientation, counselees' reproductive decision-making can be seen as an exercise in solving an equation. Counselors provide the two unknowns for the equation — the magnitude of the recurrence risk and an estimate of disease severity. Reproductive decisions can be seen as more or less reasonable in light of these two basic parameters.

The other orientation we see is one that is markedly less prevention oriented. This orientation focuses, we think, on genetic counseling as counseling, with the values and expectations of counselees, not recurrence risk and disease severity, as the basic parameters defining the situation. The clinical logic of this position suggests that it is much more difficult, compared to the more preventive orientation, to designate what is or is not rational behavior in a given situation. It is more difficult to designate a rational position, since the decision must be premised on and reflect the personal values and expectations of counselees. In addition, the task confronting counselees is less likely to be seen as one of solving an equation and more as one of arriving at a complex judgment.

This second orientation places considerable weight on the 3rd, 4th, and 5th elements of the counseling task outlined in the AJHG definition that opened this chapter. In so doing, it adds very complex and often nonquantifiable elements into reproductive decision-making based on genetic counseling. Not surprisingly, no published evaluation studies of counseling to date have embraced this view of genetic counseling, although there is one study in process which is attempting to employ assessment based on both perspectives outlined in this paper [10].

The analysis presented here is not meant to suggest that any one of the orientations discussed is superior to the other. In all probability most counseling will require a mix of information provision and psychosocial discussion, and the counselor must be able to both define the appropriate mix and see that the counselee receives what he expects and needs. Genetic counseling is at a stage of development where it would be premature to define the role and task of the counselor in a rigid fashion. It may be that the term "genetic counseling" is both inappropriate as a description of what transpires most often between expert and layman, and also is misleading in what it connotes to laymen as they approach this particular encounter [11]. Regardless, what is needed is careful attention to the problems people bring to the genetic counselor and the skills and resources counselors have at their disposal. In attempting to help people at-risk for abnormal offspring, the genetic counselor is involved in providing medical-genetic information, shaping and even changing attitudes, and, ultimately, affecting the reproductive behavior and family relations of those who come to them. We know very little at the present time about how well the genetic counselor is accomplishing these tasks. Thus, in a sense, genetic counseling is presently experimental medicine. A commitment to assessing which counseling methods work and which do not is needed now that is as strong as the commitment of genetic counselors to helping those who seek their counsel.

REFERENCES

1. Fraser FC: Genetic counseling. Am J Hum Genet 26:636–659, 1974.
2. Sorenson JR: "Social and Psychological Aspects of Applied Human Genetics: A Bibliography." Fogarty International Center, DHEW Publications No. 73-412, NIH, 1973. [Compilation of articles on genetic counseling, some of which contain definitions.]
3. Hsia YE: Choosing my children's genes: genetic counseling. In Lipkin M, Rowley PT (eds): "Genetic Responsibility." New York: Plenum, 1973.
4. Lynch HT: "Dynamic Genetic Counseling." Springfield: Charles C Thomas, 1969.
5. Sorenson J: "Genetic Counselors: Professionals in Applied Human Genetics." Russell Sage Foundation. (In preparation)
6. Albrecht J, Day N: A Survey of Genetic Counseling Facilities in Massachusetts. (Supplementary survey of physicians and genetic services which they provide.) Massachusetts Department of Public Health, 1971.
7. Bergsma D, Lynch H (eds): "International Directory of Genetic Services." 3rd Ed. New York: The National Foundation—March of Dimes, 1971.
8. Haller M: "Eugenics." New Brunswick: Rutgers University Press, 1963.
9. Ludmerer K: "Genetics and American Society." Baltimore: Johns Hopkins University Press, 1972.

10. "Proposal For A Two Year Study Of Genetic Counseling at Centers Supported By The National Foundation–March of Dimes." (Approved), Scotch NA, Sorenson JR, Swazey JP, March 1976, Boston University School of Medicine.
11. Kavanagh C, Griffin M, Sorenson J: "Genetic Information, Client Perspectives, and Genetic Counseling." Social Work in Health Care Vol 2(2), Winter 1976–77, pp 171–180.

7. Genetic Counselors Without Doctorates

Tabitha M. Powledge, MS

The field of genetic counseling is one of the best examples of "medicalization" of an area of research. The unhappy political consequences of the American eugenics movement in the early part of this century, coupled with revulsion at the Nazi horror, has made it politically very difficult to do research on applied human genetics except in a thoroughly medical — that is, explicitly therapeutic — context [1, 2]. And, as Caplan's paper in this volume also makes clear, lack of certain kinds of conceptual information for a long time made it impossible (and continues to make it difficult) for the tenets of population genetics to be applied to the human species, giving us a nonmedical science of human genetics.

The profession of "genetic counselor" therefore usually has come to mean someone with a doctorate — almost always a medical doctorate. Important recent references in major journals [3,4] speak of the profession in that manner, and it is clear that many people who study human genetics think of it as a medical specialty, essentially no different from pediatrics or internal medicine or neurosurgery [5].

It will be the thesis of this paper, however, that an appreciable portion of current efforts in genetic counseling is being performed by people without doctorates, that the trend is expanding, and that this trend may have important consequences for the profession. These assertions and conclusions are, it must be noted from the outset, based to a large extent on subjective observations and analogies from other branches of medicine, because there are available very little in the way of firm data, either on the changes in the profession or their impact. Some studies of nondoctor counselors are just beginning, but their information will probably not be available for some time. This paper, then, is in the nature of a speculation.

Informal genetic counseling, of course, probably goes back far into prehistory. The human species has been purposefully breeding plants and animals for tens of thousands of years, and it seems reasonable to assume past attempts

Birth Defects: Original Articles Series, Volume XV, Number 2, pages 103—112
© 1979 The National Foundation

to apply some of those lessons to human reproduction. Anthropologists still spend a surprising amount of time debating the origins of the almost universal incest taboo in human societies. Although many social explanations have been proposed (one argument, for instance, is that exogamy is useful in forging friendly political ties with neighbors), it seems likely that empirical observations of the occasional sad results of inbreeding, in the form of what is now established as a well-documented increased incidence of congenital malformations in inbred populations, have always played a role, perhaps a prime one. That possibility seems even more reasonable if one takes into account its opposite: the encouragement of inbreeding in certain important ritual/political situations, such as the well-known example of the Egyptian royal family, where an intent was surely to reinforce desirable leadership characteristics. All this is by way of illustrating the likelihood that a kind of folk genetic counseling existed long before its current medical framework in the West. And indeed, that kind of informal counseling goes on today, and no doubt will continue to do so. Every practitioner of medical genetics has had to cope with information (usually *mis*information) received by a patient from relatives, neighbors and even the family doctor, all ignorant of some basic fact such as Mendelian modes of transmission.

Although such informal counseling is important, in the sense that it often must be undone before people can begin to make rational choices about their reproductive lives, this paper will instead concern itself with more explicit genetic counseling that arises in three different settings. They are: 1) counseling by the clergy (and perhaps in some cases by psychotherapists); 2) counseling by genetic counseling clinic personnel without doctor's degrees, but often with master's degrees, frequently graduates of new training programs that have sprung up recently; 3) counseling by people, usually without advanced degrees but often with some brief specific training, in outreach programs such as genetic screening projects.

Genetic counseling by a spiritual adviser or someone else who is trained to counsel has the potential of being beneficial insofar as it concerns itself with exploration of the social and moral issues in a reproductive decision. Should I get pregnant if my risk of bearing a defective child is very great? What is a great risk — 5% or 25%? What are my obligations to my other children? Do I have an obligation to tell my relatives if they may also be at risk? Is it right to abort a defective child if the defect can be treated? All of these are moral, not medical (nor, in social science parlance, "psychosocial") questions. A medically trained genetic counselor may have an opinion as to the "right" answer to any of these questions, but that counselor's answer is not necessarily inherently better than a priest's, so long as both of their opinions rest on the same technical information base. The problem with the priest's answer is that it may rest on inadequate or wrong genetic information. For example, far too many people without training in genetics assume that one affected family member means a lifetime risk to others in the family, and they are all too ready to advise people against bearing children without the slightest idea of the real nature of the risks. Conversely, genetic explanations for the occurrence of a disease are often rejected by people "because it's never been in the family before." Either piece of advice can lead to tragedy.

Since the moral questions surrounding reproductive life are the proper province of the clergy, probably the only solution to this problem is to impress upon them the necessity of seeing that their "clients" get reliable, up-to-date information on the condition they are worried about, including an accurate diagnosis and facts about recurrence risks, the availability of prenatal diagnosis and supportive services, and other kinds of technical information bearing on their decisions. They should also be made aware that the family doctor can be an unreliable source for such information, which should be obtained from a specialist in medical genetics. In practice, of course, such a sequence of events will no doubt be infrequent, and the result is that many people may be making agonizing moral decisions on the basis of inaccurate or incomplete technical information. The moral problem in translocation Down syndrome is quite different from that in age-related Down syndrome, even though the two affected people may be clinically indistinguishable.

In the other two kinds of nondoctor counseling, the people performing it are adjuncts to the medical profession and, even if their technical information is satisfactory, they have no special expertise in moral questions (although some of them may have received some training in psychotherapeutic counseling techniques). But although most of them have undergone some greater or lesser degree of technical training, they also have some important differences from the doctor—counselor. These differences in training and style could have important consequences for the profession of genetic counseling.

Two major trends are responsible for the growing use of nondoctors in formal genetic counseling programs. One is the large increase in technical information about genetic disease, and the tools with which to deal with that information. The most important example of the latter, of course, is prenatal diagnosis. The genetic case load has increased as more can be done. Yet much of what can be done need not be done by a doctor. Explaining the intricacies of autosomal recessive inheritance in a sickle cell screening program can easily be done by someone with a small amount of training. That saves money because it frees the doctor's time for other tasks — and incidentally spares him a repetitive and not very interesting job. Headings and Fielding [6] observe:

> People with a number of different backgrounds may be good sickle cell counselors. Although it is helpful to be in the health field and to possess some knowledge of Mendelian genetic principles, many individuals without such backgrounds can function very well as sickle cell counselors with the guidance of a medical geneticist. Indis-

pensable characteristics are (1) sensitivity to the general problems of young adults, especially young adults from minority groups, (2) understanding of the impact that becoming aware of carrying a genetic condition can have on an individual, (3) a commitment to a non-directive counseling approach, (4) ability to assimilate the necessary factual material about sickle cell trait and anemia, including principles of genetic transmission.

The same reasoning applies, almost of necessity, to any other relatively large-scale program. A further example is prenatal diagnosis. In the programs at large medical centers which perform many amniocenteses a week, it is obviously more efficient to set up the individual explanations of the procedure on something of an assembly-line basis, and assign someone other than a doctor to do it. In situations requiring follow-up, clients' concerns will often involve issues like family strain or school placement, issues which doctors frequently do not consider their province, either by training or temperament. Adjunct personnel can, in short, be a big help to the increasingly busy doctor in a genetics clinic [3]. The whole area of postnatal counseling the parents of a child with a birth defect is just beginning to be explored, but will certainly attain more importance if the expansion of the neonatal intensive care unit and other survival techniques continues [7, 8]. Indeed, Fraser distinguishes between informative and supportive counseling, and argues that more of the latter is particularly needed in genetic health care [9].

The trend probably also owes something to the growing consumer movement and perhaps even a slight tendency toward democratization of medicine. In the emerging pattern, Barker says, "Mutuality and reduction of inequality are preferred to one-sidedness and inequality" [10]. Furthermore, we are beginning to recognize that there are things we expect of medicine for which we don't train our doctors. The lay counselor in a sickle cell screening program is often black and of similar social class and educational background as the client, which can make the exchange between them much more of an exchange between equals than the usual patient—doctor encounter. Conceivably the information transmitted could therefore be better understood and retained, both for that reason and because the information may be more likely to be transmitted in the patient's terms, rather than in medical jargon. The unsatisfactory level of understanding and remembering genetic information among clients is one of the most intractable and frustrating problems of genetic counseling, and anything which improves it should be encouraged.

In addition, there is some preliminary evidence to suggest "that physicians and nurses are more directive regarding reproductive decisions involving prevention of hemoglobinopathies than are health professionals whose roles more explicitly entail giving of information and counseling. It is hypothesized that the former are less likely to view clients as the appropriate decision-makers in these matters and thus would tend not to foster a mutual cooperation style of counselee-counselor relationship" [11]. Nondirective counseling is regarded by the majority of counselors as a desirable goal for the profession, and it can thus be argued that middle level professionals might improve chances of attaining that goal.

For whatever reasons, throughout medicine the trend is toward the physician assistant, the paraprofessional, and other such extensions of the doctor; the new kind of genetic counselor can be seen as part of that trend. For one thing, although physicians would often prefer to deemphasize it, it is cheaper than hiring an additional doctor [12]. "Several studies have suggested that physician assistants are well accepted by patients and physicians, increase the productivity of medical practice, improve access to health services and enhance quality of care. However, the ultimate test of the usefulness of the physician assistant must include estimates of the financial impact on medical practice of adding this new professional to the health-care team." The study from which this observation comes showed that physician assistants actually generated revenue beyond their costs to the practices surveyed [13]. The authors caution against generalizing their findings to other types of physician assistants (those studied were all MEDEX and all men). But it is a relatively consistent finding that practices using the primary-care physician assistant have the potential for increasing the relative number of patient encounters anywhere from 30 to 50% [14], and it seems likely that a similar situation may be true of many other medical settings, including a genetics clinic.

Certainly there seems to be very little in the way of consumer resistance to the role of the nonphysician in medical care provision. As one example, Colorado's Child Health Associates have been warmly received in settings such as a low-risk newborn nursery, where the new mothers have been very enthusiastic about the CHA's care and helpfulness. Among one group of new mothers, about 20% asked the CHA questions they said they would not have asked the doctor or the nurse, giving some hint that the relationship is indeed somewhat more egalitarian than the usual one between patient and professional [15].

The family-planning nurse—practitioner does pelvic exams and diagnoses and even treats conditions ranging from venereal disease to iron deficiency anemia, and one study reported that one group of them had never encountered either patient or physician resistance [16].

The nurse—midwife has also gotten enthusiastic notices from her obstetrician—supervisors. It is quite clear one of her chief attractions is that she spares them much of the repetitive inconvenience of dealing with their patients [17]:

> We are relieved of many telephone questions pertaining to prenatal symptoms, constipation, medications, common colds, rubella exposures, prodromal labor discomfort, 'what do I do now?' *ad infini-*

tum! An aggravation chart would show that our sleeping pattern is disturbed only about 20% as compared to a previous 50% incidence . . . you realize how patients often refrain from bringing questions and problems to their busy doctor; now we see them relating and enjoying this new team approach, where the midwife always has plenty of time to talk and respond to their whims.

It is not difficult to imagine that many similar "whims" may arise when genetic disease is involved.

As with the Child Health Associate, women apparently feel comfortable with the nurse—midwife — often more comfortable than with the physician. No one seems quite certain why this should be so, but it is a continuing finding in the literature on physician-extenders. They are less forbidding, and more accessible. Gender may play a role. These new professions all concern the bearing of children, and that in itself may constitute an experiential bond between patient and female physician-extender that the (usually male) doctor, with all his expertise, cannot match.

One problem already encountered by these new professionals, which needs to be dealt with also by the nondoctor counselor, are questions of legal liability, particularly when diagnosis and treatment are involved [18, 19]. Another problem is the willingness of third-party payers to reimburse for these services, just as they would for those of a physician. (See Reilly, this volume, pp. 291–305, for further discussion of these points and the question of licensure.)

A recent small study of both physician assistants and nurse-practitioners in several places in this country revealed that both groups were performing a wide variety of delegated tasks, including obtaining lab samples, therapy, clerical tasks, physical exams and histories, and follow-ups. In addition, the authors noted that nurse-practitioners "often emphasize patient counseling and education," which had been omitted from the list of tasks they studied [20].

As far as genetic counseling is concerned, it is important to point out here that the more egalitarian relationship may in fact not be true at all, or may apply largely to the lay counselor in the outreach program. The social worker, the graduate of the genetic advising programs and other such members of the genetic clinic team have graduate degrees. They think of themselves as professionals and their relationships with their clients may be somewhat similar to the doctor's. Since there has been a certain amount of disenchantment with mass screening as an effective and efficient form of health care delivery in general, and heterozygote screening in particular, the lay counselor may gradually disappear from the scene. At least one authority has expressed doubts about whether such programs of screening for genetic traits will or should continue in their present form [21].

The counselor with intensive training, however, is likely to be a long-term feature of the genetic counseling clinic. In some centers, such roles may be taken by registered nurses [22] or professional social workers, but more and more often they are filled by graduates of one of the five specialized academic programs that have recently been organized in the United States.

The programs themselves avoid use of the term genetic counselor in connection with their graduates, preferring such alternatives as "genetic associate" or "genetic adviser." And there is a body of physician-resistance to use of the term genetic counselor for these graduates [5]. But certainly many of the graduates think of themselves — and even speak of themselves — as genetic counselors. Some of these graduates work in laboratory settings, but most of them have found work that involves direct patient contact: taking histories, doing pedigrees, working in fund-raising organizations (such as those associated with a particular genetic disease) and counseling candidates for prenatal diagnosis. The fact of the matter is that today's genetic counseling is a complex process, often involving extensive investigational and diagnostic procedures that must of necessity be a team effort.

The "team" approach seems to have won wide acceptance [3, 5, 23] and the Ad Hoc Committee on Genetic Counseling of the American Society of Human Genetics has stated flatly [24],

> training in either basic genetics or medicine alone is not sufficient to qualify an individual as a genetic counselor . . . appropriately trained nurses, social workers and/or genetic associates within counseling units will greatly increase. These persons can effectively act as the interface between the geneticists and the patient population, making it possible for the geneticists' time and skills to be most efficiently utilized, while at the same time enhancing the process of communication and assisting patients and families in dealing with their problems. It is recommended, however, that the extent of their responsibilities for genetic counseling be determined by mutual agreement among the members of the genetic counseling team.

One counselor argues for the importance of the intake interview, particularly in raising nongenetic concerns, and says that such interviews can, from her experience, be conducted successfully by genetic advising students and public health nurses, as well as a PhD [25]. Many other aspects of the counseling process — tracing old hospital records, arranging for school placement, and so forth — are tasks with which a doctor is often delighted to have help. There are many jobs that are, or can be, a legitimate part of genetic counseling. They can be done (and in some cases perhaps should be done) by people who are not doctors. Many graduates of at least one master's program perform such functions as clinic administration, intake history, pedigree taking, supportive counseling, patient education, and teaching other health professionals [26]. The University of Oregon Health Sciences Center has employed group counseling procedures for such relatively common disorders as Down and Turner syndromes [27]; organizing and running such groups would also be an appropriate use of master's-level training. Such people have also been very useful to regional programs that must take their services periodically into small communities, such as those in rural and mountain Georgia [28] and Colorado and Wyoming [29]. Graduates of the programs have met some professional resistance, but the economic climate of recent times has also worked against them, and some clinics that might have liked to add such personnel to their staffs have not had the money to do so.

The programs in existence are all very different in style and goals, and their curricula vary accordingly. The oldest and largest of these programs is located at Sarah Lawrence College, Bronxville, New York. It began in 1969 and now has well over fifty graduates [26]. Shortly thereafter, a similar program began at Douglass College of Rutgers, The State University, New Brunswick, New Jersey. There are also two West Coast programs, both in the University of California system: the Genetic Advising program, part of the Health and Medical Sciences program at Berkeley, and another within the Department of Pediatrics, California College of Medicine, Irvine. There has also been a program located within the Department of Biophysics and Genetics, University of Colorado Medical Center, Denver.

Genetic counseling itself has been seen by its practitioners in varying ways, so it is not surprising that the programs should also vary. The curricula, naturally, contain a core of genetics and other technical subjects, training in the counseling process, and some time spent getting clinical experience. Emphases vary, however. The then director of the Colorado program, for instance, argued in a June 1975 meeting of people involved in all the programs that he thought his students should be trained not only in organic and biochemistry, but physical chemistry as well. By contrast, the Sarah Lawrence program lays strong emphasis on the development of counseling skills; in addition to their formal place in the curriculum, these skills continue to be emphasized in a series of seminars the program runs for its working graduates. These curricular differences may ultimately affect the style and goals of their graduates, and lead some, for instance, to view genetic counseling as properly consisting more of supportive attitudes than of technical information.

Is this new professional group likely to have an impact on genetic counseling? At the moment, of course, it is only possible to speculate.

The new genetic associates may have very little effect on the profession, particularly if, as appears often to be the case, they are simply absorbed into traditional dependent helping roles often characteristic of nurses and other female health professionals who are not doctors. On the other hand, to the extent that some degree of diagnosis and treatment become part of the genetic associate's job, the exigencies of decision-making and her ideas about herself are likely to make the dependent role both impractical and unattractive. The nursing profession is currently struggling with the same tensions. The very existence of the nurse-practioner as a new professional is to some extent a result of some nurses' explicit embrace of new ideas about their autonomy, and their recognition that, acknowledged or not, they have always made some medical decisions [30, 19].

The Health Commissioner of Massachusetts has argued that physician assistants and nurse—practitioners are not going to be very important in American medicine because of the way our health care system is organized, but the argument is based on the ideal of the physician assistant as a front-line worker in primary care (which is indeed the way they are used abroad) [31]. The genetic associate, by contrast, fits perfectly into his model of the U.S. health system: hospital-based (which most genetic clinics are), specialist-intensive (which genetics certainly is), and resource-rich (which many genetic technologies are). And in this sense, perhaps the genetic associate *is* someone to worry about: to the extent that she fits right in with the way our health care is organized, with all its deficiencies, she perpetuates it.

Part of the problem in defining this new role for a middle level professional in medical genetics is that medical genetics itself is an ill defined profession, changing and growing rapidly because of technology, but not yet agreed on its goals and aims. No one has put the problem more clearly than Murphy: "We undoubtedly need more genetic clinics that are simple but sound. We also need better clinics. But there is little use in wishing vaguely for better clinics unless we can first define what we mean by a better clinic; and secondly we take realistic steps to pursue this end. Of these two, the first is the more difficult — we are embarrassingly devoid of even a set of standards that we could use for quality control, though one of these days we may find ourselves having to produce them with some urgency" [32].

REFERENCES

1. Haller MH: "Eugenics: Hereditarian Attitudes in American Thought." New Brunswick, New Jersey: Rutgers University Press, 1963.
2. Ludmerer KM: "Genetics and American Society." Baltimore: Johns Hopkins University Press, 1972.
3. Fraser FC: Genetic counseling. Am J Hum Genet 26:636–659, 1974.
4. Kushnick T: When to refer to the geneticist. JAMA 235:623–625, 1976.
5. Epstein CJ: Who should do genetic counseling, and under what circumstances? In Bergsma D (ed): "Contemporary Genetic Counseling." White Plains: The National Foundation—March of Dimes, BD:OAS IX(4):39–48, 1973.
6. Headings V, Fielding J: Guidelines for counseling young adults with sickle cell trait. Am J Pub Health 65:819–827, 1975.
7. DuHamel TR, Lin S, Skelton A et al: Early parental perceptions and the high risk neonate. Clin Pediatr 13:1052–1056, 1974.
8. Drotar D, Baskiewicz A, Irvin N et al: The adaptation of parents to the birth of an infant with a congenital malformation: A hypothetical model. Pediatrics 56:710–717, 1975.
9. Fraser FC: Genetics as a health-care service. N Engl J Med 295:486–488, 1976.

10. Barker B: Compassion in medicine: Toward new definitions and new institutions. N Engl J Med 295:939−943, 1976.

11. Headings VE: Associations between type of health profession and judgments about prevention of sickling disorders. J Med Ed 51:682−684, 1976.

12. Long NW: Untitled. Am J Obstet Gynecol 123:39−40, 1975.

13. Nelson EC, Jacobs AR, Cordner K et al: Financial impact of physician assistants on medical practice. N Engl J Med 293:527−530, 1975.

14. Miles DL: Physician's assistants: The evidence is not in. N Engl J Med 293:555−556, 1975.

15. Dungy CI: The child health associate: The new image in the nursery. Am J Pub Health 65:1179−1183, 1975.

16. Manisoff M, Davis W: Family planning nurse practitioners in the United States. Fam Plann Perspect 7:154−157, 1975.

17. Gatewood T, Stewart RB: Obstetricians and nurse-midwives: The team approach in private practice. Am J Obstet Gynecol 123:35−38, 1975.

18. Abdellah F: Nurse practitioners and nursing practice. Am J Pub Health 66:245−246, 1976.

19. Bullough B: The law and the expanding nursing role. Am J Pub Health 66:249−254, 1976.

20. Glenn JK, Goldman J: Task delegation to physician extenders − Some comparisons. Am J Pub Health 66:64−66, 1976.

21. Childs B: Prospects for genetic screening. J Pediatr 87:1125-1132, 1975.

22. Ferrer TL: Counseling patients with genetic abnormalities. Nurs Clin N A 10:293−305, 1975.

23. Wilson MG: Genetic counseling. Current Problems in Pediatrics V (7):1−51, May 1975.

24. Ad Hoc Committee on Genetic Counseling: Genetic counseling. Am J Hum Genet 27:240−242, 1975.

25. Kelly PT: The role of the intake interview in genetic counseling. Am J Hum Genet 27:53A, November 1975.

26. Marks JH, Richter ML: The genetic associate: A new health professional. Am J Pub Health 66:388−390, 1976.

27. Plumridge DM: The use of groups as a genetic counseling technique. Am J Hum Genet 27:72A, November 1975.

28. Andrews LC, Bennuck I, Stansell D et al: Community based genetic counseling in north Georgia: An innovation in service delivery. Am J Hum Genet 27:13A, November 1975.

29. Matthews AL, Blu J, Riccardi VM: The team approach to genetic counseling: Expanded roles of the nurse geneticist and genetics associate. Am J Hum Genet 27:64A, November 1975.

30. Weiler PG: Health manpower dialectic-physician, nurse, physician assistant. Am J Pub Health 65:858−863, 1975.

31. Bicknell WJ, Walsh DC, Tanner MM: Substantial or decorative? Physician's assistants and nurse practitioners in the United States. Lancet ii:1241−1244, 1974.

32. Murphy EA: Clinical genetics: Some neglected facets. N Engl J Med 292:458−462, 1975.

8. A Counselor's Viewpoint

Jessica G. Davis, MD

I speak as a medical geneticist, trained in medicine, pediatrics, medical genetics, and its subspecialty, cytogenetics. My work concerns families, adults, and children; living children and those unborn. My case load has no barriers of race, caste, class or neighborhood, though race, religion and country of origin may be vitally relevant at times. I spend much time with patients, talking with them, listening to them, and observing them. Since I work in a medical center, I have daily discussions with members of a multidisciplinary genetic counseling team, medical students, house staff, colleagues, and other health care providers.

The purpose of my work is to educate and enlighten individuals who seek information about genetic disorders for themselves, other family members or future offspring. A corollary of my practice is updating the knowledge of the medical community. In doing this I have followed a direction taken by such medical geneticists as Fraser [1], Sly [2], and Murray [3] and have adopted views held by many of my teachers.* They all consistently champion a clear presentation of accurate ". . . medical, genetic and social facts related to the condition under consideration . . . " [3] as well as a full discussion of all the options available to the individual and their consequences. They stress the need for the counselor to take as much time as necessary to share this information in a calm supportive atmosphere.

My experience has compelled me to learn what happens to people during the genetic counseling process. I have observed how individuals deal with suffering and uncertainty and joy, how they relinquish old ideas and adjust to new ones, and how they arrive at acceptable but difficult decisions. This paper will describe the concerns and expectations of genetic counselors and how they handle clinical problems. The references may sometimes be to learned journals, but the most important reference is personal confrontation with the situations discussed.

There is general agreement among genetic counselors that our first con-

* I wish to acknowledge the teaching of Drs. Nathan S. Grosof, Lewis Fraad, Edna Sobel, and Lawrence T. Taft.

Birth Defects: Original Article Series, Volume XV, Number 2, pages 113–122
© 1979 The National Foundation

cerns are to establish an accurate medical diagnosis, to obtain complete genealogical information about all known family members, and to determine whether
the problem is an acquired or a genetic one. When all the essential data are
obtained, the counselor reviews the literature, assembles the relevant facts about
the natural history of the disorder, its prognosis, its treatment and the mode of
inheritance. The counselor also calculates the probability of the patient having
another similarly affected child. The next and most critical step is the effective
transmission of this information to the patient and other family members.

Genetic counseling relies on the complex relationship between at least two
people, the patient and the counselor. Counseling is a social act in which information is given and received. The counselor's primary responsibility is the sharply
focused delivery of knowledge to solve or clarify a problem. Ideally, the counselor imparts scientific knowledge compassionately, using skilled interview techniques. At the same time, ideally, the patient listens, weighs, comprehends, and
absorbs what is being said while relating well to the counselor.

This sounds straightforward. However, recent studies show that the reality
is much different. For example, in reporting on the complexities of parental
understanding of phenylketonuria, Sibinga and Friedman showed that communication of medical facts from the physician to the parents is often complicated
by the patient's limited ability to comprehend the information [4] . Leonard,
Chase, and Childs studied a group of families with well-defined genetic diseases
to learn if they understood the recurrence risks and the natural history of the
condition about which they had been counseled. Their results indicate that even
after extensive counseling many individuals had a very poor grasp of the medical
facts and probability [5] .

The counselor must determine the patient's understanding of human
biology and gear explanations accordingly. Medical terms are often technical
and foreign. Information can and should be carefully presented in a clear, simple
fashion. For instance, we doctors can get by using the term "fingerprints" instead
of "dermatoglyphics" and the patient will understand our meaning. If one works
with non-English speaking people, it is important to employ a sensitive, neutral
interpreter, one who is aware of the subtleties and nuances of the words being
exchanged.

Of particular concern to medical geneticists is our patients' understanding
of recurrence risks. Mellman points out that it has always been difficult for physicians and patients to understand and apply the theory of probability in
decision-making [6] . Many counselors believe that a family's perception of
probability may be distorted by the severity of "burden" of the genetic disorder
under consideration [5] . Motulsky further emphasizes the need to distinguish
between relative and absolute risks to avoid fear and misunderstanding [7] . I
believe that the manner and sequence of giving the odds makes a difference.

Many counselors employ a variety of techniques to help patients better understand probability. Simple visual material demonstrating the rules of chance and recurrence risks for different genetic conditions are available (Dr. Stanley Handmaker, Martin Luther King Jr. General Hosp., Los Angeles, CA). The use of aids such as dice or coins should be encouraged.

Genetic counselors soon recognize that the diagnosis of a genetic disorder constitutes a traumatic event with far-reaching consequences for the individual and the professionals concerned. While presenting the definitive diagnosis and reviewing all the findings that lead to this conclusion, the counselor must pay attention to the attitudes and feelings displayed by the affected individual and various family members. The counselor may be confronted with patients' disbelief, grief, sorrow, anger, fear, resentment, denial and even euphoria. If the medical problem is a severe one, the counselor knows that, in all probability, patients are in no condition to deal with a technical body of knowledge after being dealt an emotional knockout.

The counselor must demonstrate her capacity to accept the upsetting behavior patients may exhibit. "Upsetting" in this context can mean fainting, hysteric screaming or total lack of affect. One patient was convinced there was a mix-up in the nursery and she was given the wrong baby. We have found that in counseling patients who have just given birth to a child with Down syndrome, it is important to give parents an opportunity to talk alone and to postpone the further discussion to a more appropriate time. We find the second visit essential, because many patients are unable to communicate effectively so soon after hearing the diagnosis [8].

Each family situation is unique, but "appropriate handling . . . can turn a potentially devastating experience into the foundation for a satisfactory adjustment to the problem" [9]. The model medical geneticist should be compassionate, skillful, informed, intelligent, honest and responsive. Being able to listen and communicate the necessary biogenetic information in a calm, quiet manner is essential. I seek to create an atmosphere which encourages patients and their families to raise questions and to air fears, doubts and feelings.

Most counselors encourage several visits. More often than not there is a need for several information-sharing sessions so that all the material can be reviewed and the discussion expanded to include all aspects of the problem. Other family members at risk may wish to be seen. If an infant or young child is involved, all information must be discussed in the presence of both parents. If one parent is not available, I have found it helpful for a relative or close friend to be present. I see other concerned family members, such as grandparents and sibs, in order to reduce family conflict and anxiety. Follow-up visits afford me the time to establish a treatment plan and offer patients the opportunity of seeking additional consultation. If the services of other professionals are needed

advice is given about these specialties. Information about appropriate community resources, including parent groups, educational programs and recreational
facilities, may be supplied.

I also spend considerable time talking with referring physicians and community agencies, such as adoption and foster-care services, about individual
cases. It is important to share with them all the pertinent information about the
patient's condition, the laboratory results, the discussions in the counseling sessions and the rationale of the counseling process. Referring physicians and agency
representatives are invited to attend case conferences. The ongoing education of
the practicing physician and other health care providers is an important professional responsiblity.

All counselors send written reports to referring physicians. I send out
written reports to my patients summarizing the salient features of the counseling
sessions. Hsia states, "We cannot expect verbal communication to be remembered accurately, especially when unfamiliar, complicated and emotionally laden
information is presented all at once" [10]. The written summary prevents misunderstanding, provides valuable genetic information for other family members
and preserves the contemporaneous record for the counselor's own files. In
writing about his experiences in providing genetic services to a large indigent
non-English-speaking population, Handmaker says that "in order to understand
the nature of the disorder, patient and family must be provided with a clear,
concise explanation written up in a language they understand. Such an explanation should require no more than a sixth-grade level of education" [11]. The
response of my patients to such letters has been favorable. For most patients this
is the first time they have received a written report from a physician. It is clear
that the practice of sending reports should be adopted by all counselors.

Genetic counselors are also concerned about their own attitudes and biases.
Fraser warns that "one must beware of projecting one's own personality into the
situation. If you are the kind of person that likes to be a good guy, then you
sometimes find yourself being overoptimistic about the advice you're giving, and
if you are a hostile kind of person you may be overpessimistic" [12].

Many counselors use a directive approach. Pearson describes his recent
move to an authoritarian approach to questions about reproduction posed by
"clients facing the prospect of Huntington's Disease" [12]. He says that, in the
past, when asked, "what would you do if you were in my shoes?" he tended to
avoid a direct answer, in an attempt to adhere to the tradition of democratic
ideals and self-determination. Of late, he answers directly and without hesitation
that, on the basis of his experience, trying as best he can to put himself in the
shoes of someone at risk for Huntington disease, he would by all means avoid
procreation [13].

I side with those taking a nondirective stance. My goal is not to play God
but to present all the facts and options available to families in a neutral nonjudgmental fashion. I do not give specific recommendations about marriage or repro-

duction, but allow the patient or couple to arrive at a fully-informed free choice. I agree with Macintyre "that a really effective genetic counselor goes one very important step further in that he continues to support the patient whether he agrees with the decision arrived at or not" [14]. For example, a pregnant 44-year-old woman was sent by her obstetrician for genetic counseling about risks related to advanced maternal age. She decided not to have amniocentesis, but I encouraged her to feel free to contact me if she felt the need. She telephoned from time to time when she "felt blue."

This fundamental difference in approaches to genetic counseling is reflected in the goals and expectations of individual counselors. Nondirective counselors see genetic counseling as a service which provides a patient or parent with the necessary accurate genetic information required to make an acceptable free choice about further reproduction. Directive counselors dictate a particular course of action and, if asked, will tell patients what to do about matters of reproduction. Directive counselors apparently speak from a eugenic standpoint, wishing to reduce the number of affected individuals.

The types of problems that confront genetic counselors are diverse and complex. In the past there were a handful of medical geneticists dealing with small numbers of patients with known genetic problems, answering traditional questions about the natural history of a particular disease and its recurrence risks. The recent cascade of knowledge and the advent of technologic advances have resulted in a proliferation of genetic units and in an increase in the numbers of persons seeking genetic services. Public interest has been heightened by magazine and newspaper articles and by numerous television and radio programs on genetics. This has led to increased concern on the part of many prospective parents about the quality of their future offspring. Obstetricians, pediatricians, and family practitioners have also become slowly aware of genetic disorders. All centers in the United States report an increase in the number of patients being served and the number of laboratory tests being performed. Finally, and not least important, private and public monies are becoming available to support programs.

There is a growing concern among medical geneticists about meeting the increased demand for services. I worry about my ability to provide individualized time-consuming counseling sessions and quality laboratory studies to an ever-increasing patient load. For example, Milunsky writes about the underutilization of available facilities by women 35 years and older for prenatal genetic diagnosis. But he goes on to comment that "utilization by the majority would easily overwhelm currently available facilities" [15]. Expanded services, improved public and professional education and coordinated health care are the goals of all counselors attempting to satisfy the most immediate needs.

The genetic counselor handles many different types of problems, including pregnancies at risk for genetic disorders. Pregnancy is a time of normal crisis and growth, involving physiologic, somatic and psychologic changes. Pregnant women tend to be concerned with seemingly unreasonable fears and fantasies involving feelings of inadequacy. They focus on death and the possibility of delivering a defective child [16]. Mothers express ambivalence throughout pregnancy, wishing for a normal healthy baby and simultaneously fearing the birth of a damaged, developmentally disabled or stillborn infant. Surprisingly little attention has been paid to the pregnant father's feelings or attitudes, but I find he too has dreams, doubts and fantasies about his as-yet-unborn child.

Thus, the genetic counselor deals with a couple in crisis. Often such couples are referred to the counselor so late in pregnancy that services such as amniocentesis cannot be offered. Many couples are self-referred, and many come "against their doctor's advice." Couples known to be at risk for having a child with a genetic problem, or couples seeking genetic information about their reproductive plans, should be referred to the genetics unit prior to becoming pregnant. Certainly every effort must be made to have such couples seen early in pregnancy. Practically speaking, time may be needed to establish the definitive diagnosis. Certain laboratory tests may have to be performed. In addition much information must be exchanged, digested and assimilated before couples arrive at their own decision. Obviously, the pressures will be considerably greater when the genetic counselor is called in after conception.

The counselor must determine the couple's concerns and questions. She explores their attitudes and feelings, obtains complete genealogic data, establishes a diagnosis and draws up the risk figures. She spends additional time discussing related technologic developments, such as ultrasonography and amniocentesis, including the nature of the procedure, the kinds of information it can provide and the risks of the procedure. The counselor presents all the possible options, including abortion. The next step is to outline and review all the possible consequences and risks involved in taking each of the possible options.

I find, more often than not, that couples coming for information about prenatal diagnosis believe we can guarantee them the birth of a completely normal baby. The counselor must stress the limitations of her work and point out that only certain specific conditions can be identified through prenatal studies. Another point that must be made is that all couples have a two—three percent chance of having a child with some sort of birth defect regardless of history or parental age. Couples must understand that even if they undergo monitoring of a particular pregnancy that there is no way to be sure that the baby will be free of problems. The obvious should not be overlooked even though the obscure and esoteric are being searched out.

Counselors weigh all the above and consider all information in relation to the real or established absolute risk. They ask their patients to consider the matter thoroughly before arriving at any decision and offer further opportunity for review and analysis of the genetic data.

Decision-making in these situations appears to be affected by several factors such as past reproductive experience, religious beliefs and attitudes towards abortion. I have found that couples are more likely to choose prenatal diagnostic studies if they have had a previously affected child or are at risk for having an affected child with a known genetic disorder that can be diagnosed in utero with 100% accuracy, irrespective of religious belief or attitudes towards abortion.

Sometimes the results of the studies are unexpected. A recently married 42-year-old woman became pregnant and was referred for genetic counseling solely because of advanced maternal age. Upon learning her risks she decided to undergo amniocentesis. Cytogenetic studies were normal but routine study showed an elevated alpha-fetoprotein. The pregnancy was terminated and an open neural defect was found. Although the immediate problem may have been solved, the psychological effects on the patient were devastating. She became quite depressed about having conceived a physically deformed child. Ongoing support and counseling were necessary over the next eight months in order to deal with her feelings.

Couples are more likely to express ambivalence when dealing with sex-linked disorders that cannot be diagnosed in utero. Mr. and Mrs. B, a couple in their mid-thirties, were expecting their fourth child. Mrs. B was five weeks pregnant. The Bs were referred for counseling on the advice of their family physician because of a family history of mental retardation. Family history revealed that the Bs had three sons. One son was an honor student in junior high school. The other two sons were said to be retarded. In addition, two of Mrs. B's brothers and three of her sisters were in state institutions for the retarded.

All of the affected individuals in the family were seen and examined by a variety of specialists. Medical records were reviewed and appropriate diagnostic tests were executed. Our impression was a new X-linked mental retardation syndrome. The Bs decided to undergo amniocentesis for determination of the fetal sex, fully recognizing their risks. The result of the studies revealed that the fetus was male. The Bs wavered and decided to take their chances and carry the baby to term. Shortly after birth the baby was found to be affected. Despite intense counseling and active support, marital problems occurred, and they are now divorced. Mr. B said he "couldn't handle a bad outcome." Mrs. B feels "she did the right thing" and perhaps a miracle will occur and a cure will be found.

Another set of problems genetic counselors face stem from genetic surveys. Genetic screening programs are geared to early identification and treatment of affected individuals and carrier detection. Carrier detection involves the identification of otherwise healthy heterozygous adults who, under appropriate circumstances, may produce genetic disease in their offspring. Reliable and accurate tests must be available to make such determinations.

Genetic counseling must be incorporated into the screening process, which often involves large groups of people rounded up by publicity campaigns. If not, problems such as the following may arise. A childless young Jewish couple came for genetic counseling because they had learned through a college campus screening process that they each carried the Tay-Sachs gene. They were under the impression that they could have no children and that they each would die from a fatal neurologic disease. Several hours of discussion were necessary to undo all the acquired misinformation. They left feeling relieved and promised to return prior to the time they decided to become pregnant.

Being labeled a carrier can be stigmatizing and frightening. One patient told me he felt "unclean" when he learned he carried the sickle cell trait. Another said he was unfit to have children. Others make a good adjustment, such as the student who told us "now I know a little more about myself." When explaining carrier status, it is vital to emphasize the heterozygote's health and well-being. Carriers must learn that all individuals carry eight or nine deleterious recessive genes without ill-effects.

Special problems arise in advising women who are carriers of sex-linked disorders. Studies of parents of boys with hemophilia [17] or Duchenne muscular dystrophy [18] focus on the mother's guilt and the father's anger. "It's all your fault" shouted Dr. P at his wife when he learned his son had hemophilia. Extensive attempts at intervention and psychotherapy did help these parents.

In counseling such families, I try to alleviate guilt and anger by emphasizing that the child is a shared genetic responsibility. Couples are reminded that the expression of an X-linked recessive gene depends as much on the presence of the Y chromosome as it does on the X. I also offer an extension of genetic counseling at various developmental stages past the point of diagnosis to deal with the feelings of the affected individual himself and his sibs. Boys with hemophilia or Duchenne muscular dystrophy express feelings of rage and resentment about their mother's having caused their "affliction." Their sisters worry about their childbearing risks.

Individuals may try to conceal information and even hide physical findings from their marital partner. For example, the Ws came for genetic counseling in order to learn their risks for having a child with facioscapulohumeral dystrophy, a disorder involving progressive involvement of the muscles of the face and shoulder girdle. Mr. W's father, brother and sister all have the condition. Mr. W said he was asymptomatic but after neurologic examination I learned he'd grown a luxurious beard to "hide" his facial weakness.

A recurrent theme is the need for the affected individual to have a "normal" child. Mr. J's case is typical: Mr. J has neurofibromatosis, a developmental disorder of neuroectodermal derivatives. He learned of his diagnosis when he served in the Navy. His mother is affected and looks like "a bowl of oatmeal." Eventually Mr. J married and had seven children. All the children showed early evidence of the problem. At the time of each birth, Mr. J said he pressed his face against the glass windows of the nursery hoping to see if he "could give his wife a good baby." She in turn saw no problem, since all of the children were otherwise well.

Genetic investigations may lead to the detection of other family members at risk for genetic disease. By testing such individuals new cases and carriers will be found. The counselor must be prepared to present unexpected information to individuals who did not initially seek this advice. Motulsky approaches such situations by classifying genetic diseases into three groups. The first category includes treatable genetic disorders such as Wilson disease, a progressive disease of copper metabolism. In the next or "so-called avoidable" disease group, he feels information must be shared with the affected individual to prevent discomfort or tragedy. For example, an investigation of a pedigree of a defective child with a chromosome imbalance may lead to the detection of other translocation carriers with special reproductive risks. Such persons can be told about their risks and about amniocentesis. His last category is composed of persons at risk for untreatable diseases such as Huntington disease [7]. Some geneticists feel that this vital information should be provided, as it might change such persons' reproductive courses. Others worry about far-reaching psychologic effects and wonder if they're doing more harm than good.

Disorders of sexual differentiation frequently involve the medical geneticist. Oftentimes a newborn will be found to have ambiguous genitalia. The counselor is involved immediately, as sex assignment must be deferred until the diagnostic work-up is complete and an appropriate treatment plan is implemented. Therapy is designed to promote physical and psychologic well-being. The infant's family must be involved in all aspects of case management. Parents must be helped to understand that their baby was born with unfinished or incompletely differentiated sex organs. They need information about the appropriate medical and surgical intervention necessary to correct the problem. Diagrams and drawings are used to provide parents with the necessary data needed to arrive at an appropriate decision about sex assignment or reassignment.

If the parents feel uncomfortable, negativistic, or doubtful about their decision, these attitudes will eventually be transmitted to the child. One such patient told us she always felt "there was some terrible secret" about herself. Parents must be helped to speak comfortably with neighbors, friends and family so as to avoid fear and embarassment. It is important to tell parents faced with this problem that hermaphroditic children do not grow up as bisexual or homosexual, but typically differentiate according to the assigned sex.

In talking about my work it is clear that there are many ethical considerations. If genetic principles are neutral, facts which propel patients to particular kinds of action (such as abortion) must be tinged with the norms of the society rather than any imperative inherent in genetics. Current genetic practice includes counseling, screening for carriers of deleterious genetic traits, and intrauterine diagnosis. The benefits of these innovations include the reduction of human suffering and the increase of human joy through the birth of a healthy child.

The benefits gained from the use of present genetic technology must be carefully weighed. Where does genetic responsibility lie? What are the rights and obligations of the individual, the family, the genetic counselor and society? Do parents have the right to determine the genetic quality of their children? Do individuals at risk have a duty to undergo genetic counseling? Should the use of genetic innovations be voluntary or mandatory?

It is beyond the scope of this paper to offer conclusions or to attempt answers for the numerous ethical connundrums facing us. It is perhaps sufficient for a practitioner in the field to note her belief that the potential benefits to humankind from genetic knowledge are worth the necessary engagement in the social and moral issues arising out of discipline.

REFERENCES

1. Fraser FC: Counseling in genetics: The intent and scope. In Bergsma D (ed): "Genetic Counseling." Baltimore: Williams & Wilkins for The National Foundation–March of Dimes, BD:OAS VI(1):7–12, 1970.
2. Sly WS: What is genetic counseling? In Bergsma D (ed): "Contemporary Genetic Counseling." White Plains: The National Foundation–March of Dimes, BD:OAS IX(4): 5–18, 1973.
3. Murray RF: The practitioner's view of the values involved in genetic screening and counseling. In Bergsma D (ed): "Ethical, Social and Legal Dimensions of Screening for Human Genetic Disease." Miami: Symposia Specialists for The National Foundation–March of Dimes, BD:OAS X(6):185–199, 1974.
4. Sibinga M, Freedman CJ: Complexities of parental understanding of phenylketonuria. Pediatrics 48:216–224, 1971.
5. Leonard CO, Chase GA, Childs B: Genetic counseling: A consumer's view. N Engl J Med 287:433–439, 1972.
6. Mellman W: Discussion. In Hilton B, Callahan D (eds): "Ethical Issues in Human Genetics." New York: Plenum, 1973, p 41.
7. Motulsky A: The significance of genetic disease. In "Ethical Issues in Human Genetics." op cit, p 41.
8. Golden D, Davis JG: Counselling parents after the birth of an infant with Down's syndrome. Child Today 3:7–11, 1974.
9. Zwerling I: Initial counselling of parents with mentally retarded children. J Pediatr 171:645–654, 1954.
10. Hsia YE: Choosing my children's genes: Genetic counseling. In Lipkin M, Roweley PT (eds): "Genetic Responsibility." New York: Plenum, 1972.
11. Handmaker S: Management of genetic and allied disorders in a community with a large latino population, personal communication.
12. Fraser FC: Survey of counseling practices. In "Ethical Issues in Human Genetics." op cit, p 11.
13. Pearson JS: Family support and counselling in Huntington's disease. In "Huntington's Disease Handbook for Health Professionals." New York: Committee to Combat Huntington's Disease, 1973.
14. Macintyre MN: Professional responsibility in prenatal genetic evaluation. In Bergsma D (ed): "Advances in Human Genetics and Their Impact on Society." White Plains: The National Foundation–March of Dimes, BD:OAS VIII(4):31–35, 1972.
15. Milunsky A: Current concepts: Prenatal diagnosis of genetic disorders. N Engl J Med 295:380, 1976.
16. Deutsch H: "Psychology of Women: Motherhood." New York: Grune and Stratton, 1945, Vol 2, pp 126–201.
17. Mattson A, Gross S: Adaptational and defensive behavior in young hemophiliacs and their parents. Am J Psychiat 122:1349–1356.
18. Solow R: The emotional and social aspects of muscular dystrophy. Read at the Symposium on Muscular Dystrophy for Special Education Personnel, September 25, 1971.

9. Genetic Counseling: The Client's Viewpoint

Carol Levine, MA

Three couples recently visited the genetic counseling unit of a major metropolitan hospital. In each case the wife was pregnant, over 35, and had been referred by an obstetrician for evaluation and counseling for the risk of bearing a child with Down syndrome. In each case the counselor followed similar procedures: she took a family history, explained the genetic causes of Down syndrome, and outlined the process of prenatal diagnosis through amniocentesis. Abortion was available but was not stressed as an option should the diagnosis prove positive.

Although on the surface the couples, who came from similar socioeconomic backgrounds and were provided with similar information, might have been expected to react in somewhat similar ways, the outcomes were in fact quite different.

The first couple, who already had two normal children, decided on amniocentesis, "just to be sure." They did not really anticipate any problem, but agreed that if the fetus had Down syndrome, they would elect an abortion and try again for the third child both wanted. The results of the test — which showed that the fetus was indeed affected — came as a shock. Still, they recovered quickly and made almost immediate plans for an abortion and another pregnancy. This time the amniocentesis showed no chromosomal abnormalities, and a healthy child was born.

The second couple, who had not married until their mid-30s and who were expecting their first child, also decided on amniocentesis. The tension and anxiety that accompanied the waiting period for the results of the test exacerbated an already shaky relationship. The information that they would have a child with Down syndrome was a severe blow, especially to the husband. He had waited to marry until he found the "perfect" wife and could not accept the idea that she was carrying an "imperfect" child. Despite the counselor's explanations, he was sure that she was at fault. The wife was all too willing to accept the "blame," which seemed to her to be proof of her inadequacy as a wife and female. An

Birth Defects: Original Article Series, Volume XV, Number 2, pages 123–135

abortion was performed. The husband refused to consider another pregnancy and avoided sexual relations with his wife. By the end of the year they had separated and were planning a divorce.

The third couple, who had adopted a child several years earlier when it was believed that the wife could never conceive, decided not to undergo amniocentesis. After a good deal of thought, they decided that they were willing to take the risk of having a child with Down syndrome, and if this was to be their fate, they did not want to know about it ahead of time. The wife reasoned that she might never be able to become pregnant again, that a Down child would present problems of management but would probably be loving and amiable, and that whatever happened, the family was strong enough to see it through. Her husband, who had grown up in a large family and who as a boy had played frequently with a retarded cousin, supported her decision. He believed that her need to bear and nurture a child was so overwhelming that an abortion for genetic reasons would cause her great mental anguish. Their child was born without Down syndrome.

These cases illustrate one of the most obvious but perhaps least understood aspects of genetic counseling. Clients ostensibly seek information, diagnosis, and medical advice, but their decision-making process is influenced by many factors outside the realm of genetics — the marital relationship, the presence and needs of other children, religious beliefs, attitudes of other family members, career aspirations, financial considerations, self-images, and concepts of parenthood, to name just a few.

The counselor deals primarily in facts — what is genetically determined, and what is not; what is known about the diagnosis, transmission, and prognosis of a genetic condition, and what is not; what kinds of risks can be predicted, and what is still unexplained. The client, however, cannot comprehend these facts without translating them into feelings — relief, guilt, shame, unworthiness, self-pity, courage, hostility (against one's spouse, family, or the counselor).

Genetic knowledge is perhaps the most emotion-laden medical information that one can receive. To learn that one has hypertension, asthma, or even cancer can be overwhelming, but it is information that seems to concern primarily oneself. The knowledge that one's children may be deformed, retarded, or suffer a life of pain and dependency because of inheritance is a heavy burden to bear.

Hecht and Holmes [1], among others, have pointed out this important aspect of genetic counseling: "The counselor is engaged in a complex psychodynamic process that involves the lessening of denial, the relief of guilt, the lifting of depression, the articulation of anger, and gradually, rational planning for the future. Everyone who has provided genetic counseling has witnessed these processes. Yet little is known about the formal dynamics or results of genetic counseling."

This chapter summarizes the little that is known about how clients view genetic counseling. In the past ten years or so there have been about 30 reports [2] from individual counseling centers here and in England describing the patient's understanding and retention of genetic information, and the impact of counseling on subsequent reproduction. However suggestive their findings, these studies were based on small samples, used a wide variety of measurement and evaluative techniques, and were conducted from the counselor's point of view. Some of these studies will be cited here, but it is not clear to what extent their data can be extrapolated to other settings and other clients. Major studies that will cover a large number of centers over a period of time are just getting underway and will be described briefly. Some of the case material cited in the chapter is based on discussion with clients and observations of counseling sessions. The information that is available now is far from definitive, but it is possible to outline the dimensions of the question.

WHO ARE THE CLIENTS?

Genetic anomalies occur in all segments of the population, but not all segments are equally represented at counseling centers. Most clients are in their 20s and 30s, from middle and upper income levels, and above average in education. Carter's follow-up report of families referred to the genetics clinic of the Hospital for Sick Children in London indicated that the majority of the fathers had occupations that put them in the top two social classes in England [3]. At the Yale-New Haven Hospital, Hsia reports that a "disproportionate" number of the clients are middle-class [4]. The prospective study of midtrimester amniocentesis conducted by the National Institute of Child Health and Human Development National Registry for Amniocentesis Study Group showed that over 90% of the 1,040 subjects and 992 controls were white and middle-class [5]. However, in a ten-year retrospective study of 300 families who received counseling at the University of Colorado Medical Center, 40% were in the two lower socioeconomic levels [6]. There are few breakdowns of client population by race or religion, except in those studies specifically concerned with genetic diseases that affect a particular group, such as sickle cell anemia or Tay-Sachs disease.

Most clients are referred by physicians; those on the upper income levels by private physicians and those on the lower levels by clinic or hospital staff. A large number of clients, however, come to counseling on their own, because they do not trust or want to believe the medical advice they have already received, because they have read or heard about new methods of prenatal diagnosis, or because family and friends have urged them to seek counseling. These clients tend to be among the most highly motivated; at the other extreme are clients who are referred by physicians and do not really understand why.

Sometimes a client may be referred for one reason and actually be concerned about another. At a group counseling session I attended for couples at risk for Tay-Sachs disease, one young woman sat through the explanation with seeming indifference. When the counselor completed the presentation and asked for questions, the young woman said, with obvious anxiety, "My neighbor has a Down child. What can I do to prevent that happening to me?" Sometimes clients may not be as willing as this woman to voice their fears openly, particularly in a group. They will speak up only if some opportunity is provided for them to talk privately with a counselor to discuss disorders other than the one that appears to be the highest risk. Similarly, clients may assume, unless specifically informed otherwise, that the information that they are not at risk for one disorder, say Tay-Sachs, applies to other disorders as well.

Clients are generally married couples, although many married women come to counseling without their husbands. Some single people come for premarital advice, primarily first cousins contemplating marriage or individuals whose family histories have a strong line of genetic disease. At this point there seems to be no development of genetic counseling as a routine premarital procedure. Nor is there yet any widespread counseling or referral for counseling for common diseases such as diabetes, hypertension, heart disease, or cancer in which there are well-known familial tendencies. These conditions so far seem to be outside the mainstream of medical genetics, probably because they develop late in life, are not as readily predictable as genetic entities, and do not present the same emotional crisis as the birth of a child with a genetic disease.

Typically clients seek genetic counseling because they already have a child (or children) with a defect believed to be genetic in origin; as many as 80% of the clients may fall into this category [7].

These clients want to know several things: "What is wrong with my child? Why did this happen? What is the prognosis? Will it happen again?" These questions themselves are straightforward enough, but behind the stated reasons there are usually deeper implications. The client who asks "Why?" is not, as Griffin, Kavanagh, and Sorenson point out, just asking for a technical explanation [2]. As often as not, the question is an existential one. Parents really wonder, "Why do I have a defective gene? Why did I happen to marry someone with a defective gene? Why did this happen to my child?" Even if the counselor reassures them that it was not an action on their parts, like taking medication, that caused the defect, the deeper question remains unanswered.

In his in-depth study of 25 couples who underwent amniocentesis and abortion, Fletcher found that their motivation for coming to counseling was framed in their understanding of parental responsibility [8]. Their children's health and the well-being of the family depended, they said, on their decisions; the concept of "fairness" often was evoked in their deliberations. One mother opposed to abortion for economic or psychologic reasons still favored it for a genetic defect. "It is not fair to 'the child,'" she said, "to the family, to society, or to me to bring another child like the one I have into the world."

Although such concerns may not be articulated, they form an important background for the way in which the counselor's diagnosis and evaluation is received and interpreted by the client.

HOW MUCH DO CLIENTS UNDERSTAND?

The first step in decision-making for clients is to understand the information that the counselor is able to provide after studying the family pedigree, appropriate medical records, and results of diagnostic procedures. Here the information on clients' perspectives is particularly sketchy; we have only the interpretations based on studies conducted for other purposes, and from the counselor's point of view. These have shown a wide range of levels of understanding, possibly because they have used very different measures. Some studies stressed precise recall of risk statistics; others used more impressionistic standards. Generally studies have tried to assess the client's ability to recall genetic facts at some point (usually several months) after the counseling session. However, no assessments have been made of the client's understanding before entering counseling, so it is difficult to attribute any knowledge precisely to the sesssion.

Carter found that in general the couples in the London group had understood the risks they had been given [3]. The Colorado study also showed high levels of "adequate" understanding — 84% [6]. However, Leonard et al, in reporting a study of parents of children with cystic fibrosis, phenylketonuria, and Down syndrome compared with a control group of parents with children who had a severe but nongenetic disease, found that only about one-half of the families had a good grasp of the information given in counseling, one-quarter gained some knowledge, and one-quarter gained very little [9]. At Yale Hsia found that three-quarters of the clients who responded to a questionnaire gave "appropriate" responses to a question about their chances of having healthy children, ie these answers were considered "appropriate" because they matched the counselors' perceptions of the risks [4].

Differences in measurement aside, why do clients apparently have difficulty in comprehending genetic information? It would seem that this population, skewed toward above-average intelligence and educational levels, would be particularly apt at assimilating factual material. And it is true that those at the higher ends of the educational scale generally (but not always) show greater comprehension than clients who are less well educated.

One difficulty is that even well-educated people often have little knowledge of medical genetics; even those who have been exposed to some basic genetics in school have not kept abreast of recent developments. The terminology is strange, the concepts sometimes difficult to grasp, the implications hard to interpret. Many clients lack an understanding of elementary biology, let alone genetics.

If the counseling is initiated at a time of great stress — soon after the birth of a child with a defect or after learning that a child believed to be normal is affected with a genetic disease — understanding is further hampered.

The form in which the information is communicated may also have an effect. Information not fully understood in an oral interview may become more comprehensible in a written report. Such reports are generally considered valuable by clients, who may read them several times, show them to family members, and keep them in a safe place. On the other hand, information conveyed only in a written report may be devastating. One couple, after spending two years in a fruitless search for a diagnosis for their son's conditon, consulted a well-known geneticist. He made no comments during the examination and no follow-up interview was held. The parents received a letter stating only a diagnosis (Bloom syndrome, a rare Jewish genetic disease), the characteristics (altered chromosomes, dwarfism, sensitivity to sunlight), and a prognosis (no treatment or cure). Several years later, when I interviewed them, they still recalled the shock of this impersonal communication.

INTERPRETATION OF RISK

One of the most important aspects of genetic information given to the client is the risk factor. Counselors generally share a sense of what is a "high" risk and what is "low." To clients, however, these terms are meaningless, unless carefully explained, and even then subject to misinterpretation. A 1 in 10 risk, for example, may be interpreted by a client to mean that only if she has ten children will there by a chance of having an affected one. A couple with a severely handicapped child may not be willing to undertake even a very low risk of having another similarly affected. A mother of a child born blind says, "I wouldn't take a 1% chance of anything happening again," while parents of a 3½-year-old child with PKU, who waited until they saw him developing normally to decide on another pregnancy, feel that they can take the 1 in 4 risk of having another [10]. Sometimes clients can even be disappointed with low risk figures. Pearn reports one case of a woman with two celiac children whose family had adjusted so well to the special diet that the 1 in 10 risk that a third child would also be affected was too low. She felt that a normal child would disrupt the carefully planned regimen of the household [11].

Risk-taking is part of everyday life, but few people have a good grasp of probability concepts. Most of life's "gambles" are so trivial that the outcome is not of great consequence. How many people know — or care — what the actual odds against cashing in a jackpot lottery ticket are? Even when the stakes are higher (eg accident rates of automobiles compared to airplanes) people make choices based on personal preference or irrational fears, not probability.

Individuals differ by disposition and psychologic makeup toward risk-taking in general. People tend to think of themselves as "lucky" or "unlucky"; an optimistic person may believe, quite unrealistically, that "such a thing (a genetic disease) could never happen to me"; a pessimist may believe, just as unrealistically, that "it will be just my luck to have it happen." People who like to feel in control of their lives and who plan for major events are generally unwilling to take many risks; impulsive people who are not inclined to plan are more inclined to take risks. If two individuals of opposite bent happen to be married to each other, the assessment of genetic risk will inevitably involve conflict.

One such couple, who had come to genetic counseling at the wife's insistence, reacted to the information that there was a 1 in 4 chance of having a child with Duchenne muscular dystrophy in quite different ways. The wife was totally unwilling to consider a pregnancy and immediately consulted a physician about sterilization. The husband did not consider the risk unacceptable, particularly since amniocentesis would show the sex of the fetus. He considered abortion of a male fetus a plausible option, and found sterilization abhorrent. The conflict that surfaced in a counseling session I observed was so severe that the couple was referred to a marriage counselor to try to resolve their difficulties.

What kinds of risks do people actually take after genetic counseling? Here again the only information is based on studies that emphasize the counselor's point of view. Carter found in his study of 74 high-risk families (his definition of high-risk was 1 in 10) that two-thirds were unwilling to take such a risk and did not have any more children; it was surprising to him that as many as one-third were willing to take that level of risk. In the low-risk group of 95 families, three-quarters were undaunted by the odds, but one-quarter refused to take even a low risk. A particularly difficult group to reassure, he found, was that of families who had already had two children with unrelated conditions. They could not believe that their fate was mere coincidence [3]. One woman, who had undergone several miscarriages and a stillbirth before giving birth to a boy with an ultimately lethal disorder, said in an interview, "I just wouldn't try again. It is simply not meant for me to have a normal child."

A high risk is sometimes more acceptable if the child will have a disease that causes early death [9]. If the disease is one in which the life-span will be long but the prognosis very poor, the parents are often more unwilling to take the risk [12].

Leonard et al concluded that the client's attitude towards further reproduction was influenced more by the sense of burden (including mortality, management problems, and prognosis) implied by the risk figures than by the precise statistics. Even the control group families, whose children did not have a genetic disease, and who therefore faced no genetic risk at all in having more children, were concerned about the future; one-half took steps to prevent further conception [9].

Other elements that go into the final decision to have or not to have more children are related to family life in general. The couple may already have the number of children they want; one study indicates that couples do not have an additional child to compensate for the affected one but continue to have children as do the parents of normal children [13]. However, this attitude varies according to the specific disorder, and to the religious or cultural background of the family. In Africa parents with a child affected with sickle cell anemia traditionally had another child to compensate, and this tends to be true among black American families today as well. Parents of some ethnic backgrounds may believe that the only way to remove the "curse" of an affected child from their families is to produce a normal one. Money is clearly a factor in the decision to have another child. Another factor is the attitude of important people — family, physicians, clergy, perhaps colleagues, or friends.

On the whole, the studies conducted so far indicate that couples who have undergone genetic counseling and have been informed of some risk take it seriously. They may decide not to have more children or to postpone pregnancies. Sometimes pregnancies do occur, of course, planned or unplanned; but relatively few clients appear to disregard the counseling altogether. Among the alternatives that are considered are contraception, sterilization, abortion, adoption, and artificial insemination.

THE MORAL DILEMMAS POSED BY GENETIC COUNSELING

The decisions reached by clients are not easy ones and on the whole are not lightly taken. What may seem an unambiguous situation to a counselor — a positive prenatal diagnosis of spina bifida through amniocentesis — may present a difficult dilemma to the couple involved. Fletcher [8] found that the prevailing moral problem in the 25 couples he studied extensively was abortion. He defined a moral problem as a conflict either between the individual and the community (a Catholic mother who would be judged by the norms of the community if she decided on an abortion) or an inner conflict when a person faces sharply divided responsibilities (between exercising responsible parenthood and the desire for a child). Even though no prior commitment to abortion was required for amniocentesis, the parents felt it was a grave moral responsibility and anguished over their decision. The waiting time between amniocentesis and the results was particularly agonizing.

Even if couples do not have religious or moral objections to abortion, they may experience conflict over the decision on whether to abort a fetus with a X-linked genetic disease. Amniocentesis will tell whether the fetus is a male or female, but if it is a male, not whether or not it is affected by Duchenne muscular dystrophy or hemophilia. The couple has to decide whether to abort a fetus that has a 50-50 chance of being perfectly normal.

Even the possibility of having to face such a decision may deter some couples from another pregnancy. "I believe a woman who does not want to bear a child — for whatever reason — has a right to a safe abortion," said one mother in this situation in a interview. "But, as for me — I don't know whether I could go through with it. How could I live with the knowledge that I might be killing a perfectly healthy baby? And, if the child turned out to be affected, like my son, how could I live with *that*? The only answer for me is not to become pregnant, ever again."

For some parents choosing an abortion would symbolize a rejection of the child they already have. "If I had had an abortion the first time, then I wouldn't have my daughter," a mother of a child with a crippling defect stated in a counseling session. "I would rather have her like this — with all the problems — than not to have her at all."

Another factor that affects the decision is how an abortion will be perceived by their child who has a genetic disease. Will that child feel the abortion of a potentially afflicted sib as a personal rejection? One mother said: "He (her child) knows what's going on. I wonder what he thinks about the baby. He could think . . . they want to put me out of the way, too. And he could think, no one should have to suffer the way I do. I suppose it would be more the second" [8] .

Even after a decision is reached to undergo an abortion, the consequences may be unexpected. A study of 13 families who underwent abortion after amniocentesis showed that 11 of the wives and 9 of the husbands suffered depression, a far higher percentage than would normally be associated with elective abortion for other reasons or with the birth of a stillborn child [14] .

A woman in this study who had one hemophiliac child elected an abortion when it was learned that she was carrying a male fetus. However, she was torn by guilt feelings, especially after the nurse commented, "You would have had a beautiful boy." Even though she felt that she had done the right thing by choosing the abortion, the experience was so upsetting that when she became pregnant again and the fetus was again determined to be a male, she would not repeat the abortion. The child was born without hemophilia, and the couple now believe that the aborted fetus would have been a hemophiliac, a not uncommon reaction to this situation.

Four of the couples separated during the pregnancy and abortion period; one woman who had been a teacher gave up that job to become a secretary because she "didn't want to work with children any more" after two abortions for probable Duchenne muscular dystrophy.

One woman in the study had previously had an abortion of convenience, and reported that the depression that followed that experience lasted only a week. Subsequently she had three healthy children. However, the abortion for genetic reasons was perceived as "the worst thing that ever happened to me."

An abortion for an unwanted child is a social and psychologic choice. A stillbirth can be rationalized as an "accident of nature"; a miscarriage as a "blessing in disguise." An abortion for genetic reasons, however, seems to be accompanied by guilt for having "caused" the defect, and disappointment that the wanted child will not be born after all.

Fletcher found that parents who elected abortion and sterilization tried to justify their decision and to understand it better themselves [8]. The mothers experienced what he calls "cosmic doubt," but only one, a Catholic, expressed this in religious terms. None expressed any regrets at having used amniocentesis, however, and those who found the tests to show the absence of genetic disease were relieved and found that the pregnancy proceeded more smoothly than it might have otherwise.

RETROSPECTIVE EVALUATIONS OF COUNSELING

How clients view counseling retrospectively depends not only on the experience itself but on their expectations of it. The word "counseling" itself may lead clients to believe that they will be given advice or told what to do by a genetics counselor [2]. Some counselors in truth are more directive than others, and perhaps most, especially physicians, are somewhat directive; but a client who believes that the counselor's role is to provide information and options will not share the same expectations of the experience as one who believes that the decision will be made by others. Clients who come expecting clear-cut diagnosis and prediction will be disappointed with information that is less than complete, as it may of necessity be. Those who are told that the condition they have is not genetic or that amniocentesis shows negative results will clearly be reassured and relieved. Some situations exist for which genetic counseling still cannot provide any answers; these clients will not be satisfied with partial explanations.

The client's perception of the experience may differ from the counselor's view. The Yale questionnaire asked the clients: "Did you feel the doctor had advised you not to have more children?" Even though the counselor's goal had been to be nondirective and leave the decision up to the family, more than 1 in 3 of the clients who had not received a written report believed that directive advice had been given. Fewer than 1 in 6 of the clients who received a written report felt that the advice had been directive [4].

Sometimes the quest for genetic counseling only masks deeper problems within one member of the family or between the husband and wife. The genetic information may not be sought for its own sake, but as a weapon against the other partner, or as an excuse not to have children.

Those clients who come to counseling on their own probably have the best chance of being satisfied with the results of the experience. Those who come because a physician has said they should, or to satisfy the demands of family or others, are poorer candidates, as are those who have strong preconceptions of the risks involved — either high or low — or who tend to deny unpleasant information.

In the Yale retrospective study, Hsia found that of nearly 200 families, 90% felt that the counseling was geared to a level they could understand and their questions had been answered satisfactorily. One group — the families for whom no useful information could be given — did not share this view, but even they felt that every effort had been made to help them. Parents of babies with severe congenital malformations said: "They couldn't find the cause but they really tried, and it was comforting to know that everything had been done."

Hsia asked: "Was the counseling worth the cost?" realizing that the "cost" even in monetary terms was a false figure, since most families had medical insurance, were on welfare, or were not charged the full fee for other reasons. Of those who answered this question, 90% said that it would have been worth whatever they had been asked to pay.

The counselor may see a decision not to reproduce when there is a high risk of genetic disease as a rational one and any other decision as irrational and irresponsible. Emery puts this view quite clearly: "In the present study (of Duchenne muscular dystrophy) the majority of those at high risk avoided further pregnancies, but a small proportion seemed undeterred and we feel that the responsibility for this must lie, at least in part, with the genetic counselor" [15]. The couple involved may indeed make the "rational" decision but at a great emotional cost. They may view the counseling experience ambivalently; it gave them information, but also caused them great suffering. It is, of course, impossible to know whether that suffering would have been greater or less than that caused by the unforeseen birth of an afflicted child. And if the decision is, in the counselor's sense, an "irrational" one, it may still satisfy the client's other, more pressing emotional needs, and therefore be consistent with the family's own goals for the future.

STUDIES IN PROGRESS

Within a few years there should be a much clearer picture of genetic counseling and the client's perspective. A major two-year study designed to provide both quantitative and qualitative data on the organization, operation, and effects of genetic counseling, from the perspectives of both providers and clients, began late in 1976, after a one-year pilot project. This longitudinal study, directed by Norman A. Scotch, James R. Sorenson, and Judith P. Swazey of the Department of Socio-Medical Sciences at the Boston University School of Medicine, will analyze and evaluate the relationships between the goals, structure, and operation of counseling programs supported by The National Foundation—March of Dimes, the needs of their clients, and the outcomes of the interactions between providers and clients.

A variety of methods will be used to collect data. For example, clients who receive counseling will be asked to complete a questionnaire just prior to counseling, a postcounseling questionnaire immediately after the interview, and a six-month follow-up questionnaire. Counselors will be asked to complete a questionnaire immediately after they see a client.

In addition, a subsample of clients and counselors will be interviewed in depth, and counseling sessions will be observed and tape-recorded, so that a series of detailed counseling case studies can be developed to examine certain critical issues in counseling, such as the relationship between the client's expectations about counseling and a counselor's definition of his or her task. There may be as many as 250 counselors involved in the study, and possibly as many as 3,000 clients.

Another study, at the University of Pennsylvania's Human Genetics Center, is being conducted by Charles Bosk, Renée Fox, and Alexander Capron. It is examining selected groups from three populations over a period of five years: 1) people who come to Children's Hospital of Philadelphia for counseling after the birth of a child with a genetic defect; 2) women who use the obstetric services of the University of Pennsylvania hospital; and 3) parents of children with genetic defects who are in self-help groups. The objectives of the study are to learn about the client's and the counselor's expectations about counseling, the client's understanding of information, and, insofar as it is possible, about the process of client decision-making. Now at midpoint, the study is focusing on the determination of successful counseling from the client's and the counselor's points of view.

CONCLUSION

The little that is known about genetic counseling from the client's perspective suggests that first of all it is a highly significant process that frequently determines, for better or worse, the future course of the client's life. At many points in the counseling process differences in perception between the counselor's and the client's points of view, can affect the outcome. Because clients are frequently in a state of tension or confusion at the time of counseling, it may be difficult for them to comprehend fully the significance of the information.

Factors not directly related to the genetic risk can play a great role in a genetic decision, and these are highly individual and personal concerns.

Sheldon Reed, who suggested the label of "genetic counseling" in 1947 for what had earlier been called "genetic consultation," "genetic advice," or "genetic hygiene," [2] recently wrote, "The emotional aspects of genetic counseling have probably been its greatest weaknesses" [16]. And it is precisely the emotional aspects that are often most important from the client's point of view.

REFERENCES

1. Hecht F, Holmes LB: What we don't know about genetic counseling. N Engl J Med 287:464, 1972.
2. Griffin ML, Kavanagh CM, Sorenson JR: Genetic knowledge, client perspectives, and genetic counseling. Social Work in Health Care 2:2, 1976.
3. Carter CO, Fraser-Roberts JA, Evans KA, Buck AR: Genetic clinic: A follow-up. Lancet 1:282, 1971.
4. Hsia YE: Choosing my children's genes: Genetic counseling. In Lipkin M Jr, Rowley PT (eds): "Genetic Responsibility: On Choosing Our Children's Genes." New York: Plenum Publishing Company, 1974, p 46.
5. NICHD National Registry for Amniocentesis Study Group: Midtrimester amniocentesis for prenatal diagnosis: Safety and accuracy. JAMA 236:1471–1476, 1976.
6. Reynolds BdeV, Puck MH, Robinson A: Genetic counseling: An appraisal. Clin Genet 5:177–187, 1974.
7. Sorenson JR: "Social Aspects of Applied Human Genetics." New York: Russell Sage Foundation, 1971.
8. Fletcher J: The brink: The parent-child bond in the genetic revolution. Theological Studies 33:467, 1972.
9. Leonard CO, Chase GA, Childs B: Genetic counseling: A consumers' view. N Engl J Med 281:433, 1972.
10. Hsia YE: Parental reactions to genetics counseling. Contemp Ob/Gyn 4(1):104, 1974.
11. Pearn JH: Patients' subjective interpretation of risks offered in genetic counselling. J Med Genet 10:131, 1973.
12. Emery AEH, Watt MS, Clack E: Social effects of genetic counseling. Br Med J 1:724, 1973.
13. Sultz DDS, Schlesinger ER, Feldman J: An epidemiological justification for genetic counseling in family planning. Am J Public Health 62:1489, 1972.
14. Blumberg BD, Golbus MS, Hanson KH: The pyschological sequelae of abortion performed for a genetic indication. Am J Obstet Gynecol 122:799, 1975.
15. Emery AEH, Watt MS, Clack ER: The effects of genetic counseling in Duchenne muscular dystrophy. Clin Genet 3:150, 1972.
16. Reed SC: A short history of genetic counseling. Soc Biol 21:332, 1974.

10. The Genetic Counselor as Facilitator of the Counselee's Decision Process*

Ray M. Antley, MD

One of the most rapidly expanding areas in applied human genetics is genetic counseling. As the need for genetic counseling services has grown, the background of the individuals providing genetic counseling and viewing the process has become more varied. In addition to academic and clinical geneticists, professionals with training in psychology, sociology, and theology are now found actively involved both in the genetic counseling process and in the dialogue about its implications. This diversity of backgrounds and expertise has contributed to a sharpened awareness of counselor goals and, subsequently, to an emerging conflict among proponents of different counseling orientations. Specifically, major polarities have developed among advocates of eugenics, disease prevention, and psychosocial goals in genetic counseling.

The lack of an overall conceptual framework in genetic counseling makes it difficult to determine whether various points of view are in agreement or disagreement. For example, when counselors ostensibly agree in intent but are divergent in their practice, or vice versa, the variations may be due to differences in ethical orientations, to semantics, to contradictions between goal orientation and practices, or to a blurring of the distinction between the affective and cognitive information counselors provide counselees. Therefore, as an initial step in attempting to improve communication among the often disparate groups interested in genetic counseling, this chapter will try to clarify the decision which the genetic counselor makes about the goals of genetic counseling and in carrying out the process of genetic counseling. The decisions the counselor makes in the process of counseling are detailed in the appendix at the end of the chapter. The argument is made that the counselor decision processes should be oriented

* Supported by Genetics Center grant GM 2015401, NIH grant HEW MCHS 924, and grants from the Little Red Door, Inc. and the Riley Memorial Association.

Birth Defects: Original Article Series, Volume XV, Number 2, pages 137–168
© 1979 The National Foundation

toward facilitating the counselees making personally evaluated, informed decisions. The rationale for this approach is compared to those advocated by alternative models of genetic counseling.

COUNSELOR GOALS IN GENETIC COUNSELING

The decision of how to proceed in counseling is preceded by implicit or explicit counselor decisions about what is the desired goal or goals sought in counseling. The range of goal options open to the counselor is potentially wide. For the purpose of this model, the goals are limited to the possible outcomes of the counselee's behavior.

There are basically three categories of goal options in counselee behavior. They are goals related to: 1) cognitive behavior, ie learning the information; 2) affective behavior, ie the feelings which emerge in relationship to the genetic concern; and 3) the actual decision and decision-making behavior.

Counselee education is a limited goal for genetic counseling. The factual information conveyed usually includes an organized, selected description of the medical and genetic situation, the various options and means of dealing with these options, and the relevant probabilities. Information itself has little intrinsic value. The most important reason for information acquisition in genetic counseling is its use in decision-making; therefore, the acquisition of information is probably best seen as a valid intermediate objective in the complete process of genetic counseling.

In the process of evaluating external events, feelings are probably important in helping a person place variables into hierarchies of importance. Feelings may emanate from perceived reproductive success, degree of certainty about future reproduction, or expectations of failure. The important function of bringing a person in touch with those feelings is to make him aware of how subjective his evaluations are. Changing affective behavior itself may be a goal of counseling. "Crisis intervention" approaches may mandate the effective lifting out and discharge of feelings of guilt, remorse, or responsibility in the counselee. Feelings can thus be alarming, motivating, or paralyzing factors in subsequent decision-making.

Finally, a third category of goals for genetic counseling is that which emphasizes the decision-making itself. Decision-making includes the specification of options and the means of choosing among them. Decision-making behavior embraces both the choices and the action options. In the process, the counselee may either directly or indirectly evaluate his choice against other alternatives. When facilitating the decision-making process is selected as the goal in genetic counseling, information acquisition is a necessary part of this process. The decision-making process includes evaluation of the genetic information and the consequences of different action options. Since feelings emerge in conjunction with such evaluation, they are an important factor in decision-making. The purposes of decision-making perceived by the counselee may include avoidance of harm, maintenance of social and biologic equilibrium, and improvement of his sense of security. To approach these goals, the counselor must commit himself to dealing with both the information and the counselee's attendant feelings.

The values assigned to these goals place different weights on the counselor. An important choice is whether information acquisition, per se, is an adequate or acceptable goal. This goal is initially appealing to the counselor because it is easier and less expensive to deliver genetic information than to facilitate decision-making. The goals of information acquisition can be translated into well-defined objectives whose attainment can be evaluated.

When information acquisition for decision-making becomes a primary goal of counseling, the counselor makes the assumption implicitly that the subset of facts he provides is exactly the data base the counselee needs to make his decision. It is the counselor who determines which facts to present to the counselee and he is judge of the appropriateness and adequacy of these facts. Furthermore, if the counselor gives the information and does not enter into the decision-making process to see how the counselee applies and interprets the information, the counselor is tacitly assuming an exact communication, interpretation, and application of these facts. This appears to be an erroneous assumption, in view of the limited ability of the counselees to learn genetic facts, to interpret these facts reasonably, to personalize these facts, and to act in accordance with their chosen goals [1, 2]. If, then, the information given in genetic counseling is to be assimilated by the counselee in the manner which best enables him to evaluate situations and options, it is important to understand the dynamics of this assimilation process before the information is given.

Just as information distribution does not exist in and for itself, but rather in order that the counselee may have a data base for informed decision-making, so personal feelings cannot be dealt with in genetic counseling for their own sake, but as an integral part of evaluating the counselee decision-making process. The counselee's feelings, which are generated by the decision-making process, result from confrontation of the realities of the medical and genetic information. As he evaluates these substantive issues and personalizes their meaning, he generates attendant feelings, such as guilt, despair, or optimism. If the counselor is seeking a particular decision by the counselee, he will likely deal with feelings only insofar as they pertain to reaching the counselor's own interpretation of desirable counselee behavior. If, however, the counselor's goal is to stimulate and facilitate an effective decision process, then a major thrust of his counseling should be to help the counselee understand his feelings in relation to the new information. In this way, the counselee attains a fuller and better evaluation of his situation and choices. Thus, the counselor's decision about the way in which he will deal with the counselee's feelings is inexorably linked to his determination about the type of counselee decision he is seeking.

GOALS FOR THE COUNSELEE DECISION

Decision-making is the process of evaluating information which serves as a basis for a judgment about the desirability of a course of action. The judgment is usually rendered on the basis of a series of such evaluations. The first step in an evaluation is to choose the relevant variables which are to be used to compare the options and methods of obtaining outcomes. The evaluator chooses those variables which seem important, and attempts to quantify them for use in evaluating each potential option.

The choice of variables for comparison is based upon the decision-maker's value system. For instance, in responding to a questionnaire prepared by Professor James. R. Sorensen of Boston University, some genetic counselors indicated that they thought counselee desire for children was not important in decision-making [3]. This result indicates that some counselors are less likely to put the value of being a parent into the decision equations. Some counselees do put value on parenthood and see this as a counterbalance to their risk and burden, so that they can make a decision to have additional children [4, 5].

Ultimately, each evaluation is personal. The notions of "good" and "important" are based upon a summation of the evaluator's total past experience. The counselor should be aware of this key observation in weighing who should be the evaluator for the counselee's decision process. Where the counselor assumes control of the counseling objectives, his value choices usually range between a desire that the counselee arrive at a "proper" decision or that the counselee engage in an "acceptable" decision-making process. In the former option, the counselor may be less concerned with how the decision is made than with the correctness of the decision. For instance, the counselor may perceive his goal as preventing or encouraging a particular gene combination. To improve the gene pool or prevent the birth of an affected child, he can present or emphasize options to optimize the probability that the counselee will choose a course leading to the "desirable" gene combination. This is an externally derived decision based on a value orientation which may or may not be shared by the counselee.

In this model, the counselor may attempt directly or indirectly to persuade the counselee of the value of the choices leading to the gene combination the counselor believes to be optimal. In the medical model of physician-patient relationship, the strong precedent for the counselor's being the evaluator is based upon the assumption that the values of the physician and counselee are the same for the relevant variables, or that the scientific expertise of the counselor makes him better suited to decide. The counselor's choice is whether this is a reasonable basis for goal setting in genetic counseling or whether the alternative should be sought.

The alternative is an effort in which the counselor works for the active participation of the counselee to optimize the decision-making process. Optimizing the decision process includes facilitating the counselee's improvement in self-esteem, and explaining all relevant options and means for their attainment. The counselor works with the counselee to evaluate: 1) potential outcomes of various options in physical terms, 2) effects upon intrapersonal conflicts, and 3) consequences for social and interpersonal relationships.

Ideally, the counselor's activity is designed to promote the choice of outcome which the counselee thinks is best and important, taking all of the potential outcomes into consideration. Here the counselor's goal is for an internally evaluated counselee decision. He has opted for the counselee to be the evaluator in the context of his own value system rather than to assume control over the evaluation process itself.

In contrast, externally evaluated decisions presume evaluations of "the good" which the counselee may or may not hold. Depending on the extent to which the counselor advocates an internal evaluation process or an external one, he will employ strategies to accomplish his end. These alternative strategies are most often categorized as directive or nondirective counseling.

COUNSELOR'S DECISION ABOUT THE METHOD OF COUNSELING

In genetic counseling, the terms "directive" and "nondirective" usually imply some form of "telling" or "not telling" counselees what they ought to do. In psychologic counseling, these terms have a different meaning. The nondirective psychologic counselor is ideally nonjudgmental, using a reflexive technique to increase the counselee's self-awareness; the directive counselor is active and confrontive. By this definition, all genetic counselors are directive to the extent they perform the activities of an educator.

Because of this confusion with these terms, the following definitions are offered:

Directive — A counseling orientation in which the counselor is active in the counseling session, using educational methods and confrontation to accomplish counselor-, and/or more rarely, counselee-specified goals.

Nondirective — A method of psychotherapeutic counseling which uses as its primary therapeutic approach the creating of an accepting psychologic climate for the client. In this approach, the counselor uses reflective responses to enhance the client's self-awareness and self-esteem.

Prescriptive — The counselor is either active or passive in counseling, but seeks to achieve a specific counselee behavior.

Nonprescriptive — The counselor is either active or passive in the counseling session, and works for a goal of preparing the counselee cognitively and emotionally so that the counselee can make the evaluations and decisions for the situations he is confronting. The process by which nonprescriptive counseling is done relies on internally evaluated decisions by the counselee.

Thus, according to these sets of definitions, directive and nondirective are defined the same in genetic counseling as in psychologic counseling. Further, directive does not imply a knowledge or an imposition of the counselor's goals. Nondirective implies a strategy to enhance the counselee's self-esteem, and the implicit assumption is that the counselor goals are ultimately for an internally evaluated decision; but this approach is silent about providing the content, genetic information.

Conversely, the words prescriptive and nonprescriptive designate counselor approaches in which the counselor's goals are implied. In addition, prescriptive can be either overt or covert, depending upon whether the counselor confronts the counselee directly with the decision he is seeking. Overt prescriptiveness refers to telling the counselee what he ought to do or otherwise openly attempting to lead the counselee to a specific decision. Covert prescriptiveness includes counselor activities such as varying emphasis on the facts to affect a decision, or actions to mobilize guilt and/or reinforce authority and compliance characteristics in an attempt to prescribe counselee decisions and behavior. In the nonprescriptive orientation, the dichotomy between overt and covert is less of an issue since the acceptance of specific values themselves is not a necessary goal.

The counselor's choice of an internally evaluated counselee decision versus an externally evaluated one can be based upon either ethical or practical considerations. Gustafson has pointed out that in most specific cases which emerge in genetic counseling, multiple ethical points of view exist [6]. These ethical polarities tend to be resolved into choices between two valid, but opposing ethics, rather than between an ethical and a nonethical position. Ethical evaluation of goals is usually a complex and tortuous path for developing an argument by which consensus might be attained.

Ethical considerations of methods in genetic counseling, however, provide a more direct and convincing set of discriminating options. Because the ethical considerations of methods are related to everyday social discourse, they are also reflected in practical issues which influence the outcome of counseling at a common sense level. For these reasons, the argument for the counselee goal decision is based principally upon projected, practical outcomes.

Effects of Prescriptive and Nonprescriptive Approaches

The criterion of effectiveness in conjunction with ethical considerations can be used to evaluate the desirability of counselor goal choice. To evaluate their relative effectiveness, the counselor strategies of overt-prescriptive, covert-prescriptive, and nonprescriptive need to be examined in comparison to potential counselee reactions and probable outcomes. Each counselor strategy has the potential for engendering a range of predictable counselee responses which can be evaluated as effective or ineffective in accomplishing the counselor's goal.

If the counselor comes to genetic counseling with an agenda which dictates specific counselee decisions on some issues, then he will take a prescriptive approach. In his prescriptive approach, he will either be overt or covert in attempting to effect the prescribed counselee decision.

Overt-Prescriptive

The counselor's intent in the overt approach is to have the counselee accept the counselor's evaluation, coming to the same conclusions by directly discussing the issues. The psychologic climate perceived by the counselee may be that the counselor's opinion is more important than the counselee's, or that their respective opinions are of equal importance, with the possibility of open disagreement over their differences. If the counselee reacts as in a peer relationship, then the overt prescriptive approach is a respectful one based upon an equal power relationship between the counselor and counselee. This is not likely to be the relationship because of the expertise, authority, and social status of the counselor. Available data indicates that counselees of lower social and educational status are the least knowledgeable when they come for genetic counseling. Presumably they are also the most in need [7].

Alternatively, the intent of the counselor may be to use his power to facilitate a passive acceptance on the counselee's part. This strategy may or may not work. For the overt-prescriptive approach, the possible outcomes are independent of the counselor's intent. The technique does not necessarily increase the counselor's control over the decision process because the total responsibility for constructive use of the counselor's expertise is dependent upon the psychologic resources (or lack thereof) of the counselee alone. The possible counselee reactions are: 1) self-evaluation and acceptance of the counselor's advice for internally evaluated counselee decision; 2) reaction against the authority's advice; or 3) passive resignation to the counselor's advice.

Reaction against advice deprives the counselor of achieving his goal, ie the counselee making the "proper" decision. It can also deprive the counselee of a personally responsible or professionaly advocated decision. Resignation, another possible counselee response, accomplishes the counselor's goals, but raises major problems of counselee autonomy and responsibility. Evaluation of the human consequences of resignation by the counselee depends upon one's perception of the dependency generated. Overt-prescriptiveness may be perceived as respectful by a few counselees. Among these may be persons who are the most self-confident, the best informed, and the least in need of counseling. Those who come to the "proper" decision by passively accepting the counselor's role are similar to those who conform to the covert prescriptive approach to be discussed below.

Covert-Prescriptive

The intent of the covert-prescriptive approach is also to achieve a proper decision. It differs from the overt-prescriptive in that it does not openly require that the counselee accept the counselor's evaluation. In its purest form, the goal is for the "proper" decision irrespective of the reasons. Thus, knowledge of genetics, options, etc, are variable requisites to bringing about the "proper" decision. Information can be used insofar as it seems helpful to accomplish what the counselor deems good and important for the counselee, for the counselor, for society, or for all. The counselor either consciously or unconsciously attempts to bring about a particular counselee decision by techniques intended to be unperceived, such as selective emphasis of facts, and enhancing and/or allaying certain fears and anxieties.

If the counselor's agenda is truly unperceived and the counselor is able to affect his outcome by facts alone, the counselee will perceive that he is participating in meaningful decision-making and may even experience an enhancement in his self-esteem. If the counselor uses guilt mobilization or other implicit psychosocial threats, he may affect the decision but at the expense of self-esteem. The expected outcome is a decision which has been only evaluated by the counselor if the counselee passively follows the advice. The advice will be good or bad depending upon its consequences for the counselee, the counselor, and society. Furthermore, the externally evaluated decision usually is made in the absence of many important factors from the counselee's psychosocial arena (such as the way in which he values being a parent). The most potent and salient effects will be upon the counselee. If the outcome of counseling is perceived as undesirable, the counselee will likely be bitter towards those he identifies as having led him to the decision for which he was incompletely informed. The counselee will tend to absolve himself of responsibility for the decision to the extent that he was not informed. If he feels punished by the outcome of the decision, he may even seek compensation.

Alternatively, the counselee may reject the counselor's advice because either he senses the coercive component or because he values other options and consequences more. When this happens, the psychologic climate the counselee perceives is usually negative. For example, the counselor communicates to him that he could not be trusted to make a responsible decision. The implicit message is that he is not a responsible adult.

A few counselees will perceive the psychologic effect on themselves as neutral and attribute the occurrence to the counselor's inability to deal with the matters overtly. If the counselee rejects the counselor's advice because his targeting of the decision becomes apparent, then the counselee is usually deprived of a fully informed decision. If the counselee chooses other options in spite of the counselor's covert prescriptive approach, then he can achieve an internally evaluated counselee decision. Finally, some counselee decisions would correspond with the counselor's "proper" decision if the approach were purely informative. A disturbing, underlying problem is how many counselees fail to choose the option in keeping with their value system or the counselor's advice because they are reacting against the covert prescriptive approach.

Nonprescriptive

The counselor's intent in the nonprescriptive approach is to engage the counselee in a multidimensional, informed decision-making process. Engagement in the process is the goal. There are two interrelated problems being addressed in this approach. One is assembling the cognitive prerequisites, options, means, and probabilities for internally evaluated counselee decision. The second is to promote the counselee's psychologic acceptance of the situation and of having to make decisions. The psychologic climate set for the counselee is one of high expectation for acquisition of knowledge and evaluation of options. The potential counselee reactions are: 1) denial of all or part of the facts, significance of the facts, or feelings about the facts; 2) acceptance of the facts and abdication of decision-making; and 3) acceptance of facts, decision role, and behavior control. The potential outcomes are that the counselee makes: a) an irresponsible decision, ie consequences are not considered or accepted as a part of risk-taking; b) a responsible decision is achieved, but emotional upset leads to behavior that is disruptive of behavior control; and c) responsible decision with behavior control which stabilizes or improves the situation for those affected.

The outcome of this approach is dependent upon the counselee's resilience and ability to adapt to altered expectation in his life situation, and the skill of the counselor in facilitating this adaptation. For the counselor to facilitate this process, it is usually necessary for him to make decisions and use his full power in the counseling session to bring the counselee to at least a minimal level of genetic knowledge for decision-making; to raise the important issues which emerge from the genetic and medical diagnosis; and to enter the decision process with the counselee to clarify issues, outline options, project outcomes, and evaluate alternative consequences in the context of the counselee's sense of what is good and important. In this context, the power and authority of the counselor is used to reinforce the counselee's potency in facing and making his own decisions.

Some counselees will reject the counselor's expectations and wish for a counselor who will be prescriptive. Other counselees will progress towards decision and behavior control at a rate determined by their resilience, their relationship with the counselor, and the counselor's skill.

This is a flexible approach. The counselor's orientation can be expected to minimize the chances that the counselee will reach a random and unevaluated decision. The relationship of this approach to the prevention of affected children is dependent upon the extent to which the prevention of the affected child is a value held by the average counselee. However, it is not clear that this approach is less effective than the prescriptive in reaching the eugenics or disease prevention goals.

A portion of counselees approach counseling with significant amounts of denial. For either the prescriptive or nonprescriptive approaches to be successful for them, the counselee usually will need to accept and personalize the realities of his genetic problem; otherwise, serious decision-making and/or behavior control are moot.

In both prescriptive approaches, there are significant reactive factors which will interfere with some counselees' acceptance and, consequently, their behavior control. On a theoretical level at least, the nonprescriptive is superior because it is less likely to lead to counselee reactiveness; it also enhances the self-esteem of the counselee as he experiences himself as being capable of making his own decisions, as well as in his actually making these decisions. In addition, the strongest motivation for the counselee's complying with a decision comes directly from his participation in the process.

Given that the counselee controls his own behavior, the strongest motivation for such control is expected to emerge from one's personal involvement in decision-making, as advocated in internally evaluated counselee decision goal. In addition, there is no evidence that the prescriptive approach leads effectively to persuading counselees what course to follow. The work of Korsch [8] suggests that mothers are motivated to give their children medicine prescribed by a pediatrician as a function of their perceived participation in helping the doctor make the diagnosis. As counselees participate in decision-making, they often need to help in persuading themselves of the desirability and correctness of the final decisions.

The prevention of an affected child in a family is a different question. If there were clear evidence that overtly prescriptive approaches were superior in preventing recurrences, then this could be a debatable point. At present, it would seem that the burden of proof is upon those who would advocate a prescriptive approach since there is no positive evidence of efficacy, and, on a theoretical basis, there are some strong negative reasons against its use. In addition, if behavior control for certain individuals or families for genetic reasons were advocated, it would be fairer, more consistent, and more effective to carry these out through the legal system. These observations lead me to conclude that the orientation of genetic counseling should be nonprescriptive. A prescriptive approach, when indicated, should be based upon a formal, societal decision to effect behavioral control for genetic reasons.

Potential modes of nonprescriptive genetic counseling might include information providing only, or go beyond this stage to facilitate psychologic acceptance of the situation and help the counselee make the necessary decisions. The main argument against the former is that providing new information in the form of the genetic facts alters the conceptual framework through which the counselee views the problem. This alteration is sufficient to affect values in and of itself.

Proponents of nonprescriptive counseling beyond information transfer, like myself, argue that the counselor should help the counselee develop an effective component to handle the information addition to his conceptual framework.

The model presented in this paper outlines a nonprescriptive counseling that aims to develop what the counselor feels is an adequate basis for the counselee's confronting a given situation and for dealing with the choices presented by that situation. The counselor must first determine the resources from which he will work: the initial values of the counselee, the extent of the counselee's knowledge of general genetics and of his situation, and how he feels about it. The presentation of information must be geared to these initial conditions. During the educational process, the counselor must constantly check to insure that understanding develops along with the broadening information base. The responses of the counselee may indicate that the chosen method of education is somehow inadequate, and alternate methods must then be explored.

But the final step is the most important. The new information base must be converted into concepts which can be used for evaluation and into potential options from which he might choose. The counselor must foster the development of effective use of the new knowledge, and the ability to engage in informed decision-making. The counselee must do more than recite back the facts as given him; he should demonstrate that he can incorporate those general facts into an understanding and appreciation of his specific problem.

The counselor's most important contribution, then, is not to provide information per se, but helping the counselee to develop a way of dealing with the new information. The counselor has not prescribed an arbitrarily determined "right" set of values; rather, he has helped the counselee gain a better understanding of the problem and his view of it. (A model for achieving an optimum facilitation of counseling decision-making is given in the appendix following this chapter.)

RATIONALE

The justification for a model of decision-making is based upon showing that it affords an effective solution to the recognized goal processes of genetic counseling. The reasons why one approach is better than another depends upon both values and logic. The distinction is an important one since the counselor needs to know whether he is arguing values or logic when trying to resolve the basis for declaring one approach better than another.

The important value premises which are used as a standard for guiding the evaluation of genetic counseling are:

1) Decisions based upon fact and probability are better than intuitive decisions.

2) A person can reasonably take responsibility only for the consequences of decisions and behavior which are his own.

3) It is good and important for a person to believe he is valuable to himself and others, and he comes to feel successful as he makes decisions and acts upon them.

4) Motivation for acting on a decision is related to participation in the decision-making process.

5) It is good and important to be open to evaluating the consequences of one's behavior.

6) It is good to respond to the needs of others.

7) Credibility is valuable, and ultimately based upon honesty.

8) Humans thrive and grow in an atmosphere of respect and understanding.

These values are the basis for evaluating the relative merits of all the potential approaches to genetic counseling. The first issue is the role definition of the counselor in genetic counseling. A prescriptive role of the counselor is contrary to the stated values and is impractical as discussed under counselor's goal decisions. The three counselor roles which have been proposed as nonprescriptive are information-giving, psychotherapy, and the Decision-Making Model (see appendix).

COMPARISON OF THE PSYCHOTHERAPEUTIC MODEL AND THE DECISION-MAKING MODEL

The Psychotherapeutic and Decision-Making Models are similar in their value orientations and in their theoretical premises about human adaptation to change. These similarities are more important than any of the differences suggested below. In fact, the variance between the models is probably no greater than the difference between individual counselors. However, there are differences between the models which are highly significant when a discrimination is being made for policy decisions relative to health delivery or training of counselors.

The points of similarity are the emphasis upon the necessity for the counselor to understand the content and emotional impact of his own messages and those of others upon the counselee. In addition, these models are consistent in that they advocate the need of the counselor to use his relationship with the counselee to enable him to raise issues and confront counselees with their denial, covert obstacles to decision-making, and coping. Some of the differences are quantitative in regard to emphasis. The major quantitative difference is the emphasis on facts (genetic and medical). In the Decision-Making Model, the facts are the starting point and the necessary substrate for successful counseling. In the Psychotherapeutic Model, the facts are dealt with as a part of the process rather than with formal emphasis. The differences between the two models lie in their major focus. This is reflected in the contracting procedure. In the Psychotherapeutic Model, the counselor stresses the emotional issues as paramount in counseling. In the Decision-Making Model, the counselor emphasizes that the goals are: 1) processing a body of facts; 2) clarifying the meaning these facts have for the counselee; 3) dealing appropriately with the attendant feelings; and 4) making decisions. There are reasons why the Decision-Making Model is preferable.

The boundaries for the potential outcomes of genetic counseling are determined by the counselee's reasons for seeking counseling, by the counselor's decisions about his goals, and by societal expectation of what genetic counseling is. At a practical level, the potential for each case is set by a negotiated set of objectives that reflect both the counselee and counselor desires. In this sense, the contracting procedure is a compromise. A constraining factor on the contract is that societal expectation dictates that an important component to genetic counseling is information-giving. Counselees seek information for its intrinsic value in giving them control over their physical life. The hidden agenda is that they also come out of concern for maintaining or improving a relationship which they value, and to resolve issues regarding their self-evaluation or self-esteem. It is in recognition of the importance of these latter two issues that both models are proposed. The problem is the counselee is usually unprepared to work on these hidden issues when he comes to genetic counseling, and it is the task of the counselor to help the counselee articulate his anxiety. Through this procedure, the counselee is educated to understand the nature of other needs for which the treatment is psychotherapy.

The point at issue is an important one. In psychotherapy, the counselee comes because he is dissatisfied with himself. The therapist helps the client to explore and understand the discrepancies in his behavior and to resolve the difference between his standard for behavior and his actual behavior. In genetic counseling such a behavioral discrepancy that involves a genetic concern becomes a sensitive issue because the counselee has not sought a situation in which he will be confronted with these discrepancies. It has been hypothesized [2, 9] that many potential counselees avoid the geneticist. For those who come for counseling and for whom such issues cannot be given a primary focus, the Decision-Making Model is more appropriate because: 1) it recognizes that the average counselee's overt need is for facts and decision-making; and 2) that the best avenues for helping the counselee deal with his concern about behavior discrepancies (ie psychotherapy) develop from accomplishing the task for which he came (ie learning the facts, making decisions, and acting in accordance with those decisions).

In the Decision-Making Model, the focus is more restricted than that of psychotherapy. The thrust is to begin with the genetic issues and work towards having the counselee cope with the issues that emerge from the medical and genetic facts of his case. The model is a formal recognition that the counselor's powers are limited. There are many important problems for the counselor to address but he cannot do them all. The setting of realistic goals by the counselor is an important consideration when advocating a counseling model. Thus, the Decision-Making Model comes closer to counselee and societal expectation for genetic counseling as well as to recognizing the importance of the content of the genetic information. The contribution of counselee values and self-esteem in decision-making are appreciated as major components and are dealt with as they arise out of the process, always with the understanding that the counselor cannot be effective without the consent and active participation of the counselee.

DIFFERENCE BETWEEN THE INFORMATION-GIVING MODEL AND THE DECISION-MAKING MODEL

To illustrate reasons why the Information-Giving Model is unacceptable for genetic counseling, it will be compared to the Decision-Making Model. The difference will also apply to the Psychotherapeutic Model unless otherwise indicated. Before beginning the comparison, it is informative to examine the basis for giving information preeminence.

The first major reason that might explain support for the Information-Giving Model is a difference in values between the proponents of the Information-Giving Model and the Decision-Making Model. Examples of such differences might be: 1) the genetic counselor knows how to do other things better and should spend his time on these; 2) the process is too time-consuming for genetic counseling per se; and 3) the amount of conflict aroused will render the process ineffective. The value assumptions behind these assertions are that the counselor believes it is good and important for him to spend his time in other ways, and that it is bad for the counselor to become embroiled in situations of conflict. These are tenable values for the counselor, and what one needs to assess is what is the import of these counselor limits upon the counselee.

The second major reason for the counselor limiting his participation to information-giving is that he does not wish to impose his values on the counselee's decision. The assumption is made that by limiting himself to the facts, then the counselor will achieve impartiality and be the most helpful. This point of view is based upon the premises that counselees are ready to make decisions and cope, and that they only need information. This, in fact, is true for relatively few counselees.

The evidence which is presented to counterbalance these points of view is related to the effect upon the counselee. The contention is that the effect upon the counselee is so significant and so injurious as to make the support of the Information-Giving Model untenable. The evidence against both reasons is highly interrelated. Therefore, the counter-position will be presented as a unit.

The Information-Giving Model proposes that genetic counseling ends with the providing of the genetic facts. The arguments against this point of view are: 1) information-giving is an ineffective form of genetic education; 2) the genetic facts elicit anxiety with which the counselor must deal in order to facilitate learning these facts; 3) the Information-Giving Model involves an inescapable recommendation of values which should be explored; and 4) information-giving is less than the counselor can do in helping the counselee to reach his life goals.

COUNSELEE'S PSYCHOLOGIC REACTIONS MAKE INFORMATION-GIVING ALONE MOSTLY INEFFECTIVE

The psychologic reactions of counselees argue against information-giving as the treatment choice. To illustrate the relationship between the psychologic reactions and ineffective use of genetic information, a model for grief reactions will be used. The use of this model will delineate the effect of psychologic reactions upon genetic counseling.

The grief model is a general analogy which can be applied to all human adaptation to change; it has applicability to patient and family acceptance of genetic diagnosis [2, 10, 11].

In general, the outlook of the genetic counselee is that of a person who has suffered multiple losses or disappointments. At stake is the anticipated health of self or child [12]. In addition, a person usually assumes that he or she carries a normal set of genes. Thus, a further loss or disappointment is the fact or implication that the counselee's genes are abnormal. The psychologic reactions follow directly from the extent of the perceived loss, in relation to the degree to which the person thinks he needs that which has been ruined. The amount of loss which the counselees perceive can be understood in terms of their knowledge of the specific disease (their perception of the prognosis, recurrence risk, and stigmatization) as contrasted with their life goals and the degree to which such goals are felt to be threatened. Psychologic reactions do not emanate from the loss alone, but from the meaning of the loss for the individual's concept of self and the constructs he holds as essential evidence for his worth as a person.

To illustrate more specifically some of the underpinnings of these psychologic reactions, one can examine the implication of being genetically defective in the context of a person's and a family's self-concept. Clinical experience in genetic counseling indicates that prior to the development of a medical diagnosis, most counselees had not consciously considered that they might carry any abnormal genes. People take for granted that all of their genes are functional. In addition, the belief in romantic love and marriage in our society leads to the concept of an ideal family, or at least a normal family. Thus, for multiple reasons, expectant parents often look upon their children as self-enhancing extensions of themselves.

Rarely does a couple conceive a child with the notion of taking a one-in-twenty risk for a serious birth defect. In essence, couples plan for an ideal family. The disclosure of a genetic abnormality is in opposition to these prior expectations. With the diagnosis of a genetic disease, a new dimension to personal-self and family-self has been actualized which may be perceived as defective, and for which no previous allowance in self and family concepts had existed. Out of the disappointment, a conflict emerges between idealized self and family. The personal and family adjustment necessary to integrate and bring back into equilibrium the ideal self and the perceived self is the "grief" process. The resolution of the disappointment or conflict can be formalized in four phases. They are 1) shock; 2) denial; 3) emotional upset, struggling with the disturbing information, internal conflicts, and inconsistent patterns of behavior; and 4) acceptance, with consistent and integrated behavior. Despite the relatively few studies on the psychologic aspects of genetic counseling, there is ample clinical evidence that denial, emotional upset, and conflicting behaviors are important problems [2].

As indicated above, shock and denial are usually the first psychologic reactions to the discovery of a genetic abnormality in an individual or his progeny. This initial reaction lessens the effectiveness of genetic information. Leonard et al [5] reported that 5 out of 61 of their counselees denied ever having been counseled. An additional six denied some aspect of their child's disease such that the usefulness of the genetic information was questioned by the evaluators. Fraser et al [9] reported 40% of their counselees had one or more children after the birth of an affected child. A similar percentage had waited over two years before coming to counseling. During the interval between the birth of the affected child and the parents' coming to genetic counseling, 15% had a second child with a genetic defect. Denial is an important psychologic variable which is perhaps delaying genetic counseling unduly, thus preventing couples from receiving and using genetic information.

Denial is usually a temporary phrase, and as counselees begin to accept their diagnosis and partially understand its meaning, they experience significant amounts of distress. Langsley [13] has reported his clinical experience of a family with Alport syndrome in which a rather complete spectrum of these reactions is described in various members of a single family. In addition to clinical observation of emotional upset, psychologic measures have shown that counselees coming to the genetics clinic because of a Down syndrome child were experiencing increased anxiety, hostility, and depression [10]. The way in which this upset interferes with the success of imparting genetic information is an important and unanswered question. Experience with students has indicated that some degree of anxiety improves the performance of learners; however, anxiety which is too high has a deleterious effect on learning [14]. Depression, unlike anxiety, can be expected to have a more consistent negative effect upon learning; and a number of mothers of Down syndrome children are depressed at the time of counseling. The mother's depression and its inhibitory effect on learning, suggested in the case of Down, would appear to be generalizable to many other genetic diseases which place a high burden on a family [7].

As postulated earlier, the function of denial is to enable the counselee to maintain some level of hope or sense of well-being in the face of what is perceived as overwhelming disruption. Thus, the function of denial can be seen as a means of controlling, or perhaps putting off emotional upset. If the information given at genetic counseling is itself upsetting, then it may evoke another phase of denial, and further learning during counseling may be blocked even more effectively than among anxious students.

Self-concept is for many people at least partially defined in terms of the common assumption that they carry normal genes. Because one of the tasks of genetic counseling is to replace this assumption of perfection with more realistic information, the self-concept usually suffers as a result of genetic counseling. Another effect of defining self in terms of one's genes may be feelings of guilt and self-blame for the genetic defect of one's child. These feelings were reported by one-half of the mothers and one-third of the fathers counseled by Fraser et al [9].

To summarize, patients seeking genetic counseling are to varying degrees in the midst of sudden change in the way in which they perceive themselves and their relationships to others. This sudden change is in direct extension from their genetic concerns, or their concerns about health and wholeness in general. Evidence has been presented which indicates that these changes for many counselees constitute an emotional threat, such that management by the counselees of the physical threat is delayed or ignored, thereby reducing their effectiveness in decision-making or coping.

The genetic information one wishes to impart at genetic counseling can be part of a larger threat to personhood. Because of these psychodynamics, one cannot assume that counselees are disposed to getting the genetic facts, to conceptualizing the data in an abstract way, to applying it to their situation, or to channeling their anxiety about the threat in a way which will improve effective coping. Thus, if the goal for genetic counseling is set in terms of counselee behavior, then the evidence at this point overwhelmingly suggests that presenting the information without dealing with the anxiety it generates is going to lead to a poor learning of information, a proposition supported by the majority of the evaluation studies [1]. An ancillary point is that only by having the counselee apply the facts to his personal situation does the counselor know that genetic education was accomplished. Evidence from the evaluation studies also emphasize that even information retained correctly may not be applied to decision-making.

There is suggestive evidence of unresolved emotional upset extending beyond the initial period of adjustment to a genetic disease or threat. When behavior continues to be inconsistent with stated goals and values, one may assume the presence of stress or even psychologic disturbance. Although all humans lack internal consistency at times, that consistency may be considered an indicator of the level of psychologic function. A high degree of correspondence between stated goals and observed behavior becomes a goal of genetic counseling; however, the data available indicate that some disparity exists between the counselee's stated goals and their behavior.

The results of Leonard et al [5] demonstrated that differences between stated reproductive plans and behavior are frequent. At the time of follow-up, a number of families were using birth control which was inadequate to insure that they accomplish their stated child bearing plans. Approximately 25% of the families who claimed to have been deterred from further reproduction were using ineffective means of birth control. In addition, about one-half of the families who had not made a decision at a cognitive level were practicing ineffective birth control. From this single study in which data of this kind are available, 25% of the families were not acting to insure that their stated decision to prevent a pregnancy be accomplished, or that their choice to make a conscious decision be protected. Thus, even when families get the genetic information and apparently make a considered decision, they do not always behave in a fashion consistent with their plans. This finding suggests extended, unresolved emotional conflict or the lack of a clear decision.

These facts are compelling reasons for genetic counseling beyond information-giving. Not all counselees have psychologic reactions which they need help handling, but all need to be evaluated to find out what meaning they are attaching to the facts and how upsetting that meaning is to them. If the counselor defines himself as an information giver only, then in honesty and fairness to the counselee, he needs to state explicitly his role definition so that the counselee will know to seek additional help in attempting to make decisions and control his behavior. Or that part of the information the counselee needs is referral to counselors who can assist him in dealing with grief, emotional upset, and decision-making.

Next, a consideration of the objectivity of the content information is in order. Dichotomous views exist about whether information-giving in genetic counseling is value free. One perspective is that the geneticist can provide objectively correct and complete denotative facts and risk figures. This is one of the reasons for advocating the Information-Giving Model of genetic counseling. The antithetical view is that the counselor evaluates and chooses a subset of facts out of the full scientific description for presentation to counselees. This process renders the genetic information as connotative rather than denotative. The counselee also makes an evaluation and selection about what he incorporates into his decision process. The logical extension of this second observation is that the information assimilated after genetic counseling is based upon judgments rather than scientific description. Since the selection of facts is an undeniable part of the genetic education process, values are necessarily reflected in the information the counselor chooses to provide. Thus, on a theoretical level genetic counseling is not value free.

The second proposition is that, at a practical level, genetic counseling alters values. Values are enduring beliefs that a specific mode of conduct or end-state of existence is personally or socially preferable to alternative models of conduct or end-states of existence. Once a value is internalized, it becomes a standard or criterion for guiding behavior [15]. Values constitute the basis for making simultaneous choices about what is good and important for the evaluator. As such, values provide a person with a basis for setting up hierarchies of modes of outcome and end-states. The point at issue is, that genetic information influences this hierarchy. But this is a two-sided proposition, because ignorance influences the hierarchy also. The choice is not between influencing values or not, but between influencing values with genetic information or with ignorance. Thus, the choice is between an informed or an intuitive decision. Even a chance for good intuitive decision is significantly diminished in the midst of elevated levels of anxiety.

The information in genetic counseling is used by the counselee for defining options and for evaluating situations. It is clear that, as the information is used in evaluation of outcomes desirable and others undesirable, it reflects a series of value judgments. One reason counselees block the learning of genetic information is the meaning the information has for evaluating themselves as people. When they do this, they will begin to experience a behavior discrepancy of the same general type (either shame or guilt) that clients seeking psychotherapy have. That is, their ideal self is out of balance with their perceived behavioral self. This is the origin of the suffering self-concept. When individuals are dealing with behavior discrepancies, they are experiencing anxiety which interferes with their learning and decision-making. The genetic counselor needs to help the counselee deal with this anxiety or even the learning of facts will be blocked. Thus, it is that propensity of counselees to use the genetic facts to evaluate themselves, as to their worth and importance, that is automatically used by a proportion of counselees as if it were a value rather than a description of nature which obliges the counselor to attempt to set straight. The proportion of counselees who use genetic facts for self-evaluation is high and raises the question of whether genetic counseling should be done at all if it is to be limited to information-giving.

Genetic facts influence the way in which counselees evaluate situations. Specific consequences of various actions take on different relative meaning in the hierarchy of value judgments after having the genetic information. The couple who have been anticipating a child as an important and good event may, in the light of an unsuspected genetic risk, reevaluate the situation as possibly good, possibly bad, and definitely important. Faced with this reevaluation, and the possibility of prenatal diagnosis, individuals who have previously considered abortion untenable, shift its place in their value hierarchy to less bad and important than the risk of having an affected child.

In conclusion, there are three important reasons for the counselor's giving more than information. The first is, that out of the constraint of time, he must give only a part of all the potential genetic information available and the portion he chooses will reflect his values. A conscious awareness that it does, and then checking with the counselee that he understood all of his alternatives, is the best way for the counselor to monitor his own conscious and unconscious biases. The second reason is that a counselee frequently uses genetic information, either consciously or unconsciously, to evaluate himself as a good or bad person. The counselor needs to try to interrupt this jump in logic. Finally, genetic facts influence the counselee's evaluation of future outcome and, as such, inescapably influence his value system. The counselor has a choice of either looking at the effect on values or ignoring it. The Decision-Making Model advocates that the effect be examined so that confusion, psychologic distortion, and errors in calculation be minimized. After all, the counselor goes through the counseling process daily but the counselee does so rarely. With the combination of clinical experience and the use of a relevant model such as the Decision-Making Model, the counselor has much more to offer than the facts alone.

APPENDIX
DECISION MODEL FOR COUNSELORS

A model of genetic counseling has been developed to accomplish the goal of facilitating the counselee in an internally evaluated decision process. In trying to achieve this goal, the counselor inescapably makes numerous decisions and evaluations of his own. The model explicates the types of counselor decisions, arranges them in a sequential array, and interrelates the counselor decisions to his goals. The model is structured in three stages: 1) defining the genetic basis for concern and the nature of the contractual relationships, 2) genetic education, and 3) counselor participation in the counselee's decision-making process. The model recognizes the existence of qualitative differences within each stage while providing a conceptual framework or pattern for the counselor's decisions.

The time dimension in the model illustrates the ordering of certain events, implies feedback, and indicates the interdependency of one stage upon another.

In the counseling process, there are four categories of decision which the genetic counselor makes: 1) assessing the resources — counselee and environmental, 2) setting objectives, 3) determining tactics and strategy, and 4) evaluating outcome. The interrelationship of the three stages and the four categories is shown in Figure 1.

STAGES OF GENETIC COUNSELING

CATEGORIES OF COUNSELOR DECISIONS	A. Identifying the Genetic Concerns and Contracting	B. Genetic Education	C. Decision-Making: New Options and the Need for Counselee Education
1. Assessments			
2. Setting Objectives			
3. Determining Tactics and Strategy			
4. Evaluation			

Fig. 1. Decision-making model.

Categories of Counselor Decisions

1) Assessing Resources

The counselor assesses specific variables in each counselee. Some of the key questions which the counselor attempts to answer in his assessment are: 1) How much does he know? 2) What is his motivation to learn the genetics? 3) What is his present emotional state? 4) Is there a commitment to controlling his life? 5) What is the major need? 6) What decisions are to be made? In addition, the counselor assesses the certainty of his medical data, his own skills, and other helping resources. Perhaps most important is an interaction variable — does the counselor think that he can work with the counselee? The result of this evaluation is a series of judgments about the case which are predictors of outcome.

2) Setting Objectives

This is carried out by blending the judgments from the assessment with the counselor's awareness of the resources, the burden of the disease, and the specifics of the situation which modify or delimit the ideal goals for counseling. The aim is to formulate realistic, attainable, behavioral objectives for the counselee in the specific case. Part of a realistic formulation of objectives is ordering them in terms of feasibility of approach, from the most likely to the least likely.

3) Determining Tactics and Strategy

The counselor decides how the objectives will be achieved. The resources, people, skills, time, materials, and information are integrated with objectives for the case. An overall strategy and a set of tactics are developed out of this phase of the decision process.

4) Evaluation

The final decision category is evaluation. To achieve the evaluation the counselor makes a series of measurements or judgments about the results of counseling. These data are compared and contrasted with the set objectives. The outcome can then be judged as having surpassed, equaled, or less than the objectives. On the basis of the evaluations, counseling can be concluded or negotiated to work on remaining unfinished objectives.

Stages of Genetic Counseling (and their interrelationship with the four categories)
A) Identifying the Genetic Concerns and Contracting

In the model, the first stage of counseling is that of defining the basis of the genetic concern and attempting to develop a counseling contract. The commonality of genetic counselees is that they have a genetic concern. The counselor attempts to determine the specific genetic concerns for each counselee. For each genetic concern, the counselor would like to provide a means of validating the counselee's anxiety. The validation should be empathetic to the concern, and simultaneously advance the process of specifying the counselee's expectations. On the other hand, the counselee needs to be appraised of the counselor's agenda. By each participant's talking about his concern or purpose, the various parties clarify the multiple agendas. The purpose of this process is for counselor and counselee to determine a mutual agenda they can agree upon. When they finish, they should know if there is a basis for a contract to enter into genetic counseling. For this type of counseling, a contract is absolutely necessary. Explicit agendas that are agreeable to both parties are a necessary but not sufficient condition for establishing a counseling agreement or contract. The essentials of a counseling contract are mutual agreement on the goals. It usually includes a consensus about what content information the counselor will provide in genetic education, and how the counselor will work with the counselee in the decision-making process, the time allowed, and the cost.

1) Assessing Resources. Figure 2 is a simplified schematic representation of this first stage of genetic counseling. There are four binary decision points and three processes. The first assessment (Process A) is to define the counselee's agenda and his/her feelings about the problem. The four following assessment questions usually provide the counselor with the salient concerns and some of the counselee's feelings. They are: 1) What do you think the problem is? 2) What about this problem worries you? 3) What would you like to get from counseling? and 4) What do you think caused this to happen? One can reasonably assume that all counselees have multiple concerns and this process allows for some exploration. In addition, the salient concern is not always the most important. Hidden counselee agendas are not infrequent. Overly zealous and literal attention to the first concern may prevent counseling success. It is necessary to obtain fairly complete information as to the multiple concerns and their order of importance to the counselee.

On the basis of the information about the counselee's concerns and assessing the facts surrounding the case, the counselor decides whether to advocate genetic counseling (Decision #1). If the genetic concerns or medical work-up are assessed as being inappropriate or premature for genetic counseling, then the counselor would decide whether to advocate genetic work-up (Decision #3), and/or genetic counseling at a later time (Decision #4). Alternatively, if the counselor advocates genetic counseling, then he will confront the question of whether he and the counselee can agree upon a common agenda (Process B). An affirmative answer indicates that the counselee recognizes a need for counseling services, that some of the counselee's concerns can be dealt with, and that the counselee is judged by himself and the counselor to be psychologically prepared to attempt genetic counseling.

2) Setting Objectives. In preparing to advocate genetic counseling, the counselor makes a number of decisions. Decisions in preparation include: a) what the counselor thinks the major problem is (ie who is affected, who is a carrier, and who is responsible for care and prevention). The next stage is genetic education and the counselor decides b) what the educational needs are relative to the disease process and the counselee complaints. The counselor considers c) what counseling objectives are desired in attempting to meet the counselee's articulated needs, d) how they will be attained, and e) how they are to be evaluated.

3) Determining Tactics and Strategy. Contracting includes sharing the counselor's assessment with the counselee for discussion, clarification, exploration, and finally for a decision concerning whether mutual agreement can be reached. The counselor shares with the counselee the treatment plan, goals, methods, and procedural rules. The goal is to obtain mutual agreement. How-

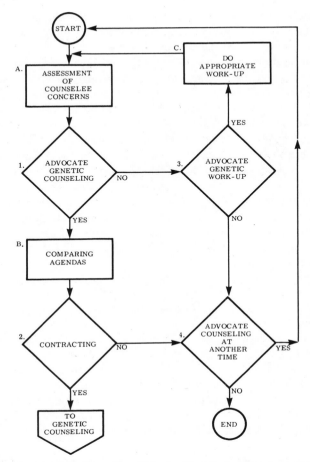

Fig. 2. Contracting in genetic counseling. This algorithm depicts four important questions (the diamonds) which the counselor decides as contracting proceeds. The rectangles are processes in which the counselors and counselees interact.

ever, the outcome can be for genetic counseling or for no agreement and no counseling.

The process of contracting is presented as occurring at the beginning of counseling and as a single occurrence. This need not be the case. Redefining the counselee's concerns and recontracting following counselor's assessment is indicated when there is no agreement on the problem to be worked on, or when the problem agreed upon is changing or has changed. As rapport and trust builds during counseling, the counselee's anxiety and defensiveness may decrease with the result that the work may shift from understanding of denotative facts to re-evaluation of the connotative meaning. If the genetic counselor is comfortable in this role, he can recontract and proceed, or it may be appropriate to recontract and refer to a psychologic counselor.

4) Evaluating Outcome. In evaluating the contracting procedure, the counselor determines how successful the contracting procedure was in alerting the counselee to his role as an active participant; whether setting counseling objectives improved the chances of realizing these goals; how successful he was in linking specific tasks to attaining concrete counseling objectives; and whether rapport was developed. As an agreement about agendas, objectives, and methods are reached, then the focus can shift to the next stage — genetic education.

B) Genetic Education and Supportive Counseling

In the educational stage, the counselor determines the counselee's knowledge and makes a series of decisions which result in the formulation of a plan which will help the counselee come to criteria for genetic knowledge. For each group of facts, the counselor should provide an educational task which will accomplish the objective. The task must be correct for the counselee and the objective. The counselor works to get the genetic information to the counselee. The goal is for the counselee to be able to accomplish predetermined behavior objectives which indicate that the educational objectives were reached. The overall goal of genetic education is to help the counselee to learn the medical and genetic facts which he needs in order to make informed decisions regarding his genetic concern. Through contracting, the counselor has attempted to establish the counselee's active participation in learning these facts. It is the task of the counselor to design, supervise, administer, and evaluate the progress in genetic education. In doing this, he makes a similar pattern of decisions in this stage of counseling as the other two stages.

1) Assessing the Educational Needs and Resources. In assessing the educational task, the counselor determines the amount of medical knowledge which is applicable to the case. He has internalized standards which tend to set a minimal level of acceptable counselee knowledge, ie the knowledge which the counselor judges necessary for an informed decision. Ostensibly, the counselee seeks genetic information from the counselor who provides access to this highly specialized body of knowledge. For each fact which constitutes an educational goal, the counselor needs to determine the counselee's present knowledge, his willingness, and his ability to learn new facts. If a counselee is trying to sustain a state of partial denial in relation to the genetic facts, new information may be incompatible with the effort to sustain denial and result in increased anxiety. The counselee tends to maintain the partial denial so that he can continue to function. The unconscious supposition in the denial is that if it were discarded, the feelings of anxiety would be unbearable. Because of the relationship between genetic education, denial, and anxiety in the counselee, the counselor often becomes the advocate of more knowledge than the counselee desires. The process whereby the counselee abandons his denial and works through the emotional upset to an accceptance is the "grief" process. This is an important factor because a significant number of counselees will be actively grieving at the time of genetic education.

The importance of this observation is that genetic education may add additional sorrow. To the extent that genetic knowledge, which implies defect, is interpreted by the recipient as change, or as implying that the counselee is a less valuable person; genetic education is not a low key, denotative process, ie this occurs when they come to feel, "I am not adequate as a person if I give my child this bad disease through my genes." Because of the connotative meaning, the counselee may deny all or part of the facts, the significance of the facts, or his feelings about the facts.

This intermixed process of the counselee who seeks information, experiences emotional upset, and attempts to control the upset by blocking further incorporation of information complicates the genetic education process and emphasizes the need for the counseling process. Furthermore, the counselee's reactions can be predicted before genetic education only within broad limits; this prediction is better for groups than individuals. The counselor makes assessments based upon limited information regarding the probable openness of counselees to various parts of the information. The major assessment of this reaction is carried out dynamically and simultaneously with providing the facts.

A final assessment is made of the counseling resources. The counselor evaluates his own skills, the expertise of his associates, and the usefulness of media for accomplishing the education objectives. In addition, he assesses the potential quality of his relationship with the counselee. In psychologic counseling, this variable has been one of the best predictors of the counselee's improvement and 'probably will be found to be important in the genetic education process.

2) Setting Educational Objectives. The counselor evaluates the counselee's level of cognitive knowledge. He borrows from the earlier assessment and collects data on what the counselee knows about diagnosis, explanation of the disorder, prognosis, recurrence risk, prenatal diagnosis, available treatment, carrier status, and fertility control. For each assessment about the counselee's level of understanding, the counselor makes a judgment as to what is the ideal level of counselee knowledge. The differential between these two levels defines the educational need.

3) Tactics and Strategy. Emerging directly from the assessments and objectives, a decision must be made as to the tactical and strategic approaches in order to accomplish the immediate and overall educational objectives. In spite of this planning, a large part of the counselor decision-making is in dynamic response to the counselee and occurs in the midst of the genetic education process. As mentioned above, assessing, setting an immediate objective, delivering the facts, and evaluating the effect is a series of short progressive encounters. The tactical and strategic decisions are related to how to engage in this or some other type of educational task. Other decisions involve the use of educational media and other personnel. Irrespective of these approaches, the process is one of giving information, evaluating the counselee knowledge, and observing the reaction. The basic evaluation in this approach is whether the counselee knows the facts. If the counselee knows the facts, then the procedure can move on to the next group of facts. Frequently during genetic education, the counselee confuses the facts, and the attendant signs of anxiety indicate emotional upset, the upset having halted the effective incorporation of information. Increase in anxiety connotes that the counselee understood the information and has been confronted with a new awareness of the threatening implications. The counselor must decide when to discontinue giving facts and work towards lowering anxiety. In the effective use of this process with a client who is not in shock but having normal anxiety, an effective rhythm of information-giving and attending to emotional upset develops.

Information-giving cannot always proceed to completion. Counselees may be unable to go on because of normal anxiety arising out of an immediate confrontation with bad news, in which case the counselor may decide to interrupt information-giving. He would then go into a posture of providing supportive genetic counseling. The treatment plan is one of empathy, support, and time. After a period of time, genetic counseling can resume. Some counselors have neurotic anxiety emanating from previously developed behavior patterns which work poorly. When the counselor recognizes this pattern, he may decide to refer the counselee for psychodynamic counseling. Treatment by a person experienced in personality and family counseling would be aimed at improving the person's overall adaptive behavior, eventually returning him for genetic education.

In conclusion, the counselor makes a strategic decision about how he plans to accomplish the educational objectives. Along the way, there are a number of tactical decisions about whether and when to offer information, reassurance, supportive genetic counseling, and psychodynamic counseling.

4) Evaluating the Outcome. The counselor makes decisions about whether and when the counselee knows the facts. The educational objectives are cognitive. They constitute the first evaluative sign indicative of progress towards psychologic acceptance. According to the grief model for adaptation to change, the cognitive appreciation of the change is accompanied by anxiety. As acceptance progresses, hostility and depression occur. They provide collateral data for evaluating the effects of the information at the emotional level. The evaluative decisions which the counselor makes in the process of genetic education are to determine the counselee's knowledge in comparison to the educational objectives. Emotional upset is ancillary information and has great importance in evaluating the application of genetic knowledge to decision-making.

C) New Options and the Need for Counselee Evaluation

At the end of genetic education, the knowledge which the counselee attains raises issues, clarifies options in a probabilistic sense, and/or provides a more accurate basis for evaluating outcomes. According to the proposed model, the counselor seeking an internally evaluated counselee decision will, conjointly with the counselee, evaluate the consequence of the alternative options for handling the situation. For a selected number of issues, the counselor needs to provide an opportunity for the counselee to rehearse his decision-making. By the time this process is finished, the counselee has had an opportunity to examine the outcome of his various behavioral options with a person who is knowledgeable with and oriented toward a series of decisions that are compatible with the counselee's value system.

1) Assessing the Issues and Resources. Evaluation at the end of the genetic education stage provides the beginning point for assessing possible counselee options. Two important categories of issues coming out of the facts are those concerning recurrence risk and self-esteem. The options for the counselee with recurrence risk are birth control, abortion, artificial insemination, alternative mating, prenatal diagnosis, sterilization, and risk-taking. The options dealing with self-esteem concern the counselee arriving at a psychologic acceptance. In addition to the issues, the counselor must decide what people, media, and other resources are available in preparing the counselee for his decison-making. A counselor evaluates his own sensitivity, aggressiveness, and the extent to which he understands his goals in exploring these issues.

The counselee's values are an important resource. As such, the counselor will need to assess these values in preparation for making decisions on how to raise issues. For example, issues for which the counselee is certain about his values will cause less emotional upset for him. It will be easier for him to discuss and share his decision-making process with the counselor. Although an assessment is indicated prior to beginning the counseling, the majority of the counselee's values will emerge in the process of evaluating the various projected consequences.

2) Setting Objectives. This is the final phase of counseling. The objectives should therefore closely parallel the counseling goals. Thus, a selected number of representative issues whose processing would illustrate that the counselee understand the information and can apply those facts to his decision-making process constitutes the counselor guidelines for setting objectives. The counselor needs to blend his judgments concerning resources and goals into a realistic set of attainable objectives. These objectives are best when they specifically define the counselee's desired behavior, albeit process behavior.

3) Tactics and Strategy: Method of Counselor Participation. In this stage, the counselor chooses a set of illustrative issues. He decides upon an order for raising these issues. In turn, each issue is introduced for counselee evaluation of

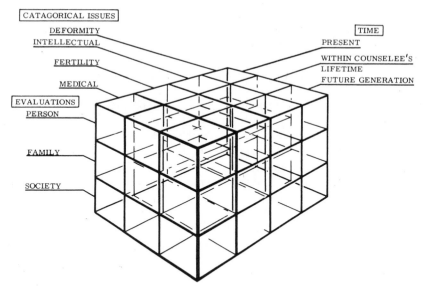

Fig. 3. Evaluation of genetic information. The paradigm illustrates the interrelationship between the disease specific variables summarized into categorical issues, the various orientations from which the categorical issues can be evaluated and the time frame over which
the evaluator(s) can base his/her decision-making. Obviously, different decisions will be
reached depending upon the orientation of the decision maker in choosing which spaces
in the paradigm are most important to consider.

the options, of the method of intervention, and of the consequences. The counselee rehearses his decision process with counselor serving as the catalyst for a
multidimensional, internally evaluated counselee decision. The counselor explores, clarifies, and supplements the data base as they work together. The process is repeated until a representative set of issues are reviewed or the alliance
with the counselor is discontinued.

There is a complicated layering effect of issues emerging from genetic
counseling. The parameters are categorical issues, time-modified projections,
and the multiple evaluation orientations on each issue over time. The categorical
issues are medical (ie health and treatment), fertility, intellectual function, and
anatomic deformities. The issues carry extended meaning in time, modifiable
outcomes with various interventions and alternatives, and interrelationships with
other events occurring along a parallel time dimension (Fig. 3). The third dimension of issues are those which result from the interpretation of the categorical
issues and their future projections through the evaluations of the counselee, his
family, and society. The counselor chooses from this universe of potential issues
a subset which he thinks can serve to rehearse relevant decisions illustrative of

the amount of knowledge applied, the weighing of their information, the degree of decisiveness, and the reference orientation of the evaluation.

Having defined a subset of issues, the counselor chooses an order of presentation. The order could be based upon estimates of relevance. The counselor must decide whether to raise inescapable issues first or last. The counselor may wish to begin with an issue of low threat to demonstrate the overall approach before raising those that he judges will be the most upsetting. The usual approach is saliency. The counselor can choose to begin with the issues which reflect the counselee's anxiety and guide the process in time towards other potentially important decisions. An important counselor decision is when this type of work can be initiated with the counselee. The quality of counselor-counselee relationship or the basic security of counselee's identity provides the basis of such timing.

When it is doubtful that the counseling is going to continue through a logical sequence until most of the important issues will be covered, urgency based upon limited time exposure determines the order. Under these conditions, counselee's decision points are evaluated and ranked as to whether they lead to long-term, irreversible decisions or short-term, reversible ones. Based upon this ordering, the counselor arrives at a reasoned approach for the limits of the situation.

Any facet of any subject chosen from the paradigm can be processed. Although the counselor use his authority and credibility to raise various issues, ultimately he and the counselee need to jointly agree upon a common issue.

Methods for Raising Issues. A logical starting point is with the physical category. For each category, there is a finite number of classifiable options. For example, if fertility is the issue, the options are two: uncontrolled and controlled. In the latter, three subcategories exist: there can be no control over reproductive behavior; there can be selected control of birth or some unselected births. To attain the various categorical fertility options, there are a set of procedural options with both desirable and undesirable consequences. The procedural fertility options are: sterilization, selective mating by artificial insemination, remating, amniocentesis and abortion, and quantitative birth regulation. The next step is for the counselee to evaluate all the categorical fertility options and procedural options. Seeking an internally evaluated counselee decision, the counselee attempts to judge what is of value to himself. The counselor works to facilitate this process. The internal orientation does not imply either a selfish or selfless decision. To the extent that the counselee thinks and feels himself in relationship with others, he will probably incorporate his value of them in his decision. The internally evaluated counselee decision implies a personal commitment to the value of the chosen alternative and acceptance of personal responsibility for the consequence.

The counselee may be unable to evaluate the choices. For example, the counselee comes to genetic education with a set of perceptions about what ends and means are good and important for himself.

The information he receives may change that. Having a child, a situation both important and good, can change to important and bad when a genetic diagnosis is made. In turn, potential recurrence of this bad and important situation must now be simultaneously judged versus a previously untenable option such as sterilization. This example goes to illustrate why genetic counseling cannot be value free. According to the proposed model, it is the task of the counselor to work with the counselee on delineating his options, evaluating each, and either making a decision or setting up the proper equation for evaluating the choices.

The final step in this process is for the counselor to evaluate the counselee's behavioral intent. The counselor compares the counselee's behavioral intent to stated and implied values for consistency. Inconsistencies point to either misunderstanding the facts, choices, and consequences or to inability to subordinate lesser values. The counselor retraces the steps in the decision process to find the origin of the inconsistency. The remedy is either genetic education or value clarification. The counselor and counselee repeat the process until the set of relevant issues is exhausted or until there is failure to agree upon a contract.

4) Evaluating Outcome. One of the advantages of the counselor participating with the counselee in formulating and making decisions is that it provides a thorough evaluation of genetic counseling. The success of genetic education in apprising counselees of the genetics, the options, and the consequences becomes apparent. Finally, it provides perhaps the only practical way of evaluating whether the goal of an internally evaluated counselee decision was reached.

ACKNOWLEDGMENTS

I am indebted to George Siskind, PhD, who has carefully and constructively criticized the development of this model and suggested many helpful avenues of approach over the six years of its development. Kenneth E. Reed, PhD, and Keith Kinney, ThM, have given intensive assistance in actualizing and refining the model. Mary Ann Antley, Alex Braitman, and Philip Lowry have given able assistance in reviewing drafts.

REFERENCES

1. Shaw M: Review of published studies of genetic counseling: A critique of methodology. In de la Cruz F, Lubs HA (eds): "Genetic Counseling." New York: Raven Press, 1977, pp 35–49.
2. Antley RM: Variables in the outcome of genetic counseling. Soc Biol 23:108–115, 1976.
3. Sorenson JR: Counselors: A self-portrait. Genet Counseling 1:29–33, 1973.

4. Carter C, Evans K, Fraser-Roberts JA, Buck A: Genetic clinic: A follow-up. Lancet 1: 281–285, 1971.
5. Leonard CO, Chase GA, Childs B: Genetic counseling: A consumer's view. N Engl J Med 287:433–439, 1972.
6. Gustafson JM: Screening and counseling: Some ethical issues. Presented at the American Society of Human Genetics, Atlanta, Oct 25, 1973.
7. Antley RM: Factors influencing mother's response to genetic counseling for Down's syndrome. In de la Cruz F, Lubs HA (eds): "Genetic Counseling." New York: Raven Press, 1977, pp 97–108.
8. Korsch B, Freemon B, Negrete V: Practical implications of doctor-patient interaction analysis for pediatric practice. Am J Dis Child 121:110, 1971.
9. Fraser FC, Levy EP, Wright S: Follow-up of a genetic counseling program. Am J Hum Genet 24:30a, 1972.
10. Antley RM, Hartlage LC, Kopitzke CA: Factors related to seeking and responding to genetic counseling. Am J Hum Genet 24:27a, 1972.
11. Falek AJ: Use of the coping process to achieve psychological homeostasis in genetic counseling. In de la Cruz F, Lubs HA (eds): "Genetic Counseling." New York: Raven Press, 1977.
12. Solnit AJ, Stark MH: Mourning and the birth of a defective child. Psychoanal Study Child 16:523–537, 1962.
13. Langsley DG: Psychology of a doomed family. Am J Psychother 15:531–538, 1961.
14. McQuire WJ: The nature of attitudes and attitude change. In Lindzey G, Aaronson E (eds): "The Handbook of Social Psychology." Reading MA: Addison Wesley, 1968, p 136–314.
15. Rokaach M: "Beliefs, Attitudes, and Values." San Francisco: Josey-Bass, 1968.

11. The Genetic Counselor as Information Giver*

Y. Edward Hsia, BM, MRCP, DCH

Informing a client with a genetic problem about genetic facts and options is the *essence* of genetic counseling [1]. The other responsibilities of a genetic counselor, whether a physician or a nonphysician, are essential adjuncts, but these other responsibilities are not genetic counseling. In this chapter the theme will be that the focus of genetic counseling should be to inform. My own attitude, built on my experience as a medical geneticist and as a genetic counselor, strongly favors this concept of genetic counseling as a communicative process with an educational aim [2]. I advocate the responsibility of genetic counselors to be nondirective, nonpsychoanalytic, and nonjudgmental. Discussion of these positions will be preceded by a discussion of the quality of information to be given, the type of information sought by the counselee, and the process of delivering or communicating genetic information [3].

For simplicity, these discussions will focus on the example of a couple's experience with the unexpected appearance of a possible genetic problem in their child. The topics covered will clearly apply to other situations too, such as when one of the couple is the one with a genetically caused disorder, when another relative is affected, or when the risk is of a condition totally outside the counselee's experience. (This occurs when older mothers are counseled about age-related risks of chromosomal abnormalities [4], and when populations are screened for parents at special risk of having children with a genetic disorder [5]).

*Supported by Human Genetics Center grant GM 20124-04 and The National Foundation—March of Dimes service grant C-143.

Birth Defects: Original Article Series, Volume XV, Number 2, pages 169–186
© 1979 The National Foundation

INFORMATION TO BE GATHERED BY THE COUNSELOR

In addition to objective medical diagnosis and pedigree analysis information, information about a family's preconceptions and subjective attitudes are also vital for effective genetic counseling. The genetic counselor must become aware of and remain sensitive to these factors because the way in which these are addressed will determine whether the delivery of genetic information is successful or unsuccessful.

Prior Understanding

The genetic counselor should probe the prior understanding of counselees about their genetic problems and must also know the level of sophistication of the counselee before embarking on any explanations.

Misconceptions about the nature of their problems are the rule in people who seek genetic counseling. For instance, it is difficult for a lay person to accept that a problem can be inherited when the problem has heretofore never appeared in other relatives. Other common misconceptions are that relatives with closer resemblances are more likely to share a genetic problem, or that a problem which had previously appeared in one sex is prone to affect only relatives of the same sex (although true for male maternal relatives with X-linked recessive disorders). Any such misconceptions have to be uncovered and corrected, otherwise the client may be no wiser after genetic instruction, because false foundations will undermine the interpretation of facts.

The approaches used in genetic counseling should obviously be pitched at a level appropriate for the individual client's educational level, so that explanations are neither too elementary nor too complex.

Stability

The emotional, psychiatric, socioeconomic, and family stabilities of counselees have to be ascertained, lest genetic counseling do more harm than good. If a family is more in need of psychotherapy, social rehabilitation, family or marriage counseling than in need of genetic counseling, they should be referred to the appropriate resources. Genetic counseling is best postponed or even abandoned when it is untimely or unlikely to be beneficial.

Recent family crises, such as the discovery of a genetic problem or the death of an affected child, will lead to a natural period of acute grief. In such a state, a counselee may be unwilling or unable to consider genetic information, even though the same information may offer immediate consolation and be instrumental in resolving his or her grief. Thus a sensitive counselor has to assess the receptive state of a counselee, and when counseling is likely to be most beneficial.

Psychiatric disturbances can render a person incapable of rational decisions about genetic data. These disturbances may require the professional attention of a psychiatrist; genetic counseling would be futile for an irrational person.

Socioeconomic problems are sometimes so pressing that a counselee is unable to concentrate on other matters. Finding means to ease these problems would be an essential service for the family, without which genetic counseling may be meaningless.

Marital instability is often an important "hidden agenda." In many current cultures, marriage breakdown is not uncommon, but any preexisting stresses can be seriously aggravated by a handicapped child or other genetic problem, or the genetic problem can precipitate instability in a formerly stable marriage. Without becoming embroiled in marriage counseling, the counselor should try to determine whether the genetic information and reproductive options available will be detrimental or have a constructive effect. This will guide how or when genetic information should be given, if at all.

Attitudes

The emotional attitude of a person asking for genetic counseling may include elements of apprehension, confusion, or suspicion. These will strongly influence how a geneticist's information is received [6].

Awareness of a counselee's attitudes and foibles will guide a genetic counselor to adopt the best approach for an individual counselee or family.

A self-made executive had impatiently sought out a succession of specialists in various medical centers for his only daughter's problems but rejected each of their preliminary opinions. Our adoption of a brutally frank approach proved to be effective, especially when our diagnosis was confirmed by further testing. When he was finally presented with incontrovertible facts, he became convinced that nothing was being concealed from him.

In this example, the father, who was accustomed to dealing decisively with difficult situations, coped best when allowed to face the grim truth.

If the attitudes of families are not sympathetically considered, it may be totally impossible to win their trust or to help them.

A mother came from Europe to seek our help for her daughter's genetic problem, despite our strong endorsements of her daughter's own physician in Europe, who was internationally respected. He had been authoritarian and had seemed aloof in his dealings with this family, and so this mother came far afield for a second opinion, because that specialist had totally failed to respect her attitudes and did not have her trust.

Reproductive Attitudes

Because one of the primary objectives of genetic counseling is to help families make reproductive decisions, the reproductive attitude of a counselee is an important determinant of how he or she receives genetic information. Unfortunately even the reproductive attitudes of the general population are still poorly understood. These attitudes are influenced by social background, economic status, marital stability, family pressures, and many other factors [7]. Reproductive attitudes are also unstable, being subject to change as the life experience of a couple changes. Specifically, if a handicapping condition appears in a child, this can have unpredictable repercussions on a couple's reproductive desires. After a child has died, many couples express strong motivation to have another child as soon as possible. Often a handicapped child will demand so much love and attention that reproductive drives wither.

> One couple confided that after the birth of a severely handicapped child, although they had been drawn closer together, they had lost all interest in sex.

Individual families' reproductive decisions occasionally are based on unusual rationalizations.

> An older couple, whose only child had Down syndrome, wanted very much to have another — unaffected — child, because of their desire to have someone to care for their child with Down syndrome after they themselves have passed on.

One of the major advances in genetics is the recent development of antenatal diagnosis for many genetic disorders [4]. Because this carries with it the implication that an affected fetus can be aborted, a family's opposition to abortion can close this option for them. Sometimes this opposition is immutably based on religious grounds, but even a family's staunch beliefs can be modified when this test alone can assure the birth of an unaffected child. A family's reproductive attitudes must be respected, but the counselee should be encouraged and helped to resolve any conflicts he or she may have about the issue of aborting an abnormal child, preferably long before the time for the test.

> A pregnant teenager had two brothers with Duchenne muscular dystrophy. By the time she sought genetic counseling, amniocentesis could not be delayed and was performed with little chance for her to reflect on its implications. While waiting for the result of the test, however, she became increasingly distressed about aborting a male fetus on the hypothetic risk (25%) that a male fetus of hers might develop muscular dystrophy. When told that the fetus was male, she decided to continue the pregnancy. (Happily, after birth her son was found to be unaffected.)

A second example illustrates even more forcibly that full explanation of genetic options and their implications must precede procedures such as amniocentesis.

A 40-year-old woman had amniocentesis performed by her obstetrician with routine explanation. The specimen was barely adequate, but a diagnosis of trisomy 13 was made. When referred for counseling, the mother turned out to be adamantly against abortion for any reason, and so the test was of no benefit to her [8] .

INFORMATION SOUGHT BY THE COUNSELEE

However earnest the genetic counselor might be about giving genetic information, when nongenetic concerns are uppermost a family will not be receptive to this information. A counselee's motives for seeking consultation can include any or all of the following:

What is the Cause?

There is a natural tendency to seek an explanation for any problem, and if a person has insufficient facts on which to base a reasonable explanation, he or she may fantasize an unrealistic one. When parents have a handicapped child, they often conclude that the condition arose from a "sin" of commission or omission by one or both parents [9] . This results in an overwhelming sense of guilt that may cloud their judgment and prevent them from making the wisest decisions for themselves or their child.

When the sense of guilt or responsibility is built on correct understanding of facts, the genetic counselor cannot deny these facts, but when it is built on fantasy, a factual, naturalistic explanation for genetic disorders can be very therapeutic.

Some counselees are morbidly curious about their problems. Occasionally they will have read extensively about it in whatever literature is available to them. Such excessive fascination can divert a parent from his or her other responsibilities, and so the charge for a genetic counselor is not only to explain about a genetic problem, but also to put it in perspective without underemphasizing it or overemphasizing it.

What Care Can Be Given?

Often families seek a geneticist not because they want to know about genetic causes or risks but rather because they seek management resources for their children's problems. These may include medical supervision, physical rehabilitation, special education, etc. Such families may be concerned exclusively about care, and may have fixed procreative attitudes, with no interest in knowing about reproductive risks or options.

The geneticist clearly has an obligation to respond to this type of enquiry, but provision of care, or referral to appropriate resources for care, is not genetic counseling. This service is an essential part of what every geneticist should offer, although it is outside the strict definition of genetic counseling.

What Will Be the Course?

A family with a handicapped child may be most concerned about the anticipated course of the child's condition. Depending on the family, there may be deep ambivalence between the parents' natural affections for their child and suppressed feelings of rejection or hostility toward the child. It is rare for these negative feelings to be openly admitted or even recognized by a family. Nonetheless, these may be ulterior reasons for concerns about the child's quality of life and life expectancy.

The geneticist will seldom be able to predict survival accurately, but he or she should strive to explain simply and objectively what may lie ahead for the child and how this may affect other members of the family [10].

What Family Planning Choices Are Available?

This is the central question in genetic counseling. People coming for genetic counseling often expect an absolute answer; many counselees expect to have a single course of action recommended to them, with certainty of a happy outcome.

It is not unusual for people to be referred for genetic counseling without any realization of what genetic counseling can offer. An unexpected nondirective explanation of risks and options can be unsettling and confusing to them, because they are left with the task of making their own decisions, despite the fact that they can now make an informed choice.

INFORMATION TRANSFER FROM COUNSELOR TO COUNSELEE

The challenge of effectively conveying complex information is what makes genetic counseling as much an art as a science, because all of a family's other concerns have to be considered as well. Although the essence of genetic counseling is merely to convey a numerical prediction and a list of options, it rarely suffices simply to state this information in a few sentences. The counselee may have many questions and misconceptions that need to be resolved, and even the most straightforward of statements can be misunderstood, misinterpreted, forgotten, or rejected as untrue or unacceptable [11].

In order to have information transferred, a rapport must be established between the counselor and the counselee. This relationship must be based on the counselee's trust that the counselor knows the facts and will be open and truthful about what he or she knows and does not know. If a counselee perceives that all personal concerns have been sympathetically considered, the counseling session(s) will proceed much more smoothly and constructively.

The Time, Pace, and Place

The timing of genetic counseling can be inopportune, as discussed in the previous section, but also its duration can be too brief and hasty, or too drawn-out and exhausting. Optimal timing depends on when the counselee recognizes the need for genetic information [12]; when he or she is best prepared to receive it; and when it can be best conveyed free of other distractions or time conflicts. Those responsible for the primary health needs of a family are in a key position to alert a family to the possible benefits of genetic information, but then the initiative should pass to the family, to decide when they wish to pursue the matter.

If there are practical or emotional reasons for urgency, these should certainly be met. Otherwise, preparations for genetic counseling ought to be paced so that all necessary prior information is collected and analyzed without undue haste.

The time needed for genetic counseling is difficult to gauge beforehand. A single brief session may suffice for one counselee; another may need prolonged, repeated sessions before the genetic information can be satisfactorily absorbed. Regardless of the duration, there should be an unhurried atmosphere, and the session should not proceed beyond the limits of physical or emotional endurance. It is far better to arrange for a later meeting than to attempt to continue when the counselee is overly upset or tired.

The locale for genetic counseling need not be luxurious, but it must convey a sense of uninterrupted privacy. A busy clinic office or hospital room is far from ideal, and the constant intrusion of telephones or extraneous noises can distract seriously from the atmosphere. Even the decor and furnishings can influence genetic counseling. A room that is too large or too small; chairs that are set too far apart or too close together, or are too hard or too soft; and decorations that are too distracting can all hinder the receptiveness of a sensitive counselee.

A lady, while waiting to be seen, was deeply offended by the garish cover photograph of a weekly magazine left lying on a chair. This so incensed her that she rejected or misconstrued everything else that happened that day.

The Persons

There is no single answer to the question of who should be present at a genetic counseling session. In some situations, a counselee is best seen by himself or herself. In others, a married or engaged couple should be seen together. Usually it is better for them to be seen without the distracting presence of a young child or of other relatives. Occasionally, however, a larger family gathering is best. Group sessions, for several individuals or couples who have similar problems, might be a very effective way of conveying genetic information [13]. The interaction of the individuals with each other, the sharing of common concerns, and the raising of common questions can often be of great benefit to all members of such a group, but the fragile relationships of a group session can be easily shattered if one member is deliberately or inadvertently destructive.

The person and qualifications of the counselor are discussed in other chapters, but the important requisites are that the counselor knows both the facts and the counselees, is experienced in counseling, and is respected and accepted by the counselees. It is unwise for the number of counselors greatly to outnumber the number of counselees, but two or more members of a harmonious counseling team can be very effective, particularly if each of the members can be identified by the counselees as having something to offer. In our experience of using a social worker to help collect prior personal information from families, the presence of the same familiar social worker during the later session with the genetic counselor can be reassuring [14]. The social worker can fulfill another role, too, in ensuring that the discussion will include unasked questions in areas of special concern to the counselees.

Other participants and observers are seldom helpful and may be harmful, although their presence is often unavoidable, for instance, in training situations. Nonetheless, the worst example to give trainees is to insert them obtrusively into a delicate counseling situation without the prior consent of the counselees.

The Manner and Content

For most clients, genetic counseling is best accomplished in face-to-face confrontation, which allows a free exchange of questions and answers and the use of both verbal [15] and nonverbal communications [16]. Sometimes genetic counseling is possible only by letter or telephone, both of which can be reasonably adequate means of communication.

Telephone conveying of genetic information, however, can be fraught with hazard.

A young couple insisted that they be given the test results of a genetic test on their daughter by telephone, refusing to travel an hour to discuss the results with us. Against our judgment, they were told their daughter's test indicated the presence of a genetic disease which would not cause any detectable problems for several decades. They thanked us for the information, assured us they understood, and declined to discuss it any further.

The next day the father telephoned us very concerned that their pediatrician would not see their daughter that very day. It took much persuasion to assure him that his daughter was in no immediate danger.

Eventually this couple did come to a better understanding of their problem, yet the initial shock of the information might have been mitigated if it had not been transmitted by telephone.

The counselor's manner should be simultaneously authoritative and sympathetic. A total lack of sympathy can antagonize a counselee, preventing effective transfer of information. Too sympathetic or reassuring a manner can be equally misleading, because the purpose of the counseling is to convey facts and to reassure only when the reassurance is compatible with reality. With experience it will become quite clear to the genetic counselor that the approach which is most effective for one client will be quite different from the one that works well for another, but the adoption of different manners for different families must never be unnatural or contrived.

The counselee inevitably is in a state of tension. This can be so excessive as to impede his or her ability to assimilate any offered genetic information. If a conversational manner or other attempts at reassurance do not succeed in reducing the state of tension, information transfer may fail, at least for that session.

The content of material to be covered should be planned, with a prepared but flexible agenda. Appropriate responses should be given to the questions of major concern to the counselees, and an explanation of the genetic risks and reproductive options open to them should be given in a manner that is acceptable and at a level that is comprehensible.

There is a tendency for inexperienced counselors to include a miniature discourse on the whole of genetics in their explanation of recurrence risks. This is an understandable temptation that should be consciously repressed. For instance, when discussing a chromosomal problem, there is no need to explain about fundamentals of Mendelism; if a family is unsophisticated, it is unimportant whether they know the normal number of chromosomes in a human cell. Similarly, in explaining the X-linked recessive pattern of inheritance, it is usually unnecessary to explain about X and Y chromosomes, let alone lyonization, unless specifically asked to do so. Mathematical models of polygenic inheritance should be avoided in presenting empiric recurrence risks unless the counselee is a mathematician or a quantitative geneticist.

Verbal. The use of repetitive or flowery phrases is a failing of minor importance in social communication, but may clutter up information transfer in genetic counseling. The use of technical jargon is a much more serious offense commonly committed by geneticists and physicians. It should be studiously avoided. Certain words have emotionally-laden meanings — "leprosy" or "cancer" sound much more sinister than "dermatitis" or "stomach ulcer," though the former conditions are not necessarily more serious. Similarly it is inadvisable to talk about "bad genes," or about whose "fault" it was, or to use words such as "dwarf," "moron," "madness," or "ugliness" when referring to the condition of an affected family member. The purpose of counseling is to inform without upsetting; so euphemisms are perfectly acceptable, provided they do not obscure meaning. The word "abortion" is a special case. To many lay people it denotes a medical or criminal procedure, whereas physicians often use it to refer to any miscarriage. Also, when talking about "termination of pregnancy," euphemistic phrases are less likely to cause offense, and the basic issues can be confronted more objectively.

Difficulties in dealing with clients who speak English poorly or not at all should never be minimized, and a good interpreter should always be used whenever possible. The best interpreter is a knowledgeable neutral person, because even in an unfamiliar tongue one can often sense that a relative or other biased interpreter is embellishing or critiquing the genetic information.

Numerical. Precision in calculations and accuracy of numbers are absolute necessities for theoretic analysis of genetic mechanisms or estimations of prevalence and incidence of genetic disorders. To the counselee, however, the numbers are only helpful in giving an impression of the relative probabilities of different outcomes [17]. An expectant mother only cares about whether a condition will affect the fetus she is carrying, regardless of its precise statistical probability. Therefore in genetic counseling the counselee must be made to understand that a counselor can only provide a sophisticated guess of genetic risks, and can *never* guarantee that a child will be normal. This is because of the predictable but undiagnosable chance (approximately 3%) that any child may be born with a major malformation, besides dangers of prematurity, birth injury, and other hazards.

> A young couple were extremely angry when their second child in-
> herited the same genetic condition afflicting their first child. They
> had understood their risk was one in four, and expected to have
> three normal children after their first affected one.

The concept of statistical risks vs the willingness to gamble are two poorly appreciated idiosyncracies which interact in very different ways in different people to determine their attitudes and behavior [1, 17].

Nonverbal. In addition to verbal inflections, nonverbal messages are conveyed by eye contact, demeanor, and the counselor's clothes or uniform [16]. These messages can support or undermine the counseling information.

Written. Articles from newspapers and periodicals can be very informative to certain families. Many special-interest organizations have explanatory pamphlets which can be very educational and helpful, but these should be systematically screened before use, because some well-meaning agencies produce frightening, obscure, or inaccurate material.

In our own counseling service and in many others, a personally written letter is used to reinforce the verbal counseling session [18]. This approach is likely to reduce misunderstandings and to correct confused memories about verbally transmitted information. I have doubts about the utility of tape-recorded material [2], but this may prove suitable for some situations.

Reservations and Promises

The genetic counselor should explain about the limitations of his or her knowledge and ability to promise that a future child will be born healthy and normal. This includes limitations in the accuracy of diagnostic tests such as amniocentesis.

Listening and Observing

Throughout the entire genetic counseling process, including both the gathering and the giving of information, the interviewer must be receptive to nonverbal signals from the counselee and must be willing to be interrupted whenever the counselee wishes to ask a question. Even with the most thorough of preparations and the most attentive of counselees, the counselor must always be ready to listen.

Very crucial information can be conveyed by the attitudes of a couple toward each other during a counseling session. How they sit, whether they touch each other, the tone of voice used, all give revealing clues to the marital balance and to who tends to lead the partnership. A change of expression, a glint of moisture in the eyes, and a shift of posture can all be strong indications to change the pace of the counseling session.

The unasked question is often of far greater importance than that which is readily expressed.

> The young sister of a boy with Duchenne muscular dystrophy was counseled very gently and carefully about the risk of Duchenne muscular dystrophy appearing in any of her future sons. At the conclusion of the counseling session, because she still looked worried, she was encouraged to ask further questions, whereupon she asked, "Is it catching?"

In this illustration the counselor had failed to ascertain, until it was almost too late, that this girl's major concern was an unrealistic fear that she might contract her brother's condition.

Silences must be carefully attended to also, especially when one member of a couple fails to take part in the discussion. At times this may signify anxiety or confusion, which needs to be resolved; at other times this may signify hostility or rejection.

> A young pregnant woman was extremely anxious about the risk of bearing a child with spina bifida, because her sister had had the devastating condition. At genetic counseling she was told her risk was small, but that the condition could be tested for by measuring amniotic fluid alpha-fetoprotein. Her husband, who had majored in biology, sat silent throughout the session. After counseling, she telephoned to cancel her appointment for amniocentesis, because her husband felt the risk was too small to worry about.

For this woman, the counseling session had failed to provide any relief of anxiety because the counselor had failed to include her husband more actively in the discussion. If his dismissal of the risk had been appreciated, the couple could have been helped to discuss and perhaps resolve the discrepancy between his cold objectivity and her subjective fears, which were strongly colored by her intimate acquaintance with the condition.

To ensure that an *exchange* of information has occurred, the counselor should refrain from talking incessantly. He or she must listen attentively, stop at times to allow questions, and not feel uncomfortable with periods of silence, since shared silence is an integral part of a communication process.

Reinforcement

Genetic information can be reinforced at the time of initial transfer by restating it in different ways and by having different members of a counseling team endorse each other's statements. Later reinforcement can be by repeated sessions, endorsements from the primary physician, use of written information, or use of telephone or questionnaire follow-up.

Recruitment of other key individuals, apart from the counselee's physician, including social workers, relatives, and ministers, can sometimes be very supportive for a family with special genetic problems or with special difficulties in accepting genetic information.

WHAT TO AVOID

When explaining such distressing problems as those about a seriously handicapped child, dealing with such intimate topics as a couple's reproductive attitudes, or discussing such controversial topics as abortion of an abnormal fetus, there are many treacherous pitfalls where inappropriate statements can produce serious misunderstandings, cause offense, or, worse still, mislead a family into an unwise course of action.

In contrast to the positions of the following chapters, I will emphasize the negative and dangerous aspects of assuming an interventionist role.

Decison-Making

Counselees occasionally ask specifically that a counselor advise them about what to do. They may be surprised or even disappointed if the counselor declines to be directive. The genetic counselor is in command of all the medical and genetic facts, and has paid careful attention to all of a family's other concerns. Why should he or she not be directive?

Dr. Cedric Carter, one of the most respected and most wide-read genetic counselors in the world, has become disenchanted with the failure of his counselees to respond to genetic risks the way he himself would have done, and has progressively come around to the practice of offering his opinion about the course of action he considers best for a couple [19].

There are hazards to being directive in this way. If a family has ambivalent feelings about the advice, they may opt for a contrary course and discover that the consequences are quite acceptable, resulting in loss of respect for the counselor. More importantly, a family may follow a prescribed course and find that the outcome was either different from what had been predicted — to the discredit of the counselor — or the predicted outcome had consequences that eventually became unacceptable to the family — to their own detriment. These unhappy complications should be avoided by the prudent counselor, for the sake of the counselees and their long-range peace of mind.

It may be argued that if the counselor did indeed know best, he or she would be shirking responsibility by failing to direct a family's decision. The issue is who *does* know the best course for a family to take. The counselor will make the better genetic prediction because of his or her professional skills. The procreative drive of counselees, however, its intensity, constancy, and durability are beyond the professional ken of the geneticist [1, 7]. Other aspects of the personal vagaries of counselees are equally imponderable, such as the willingness or ability of a person to accept and adapt to a compromise solution, and the strength of character needed for a person to cope with stressful life events [20, 21].

For all of these reasons, I judge it more advisable to give clients the genetic facts as objectively as possible and to refrain from giving the final recommendation of how these facts should be spliced into their personal equations. The clients themselves are the ones who must decide how best to weigh their own personal factors, and are the only ones who can judge when the burden of these personal factors [22] has shifted sufficiently to justify a change of mind. I do concur that the counselor should not withdraw from an ambivalent couple, but rather that the couple should be encouraged to find the best course of action for themselves. Whatever the decision, the counselor should help the couple to live with it, and must be very careful not to impose his or her own judgment, especially if it differs from that of the couple [23].

Rational decision-making is not a decision judged to be rational by the counselor. Rather it is a decision made by a counselee who has pondered genetic facts and reproductive options [1]. Hence the final decision may be one that appears unorthodox or illogical to an outside observer, but if a counselee chooses a reproductive option after careful deliberate thought, the decision is rational. The charge of the genetic counselor is not to persuade a client to adopt a certain course, but to enlighten the client about the various available courses and the predicted consequences of each course [6].

Similarly, a counselee should be made to realize that postponement of a definitive decision is often a prudent decision in itself. Furthermore, unless a decision has irrevocable consequences, the counselee always retains the option of changing his or her mind in the light of later developments. However concerned (or curious) the counselor is about the decisions of a counselee, the privacy and right of reversal of the counselee has to be respected.

Psychotherapy

Inevitably the personal and intimate nature of the information given in genetic counseling has strong psychologic implications. The counselor must tread warily in dealing with counselees, lest untoward and serious psychologic disturbances be triggered.

Since most genetic counselors are not trained in psychotherapy, I am of the opinion that, in general, they should not probe too deeply into a client's psyche. If unusual or unhealthy psychologic disturbances show up in a counselee, for the sake of both the counselee and the counselor, psychiatric consultation would be a far better course than amateurish attempts at psychotherapy by the counselor.

Guilt. The high probability that counselees have developed a sense of guilt about their genetic problems has already been discussed. The counselor should certainly realize that a counselee might harbor a sense of guilt, and should strive to relieve any blame by providing a factual explanation for the appearance of genetic problems. In providing genetic information, a counselor should be alert to the danger that the type of information to be given, or an inadvertent remark, could worsen a counselee's feelings.

Defense mechanisms. When people are faced with overwhelming stress, their natural psychologic defense mechanisms become operative, successively passing from shock through denial, and depression, eventually to resolution [9]. Frequently, factual genetic data may be instrumental in accelerating this process, but sometimes deep personality weaknesses are bolstered by resistant defense mechanisms which are best left intact. The excessive probing or undermining of an individual's defense mechanisms can cause irreparable harm if the underlying problems have no solution. Therefore, if a counselor blunders into these sensitive areas, the counselee may be forced into a less realistic, more withdrawn, or even suicidal frame of mind.

The son of a Jehovah's Witness had severe retardation and the deformities of Hunter syndrome. When referred for genetic evaluation, the father insisted that his son's problems were due to chronic sinus infection, and stubbornly held to the conviction that cure of his son's sinusitis would result in a dramatic return to normality. The father refused to bring his son back for confirmatory tests or to return for counseling because he felt it would have undermined God's plans for his son.

In trying to help this family, the geneticist and the family physician only succeeded in driving the family away from all sources of medical help, and deeper into their world of denial and unreality.

Moralizing

Nothing can alienate a counselee more rapidly than an impression that the counselor feels morally superior. Sometimes people with genetic problems, like other people, have bizarre attitudes and life experiences. Any hint of derision or condemnation on the part of the counselor may destroy prospects for effective genetic counseling. This does not mean that antisocial or self-destructive attitudes and actions are to be condoned, but the counselor is far more likely to succeed in helping his or her clients if these undesirable attitudes and acts are treated dispassionately. A counselee may be immutably entrenched in a fixed life-style, but the most promising way to help the counselee is by an objective discussion of the consequences of a course of action and the alternatives to it.

Another aspect of moralizing to be avoided is the overt or implied disapproval of other physicians or nonmedical resources relied upon by the counselee. Physicians are not always perfect, and there may have been inappropriate treatment or imperfect communication between counselees and their physicians, but no useful purpose is served in weakening any trust that the counselees may still have in their physician. If there are serious differences of opinion with the physician that cannot be resolved by direct discussion, the only reputable and ethical recourse is to reveal these differences to the counselee. When a counselee has already broken off from a physician, there is no point in even revealing any such differences, and the only responsibility is to help give the counselee some general guidelines about how best to seek a new physician. Many other resources are relied upon by counselees. These range from educational authorities for their children to community workers, psychologists, ministers, and relatives. Some of these provide splendid support, but others may be less than adequate. The same principle of avoiding overt disapproval while helping to guide the family to a best possible solution still applies.

A more difficult situation arises when a family wishes to invest in quasi-fraudulent treatment regimens. They may have heard about a miracle cure offered by faith healers, unorthodox health systems, or medical practitioners of questionable repute. When such a situation arises, it generally does little good to condemn the "miracle cure" outright. This will only result in a confrontation where the family is forced to make a choice between a rational approach and a cultist approach. If families can be offered little realistic hope by physicians, they are susceptible targets for cultism. They can be protected from the allurements of such cults by being forewarned and by being given some guidance as to whether the hope offered by a cult is inordinately expensive. A few families, however, will wish to explore any avenue that offers hope. When this occurs, the counselor can only seek to enlighten, and should still avoid being overtly directive, because it will not work.

The Myth of the Unbiased, Nondirective Counselor

It is obvious that the ideal of nondirectiveness is an impractical counsel of perfection. Whenever a counselor presents information, however sincerely he or she may strive for objectivity, the tone of voice, choice of words, and nonverbal body language will all add subjective color to the objective facts.

One very pertinent example is the issue of abortion embodied in the option of prenatal diagnosis. The mere discussion of prenatal diagnosis implies endorsement of the procedure and of abortion for an abnormal fetus.

When the genetic counselor has strong personal attitudes or biases, such as about therapeutic abortion, these are less likely to interfere with the counseling process when they are openly revealed [24] than when they are deliberately or unconsciously hidden by the counselor.

The influence of the counselor's background on counseling is discussed in the chapter by Sorenson and Culbert. My attitude is that the inevitable differences in background between the counselor and the counselee mean they cannot share the same biases. This is to me a cogent argument for the counselor to refrain from being overly directive. While recognizing that the perfect nondirective counselor is a myth, I maintain that the best interests of the counselee are served when the counselor sincerely avoids at least being overtly directive.

CONCLUSIONS

In conclusion, in order for the genetic counselor to function as an information giver, he or she has to take careful measures to ensure that the information to be given is accurate medically, adequate genetically, and appropriate psychologically to meet the questions and concerns of the counselees.

The process of transferring information should be an interactive process. The counselees should be encouraged to participate actively in seeking answers to their questions, and solutions for their problems. For optimal information transfer the counselor should ensure that the timing is propitious, the place is acceptable, and all the participants are compatible. The transfer of the information should make use of verbal, written, and nonverbal communication modalities, and ideally should be with reinforcement.

If counselees are to utilize genetic information effectively, they must make their own decisions, free from any interference or pressure by the counselor. Because the most perceptive and sensitive counselor can still misjudge the best reasonable course of action for a counselee, the counselor should not express personal opinions or attitudes that might unduly influence a counselee's decisions.

REFERENCES

1. Hsia YE: Approaches to the appraisal of genetic counseling. In Lubs H, de la Cruz F (eds): "Genetic Counseling." New York: Raven Press, 1977.
2. Fraser FC: Genetic counseling. Am J Hum Genet 26:636–659, 1974.
3. Hsia YE, Hirschhorn K, Silverberg RL, Godmilow L (eds): "Counseling in Genetics." New York: Alan R Liss. (In press).
4. Milunsky A: "Hereditary Disorders and the Fetus: Diagnosis, Prevention and Treatment." 2nd Ed. New York: Plenum Press, 1978.
5. Childs B, Simopoulos AP (eds): "Genetic Screening, Programs, Principles, and Research." Washington, DC: National Academy of Sciences, 1975.
6. Waitzkin H, Stoeckle JD: The communication of information about illness: Clinical sociological and methodological considerations. Adv Psychosom Med 8:180–215, 1972.
7. Hass PH: Wanted and unwanted pregnancies: A fertility decision-making model. J Soc Issues 30:125, 1974.
8. Elias S, Mahoney MJ: Prenatal diagnosis of trisomy 13 with decision not to terminate pregnancy. Obstet Gynecol 47:75s–76s, 1976.
9. Livsey CG: Physical illness and family dynamics. Adv Psychosom Med 8: 237–251, 1972.
10. McCollum AT: "Coping with Prolonged Health Impairment in Your Child." Boston: Little, Brown & Co, 1975.
11. Raimbault G, Cachin O, Limal J-M, Eliacheff C, Rappaport R: Aspects of communication between patients and doctors: An analysis of the discourse in medical interviews. Pediatrics 55:401–405, 1975.
12. Zola IK: Studying the decision to see a doctor: review, critique, corrective. Adv Psychosom Med 8:216–236, 1972.
13. Bracken MB, Grossman G, Hachamovitch M, Sussman D, Schrier D: Abortion counseling: An experimental study of three techniques. Am J Obstet Gynecol 117:10–20, 1973.

14. Hsia YE, Silverberg RL: Response to genetic counseling: A follow-up survey. (Abstract) Pediatr Res 7:290, 1973.
15. Leventhal H, Fischer K: What reinforces in a social reinforcement situation — words or expressions? J Pers Soc Psychol 14:83–94, 1970.
16. Fast J: "Body Language." Philadelphia: JB Lippincott, 1970.
17. Pearn JH: Parents' subjective interpretation of risks offered in genetic counselling. J Med Genet 10:129–134, 1973.
18. Hsia YE: Choosing my children's genes: Genetic counseling. In Lipkin M, Rowley PT (eds): "Genetic Responsibility." New York: Plenum Press, 1973.
19. Carter CO, Roberts JAF, Evans KA, Buck AR: Genetic clinic: A follow-up. Lancet 1: 281–285, 1971.
20. Hsia YE: Parental reactions to genetic counseling. Contemp Ob/Gyn 4:99–106, 1974.
21. Dohrenwend BS, Dohrenwend BP: "Stressful Life Events: Their Nature and Effects." New York: J Wiley & Sons, 1974.
22. Leonard CO, Chase GA, Childs B: Genetic counseling: A consumers' view. N Engl J Med 287:433–439, 1972.
23. Kaplan DM, Smith A, Grobstein R: Family mediation of stress. Soc Work 18:60–69, 1973.
24. Gordon H: Discussion. In Porter IH, Skalko RG (eds): "Heredity and Society." New York: Academic Press, 1973, pp 189–201.

12. The Genetic Counselor as Psychotherapist

Seymour Kessler, PhD

In the pages that follow, I will consider and, at times, attempt to reformulate some of the issues of genetic counseling from the viewpoint of a psychotherapist whose background includes training both in genetics and in clinical psychology. The views expressed here are not necessarily shared by all psychotherapists; others might emphasize different points, or the same ones in different ways. Nevertheless, the line of argument will be familiar to a vast number of mental health professionals. Also, virtually all major problems of genetic counseling — ethics, its goals and techniques, counselor-directiveness, the assessment of counseling outcome, the question of who should counsel — are issues already familiar to the mental health worker.

PSYCHOTHERAPY AND COUNSELING

A brief consideration of psychotherapy is in order. The term psychotherapy has many meanings and describes diverse activities. Harper [1] has described 36 psychotherapeutic systems and, assuredly, this is an underestimate of the number currently being practiced. Although adherents of each system may define psychotherapy differently, virtually all would agree that their work is aimed at helping the client live more effectively. Simply put, psychotherapy is "a situation where two people interact and try to come to an understanding of one another, with the specific goal of accomplishing something beneficial for the complaining person" [2].

Psychotherapy is often associated with the treatment of psychosis and other behavioral disorders. However, a substantial number of the individuals who seek and receive psychotherapy simply need help in dealing with a life crisis or in

Birth Defects: Original Article Series, Volume XV, Number 2, pages 187—200
© 1979 The National Foundation

obtaining greater satisfaction out of their activities and relationships with others. For some, psychotherapy is a healing, restorative experience. For others, it is a means by which the person may grow intellectually and emotionally and/or effect profound changes in one's life. On one extreme, psychotherapy might consist of an intensive course of visits to a therapist over a period of several years or, on the other, of a onetime brief telephone conversation. It is the similarity of the process in both these encounters that identifies them as psychotherapy and makes it possible for enduring consequences to occur.

Frequent attempts have been made to differentiate counseling from psychotherapy. Despite differences in therapeutic attitudes, length of treatment, treatment setting, type of problems, type of patients, techniques, and other variables, these are trivial as compared to their similarities. Psychotherapy and counseling contain the same core dimensions [3]. In this regard, genetic counseling might be considered a kind of psychotherapeutic encounter, or, at the least, an interaction with psychotherapeutic potential. The psychotherapeutic modles most pertinent to the genetic counselling situation are those of brief therapy, crisis intervention, and /or family therapy.

Psychotherapists view the human panorama from a vantage point different from that of the medical geneticist. To the psychotherapist, the process or means by which the goal is achieved is as important as the goal itself. Differing means have differential consequences for the counselees and for the counselor as well.

Because of different interests, training, and, possibly, personality styles, medical geneticists and psychotherapists sometimes assess the same circumstances differently. The former have an overriding concern with the accurate diagnosis of genetic disease, the precise calculation of genetic risk, and other content matters. His/her focus is generally oriented along a past-future dimension; the past reflected in pedigree information, the future in predictive risk figures. Often, he/she approaches the genetic counseling encounter as a self-contained problem-solving situation, an end in itself. The psychotherapist, on the other hand, may have a greater concern for the subjective meaning of content issues, as well as for their intrapsychic and interpersonal consequences. His/her central focus may be on here-and-now issues. Many psychotherapists would view the problems with which counselees come to genetic counseling as life crises, understandable only in the context of their overall life histories as individuals, as members of a family, and as members of a specific social group. They might see genetic counseling as an opportunity to further the cognitive and emotional growth of the counselees.

GENETIC COUNSELING AS PSYCHOTHERAPY

Genetic counseling has all of the essential characteristics of the psychotherapeutic situation. In both situations, the individual seeking help (the counselee) asks for help from a person trained to provide that help (the counselor). Genetic counseling is an encounter between a counselor(s) and counselee(s) in which the former helps the latter understand the nature of a genetic or congenital disorder, deal with its psychologic concomitants, and respond to the challenges that such disorders pose.

Like psychotherapy, genetic counseling is directly concerned with human behavior. Specifically, genetic counseling deals with reproduction, health, and parenthood, as well as the behaviors involved in making decisions and maintaining relationships within a family. Also, as in psychotherapy, the role, beliefs, values, and counseling stance taken by the counselor will influence the behavior of the counselee. This point might be contested by some counselors and geneticists, particularly by those who would like to believe that they are merely conduits for information or are otherwise being nondirective with respect to influencing counselee behavior. It is difficult to believe that such an influence does not occur because there are many subtle means, both verbal and nonverbal, by which the attitudes, beliefs, and decisions of the counselees might be influenced. The stance of maintaining that one is being nondirective, while in reality one is being directive, is an important psychotherapeutic strategy (as, for example, in psychoanalysis) [4]. Parenthetically, data suggest that in genetic counseling there is a substantial gap between the professed ideals of nondirectiveness and the actual practices of genetic counselors [5].

Genetic counselors and psychotherapists both make multiple assumptions about the development and dynamics of human behavior, about human personality, about the nature of man, about what constitutes the "good life," and about the goals of counseling. The counselor who believes that human behavior operates according to stimulus-response principles or one who believes that behavior is largely dominated by unconscious impulses is not likely to counsel in the same way as a counselor who believes that man basically strives toward self-motivation and self-actualization. Similarly, the counselor who believes that he/she has some superior wisdom to impart as to the decisions others should make is likely to behave differently in the counseling situation than the counselor who has faith in the counselees' ability to find their own answers.

THE PROCESS OF COMMUNICATION

The basic vehicle of the genetic counseling encounter is communication. It is important to understand the essential components of human communication. The key features may be summarized as follows:

1) Human communication occurs on multiple simultaneous levels [6, 7].

2) "One cannot *not* communicate" [7] (ie a nonresponse to a message is a communication).

3) When the sender of a message experiences anxiety, the messages being conveyed are likely to be incongruent, ie the messages on the differing levels of communication will not jibe with each other. This is the means by which the counselee may defend him/herself from a loss of self-esteem or from overtly expressing his/her feelings of guilt, shame, or depression.

4) When the receiver of a message experiences anxiety due to actual or anticipated threats to his self-esteem, he/she will defend him/herself by discounting or distorting the message, through selective inattention, by hearing one rather than another level of communication, and by other self-protective strategies.

There are two major levels of communication, the denotative and the metacommunicative. The former encompasses the literal content of communication, whereas the latter is the main route by which the sender conveys messages about needs, feelings, and states of awareness less available to consciousness. It often takes the form of nonverbal behavior (eg posture, gestures, the way one breathes) and is also expressed in the way the voice is used (eg quality, volume, tone). Metacommunication is a commentary on the denotative message. It conveys the sender's attitudes toward the message, him/herself, and the receiver. Satir [7] writes that metacommunication ". . . is a message about a message . . . (and that) humans cannot communicate without, at the same time, metacommunicating. Humans cannot *not* metacommunicate."

Another major aspect of human communication is the syntactic, physical, and social context in which it takes place. The meaning of the question "What are our chances of having a normal child?" is different when it is asked soon after the counselor has already quoted a risk figure (a not uncommon situation) than when it precedes the counselor's statement. Also, the same message is experienced differently depending on the context; the same information conveyed by telephone has a different ring than when conveyed in person. Lastly, the fact that the counseling is carried out on the genetic counselor's home territory, surrounded by the auras and trappings of Authority and Science, has a major influence on the communication process that occurs as well as on the behavior of the participants. The milieu virtually guarantees cooperativeness, subservience, and, at the least, an outward show of compliance on the part of the counselees. Patients and counselees who do not behave according to the expectations of medical and paramedical personnel tend to be quickly labeled as aggressive, obstructive, or uncooperative [8].

The model of communication outlined above has several implications for genetic counseling. First, it points out that there is a continual concurrent interplay between content material and underlying psychologic processes. It is impossible to convey a recurrence risk to counselees without simultaneously conveying multiple other messages, including the counselor's own feelings about the disorder and his/her attitude toward the genetic risk.

Second, it indicates the need for a holistic approach in which the problems and concerns of the counselees are not seen as isolated from other aspects of their lives and in which the counseling integrates both content and process issues. The model also suggests that an emphasis on fragmentation or specialization as, for example, in the so-called team approach to genetic counseling will probably be less effective than one emphasizing an integrative approach and provided by a single professional.

Third, the model suggests that the focus on content issues at the expense of psychologic ones may unwittingly convey messages to counselees that their feelings are either not being understood or are being rejected by the counselor. Thus, the counselor who responds only to the denotative level of the counselee's messages is taking a stance in which the emotional rejection of the latter is likely to occur.

Fourth, the model accounts for the distortion and poor understanding of medical and genetic facts seen in a substantial number of counselees following counseling [9]. Such distortions may be responses to material perceived as threatening to the counselees' self-esteem.

INTERPERSONAL EFFECTS OF GENETIC DISORDERS

The occurrence of a genetic or congenital disorder is known to have a major impact on family functioning [10]. To fully appreciate this point, a knowledge of family dynamics is necessary. Families are systems bound together, usually, by intense and enduring bonds of past experience, social roles, mutual support, and expectations and in which continual transactions occur between the component parts [11]. A change in one component of the system will usually affect all members of the family. As a system, processes are at work to maintain a relatively stable state in the family, such that when a perturbation occurs, the system will function to restore the preexisting equilibrium. This is referred to as family homeostasis. Inevitably, however, events occur which direct the family toward development and differentiation. Some of these events are expectable, ie most families go through them in a fairly standard sequence during the family life cycle. "To some extent, every family has difficulty in mastering expected phases of the family cycle . . . however, even more difficulty may be experienced when traumatic, excessive, and out-of-order changes in the family life cycle take place. Unusual, unexpected events in the family life cycle may overwhelm the coping capacities of family systems that might otherwise have been relatively well able to handle development changes, had they occurred expectedly, in the usual sequence, and over an extended period of time" [11].

Marital discord, separation and divorce, sexual dysfunctions, and depression are common sequelae of the birth of a child with a genetic disorder [10]. To a large extent, the response of parents to a genetic disorder are contingent upon their individual personalities, past responses to stressful events, the stage of the life cycle of the family, the presence (or absence) of a supportive social system, and other important variables. Each couple will adopt a strategy of coping designed to keep distress within manageable limits, maintain a sense of personal worth, and maintain relations with significant others. Following the diagnosis of a genetic disease, some couples may seem to act decisively with respect to further reproduction. The rapidity of such responses may give them little time to reflect or experience the distressing feelings evoked by the diagnosis. Not infrequently, contradictory behavior may be evoked. For example, following the diagnosis of Werdnig-Hoffman disease, the parents of one affected child actively set about educating themselves about genetic engineering and the principles of heredity. Concurrently they sought out the advice of faith healers. Irrespective of our attitudes toward the latter behavior, these individuals were engaged in an important aspect of coping, ie the seeking of information [12] . In this quest, they made use of multiple sources of information: friends, family, librarians, etc. Their search was in the service of maintaining hope and of avoiding the emotional pain involved in accepting the inexorable nature of the disease. Hamburg and Adams [13] describe this coping strategy as follows: "For a while, the depressing impact of the event must be controlled, and this is often accomplished by extensive denial of the seriousness of the illness. As time goes on, there is an increase of depression, which now is better tolerated. The dismal truth is perceived only as rapidly as one can stand it."

The unaffected sibs in a family sometimes bear a disproportionate share of the burden of a genetic disorder. For example, one young woman I saw in psychotherapy had several older brothers affected with muscular dystrophy. In their reaction to these children, as well as to their own feelings of guilt and shame, the parents handed over major caretaking responsibilities to their then preadolescent daughter. Understandably, she perceived her responsibilities as a burden, but the resentments she felt were not allowed to be expressed at home. She eventually fled her parents' home into an early marriage, in which she continued to play the caretaker, nurturing role.

UNCONSCIOUS AGENDAS

Traditional genetic counseling places a strong emphasis on the rational aspects of decision-making regarding abortion, procreation, child rearing, and family planning. However, it is doubtful that decisions concerning these emotionally-laden issues are or can be made entirely in a rational way. Nonrational and unconscious motives and needs play a major role in determining the decisions made about these aspects of human life. Because the counselees are not usually aware of these motives and needs, it is even more important for the counselor to be conscious of them, even though he/she may not need to uncover them in the genetic counseling session.

Counselees will bring to the genetic counseling situation many questions and concerns that go beyond their need to obtain information from the counselor. Frequently, counselees will ask for reassurance regarding the safety of a medical procedure, like, for example, amniocentesis ("Is it safe?" "Will the needle harm the fetus?") or that their baby will be born healthy. Underlying the need for such reassurances are deep-seated fears regarding one's personal survival and the survival of one's children, born and to be born. Some requests have the quality of a demand for a guarantee from the counselor that no harm or defect will occur. Realistically, the counselor does not control fate and cannot give such guarantees. Not infrequently, such requests are based on "magical" thinking, ie the counselor has extraordinary powers to remedy or avert some awful outcome or to drive away the distressing thoughts the counselees may have. Underlying such insecurities may be strong dependency needs to be protected and cared for.

Concerns about one's capacity to reproduce and to produce a normal member of the species are intimately associated with feelings of personal worthiness. The loss of self-worth (which often follows the birth of a child with a genetic disorder) is frequently accompanied by feelings of shame, which, in turn, tends to provoke one to find and assign culpability in another, generally one's spouse. This strategy may bring a temporary restoration of worthiness. However, in the long run, because the spouse is generally of one's choosing and is thus also tied up with self-worth, blaming another offers little solace for the blamer.

In the seeking of genetic counseling or merely being in the role of needing assistance, the counselees are often placed in a vulnerable position in which their self-esteem is in doubt. Differences between the counselor and counselees in education, ethnic background, socioeconomic status, age, and sex may exacerbate concerns about the loss of self-esteem. The counselor needs to be sensitive to this issue. A counseling strategy that overemphasizes these differences is not likely to bolster the counselees' self-esteem.

In coming for counseling or in the process of counseling, long-held secrets regarding an illegitimacy or a therapeutic abortion or some other skeleton in the family closet may be divulged. The exposure of such secrets generally is accompanied by a mixture of intense feelings, often involving anger and a sense of relief from the shame and guilt involved in the concealment.

How the counselees receive and assess genetic facts and information is largely determined by unconscious factors. For example, a person may have the need to expiate guilt feelings generated by a "martyr" mother and may thus experience a 25% risk figure as acceptable and relatively low, whereas another person, who might have strong feelings of inadequacy as a nurturing or giving parent, might view the same figure as an enormous risk.

PSYCHOLOGIC DEFENSES

Genetic counseling deals with important life issues, including survival, security, self-worth and self-esteem, one's adequacy as a parent, maturity, dependency, and the loss of loved ones. These issues generate intense feelings and concerns which are often experienced with discomfort and distress and thus bring into operation psychic mechanisms that dampen out and defend the person from being overwhelmed by these feelings. These psychologic defense mechanisms are discussed in detail by Anna Freud [14] (see Brenner [15] for a shorter treatment). The major psychologic defense mechanisms include repression, denial, reaction formation, projection, isolation of effect, undoing, intellectualization, and others. I will briefly focus on the first two of these defenses here; a more detailed discussion will appear elsewhere [16].

Repression consists of actively barring from consciousness such inner stimuli as unwanted memories, emotions, desires, and wishes. For example, parents sometimes have infanticidal wishes against their "defective" child [17]. Few, however, actually act on their impulse because the wish is repressed and, with the help of other defense mechanisms, is converted into more socially acceptable behavior.

Denial consists of repressing an unpleasant or unwanted piece of external reality. For example, I alluded above to the fact that counselees frequently repeat a key question regarding the safety of a medical procedure or the magnitude of a genetic risk *after* such information has already been provided by the counselor. This "lapse of memory" presumably occurs because the information has been denied access to awareness.

Although some geneticists treat the psychologic defenses as if they were impediments to the counselor's work, it needs to be remembered that these psychologic mechanisms play important adaptive roles in the process of coping with a medical disorder. Psychologic defense mechanisms are mental maneuvers, almost entirely unconscious, by which the person both protects him/herself against feelings of anxiety and fear and provides a sense of security. Freud conceptualized these psychologic mechanisms as an ego function operating to contain anxiety-provoking affects and wishes. Defense mechanisms also serve to protect the individual against threats originating from the external environment. Contemporary views tend to focus on the cognitive operations by which internal and external information is distorted, modified, or blocked from cognitive processing [18].

The diagnosis of a genetic disorder usually poses a threat to the integrity and self-esteem of the person. The responses to such threats are similar to those observed by clinicians in studies of persons facing other major life stresses [13]. One of the common initial responses to major unanticipated stress events is a period of denial, generally accompanied by a feeling of numbness, behavioral constriction, and the avoidance of thoughts and ideas which would remind the person about the event or its implications. The impact of the event is lessened, thus preventing the person from being overwhelmed by intolerable thoughts and strong emotions. Also, by helping to concentrate awareness selectively, the process of denial assists the individual to prepare, physically and emotionally, for the work of dealing actively with the event. Denial serves an adaptive function in that it permits the person to buy time in order to mobilize his/her resources to deal with the stress.

The denial phase of coping with stress events may be followed by a period in which intense affects (anger, depression, fear, guilt, sorrow, etc) emerge both in thought and overtly. In turn, this may evoke further periods of denial. Eventually, as the person subjects the original stress event to repeated cycles of cognitive appraisal and reappraisal [18] and, often, when he/she begins to take action to deal with the consequences of the event, a phase of acceptance sets in. Thus, defensive operations are the major means by which the individual adapts to, copes with, and eventually masters life stresses.

COUNTERTRANSFERENCE

Some counselees have the capacity to elicit specific responses from others, sometimes of a protective nature but not infrequently a rejecting one. Often the counselees are unconsciously expecting the counselor to respond to them in the way significant others in the past have responded to them. This has generally resulted in their experiencing a lowered self-esteem and a damaged sense of competence in their ability to make life decisions. Counselors are not immune to this process. They too may respond to the counselees on the basis of unconscious expectations derived from their past. This is countertransference.

The unconscious projections of the counselor, consisting of the attitudes, beliefs, anxieties, and fears stimulated by the counselees and the issues with which the counselees are dealing, constitute the countertransference. So long as the countertransference remains unconscious, the counselor is likely to misunderstand and distort the counselees' needs. Once they are brought into his/her consciousness, the counselor can begin to use his/her own feelings as a vehicle for understanding the counselees. Moreover, through the awareness of these feelings, the counselor will be able to demarcate clearly the differences between his/

her own responses and those of the counselees. This is not a trivial matter because counselors and counselees do not always appraise the same set of circumstances and facts in the same way. If the counselor does not have a clear sense of psychologic boundaries, he/she is liable to become judgmental, patronizing, or otherwise unaccepting of the counselees' feelings.

SOME THOUGHTS ON COUNSELING AND THE COUNSELOR

One gathers the impression from the genetic counseling literature that providing massive doses of information, facts, statistics, and rational arguments will overcome psychologic defenses, allay fears, and assuage guilt. In my experience, this approach does little toward that end and seldom has the effect the counselor consciously intends. For example, telling counselees that they should not feel guilty or reassuring them that there was nothing that they might have done to avert the birth of their "genetically defective" child, also conveys messages that what they are currently feeling is inappropriate and, perhaps, abnormal. Thus, paradoxically, reassurances are statements of rejection.

Too often, in his/her efforts to be complete and precise in providing information on the details and risks of medical procedures, the counselor may succeed in heightening already existing anxiety. (Sometimes, such tactics are unconscious attempts to bias the counselees' behavior in a direction consistent with the counselor's own beliefs and values.) Also, the counselor unwittingly may be attacking needed defensive structures which help the counselees make sense out of their experiences and provide them with hope regarding the future.

Responses of the counselor which are totally on a content level of communication address themselves to an extremely limited range of the counselee's inner world. The task of the genetic counselor is to shift mental gears, quickly and flexibly, between content and various levels of process during the course of the counseling session (it's not easy!). For example, following the provision of the recurrence risk for cystic fibrosis to a couple who had two affected children, one of the counselees asked, "Are you *sure* it's only 25%?" Her tone seemed sarcastic and disbelieving. I replied yes and immediately explored the meaning of the question. The counselee reiterated that she had two affected children. To have attempted at this point to reaffirm the principle of independent probabilities for each pregnancy would not have been helpful for this couple. Rather, I chose to respond to her sense of having gotten more than her just share and to the burden that she evidently was experiencing as a parent of two energy-draining children. This approach opened the way for both counselees to experience and share with each other their respective frustrations and disappointments. Only later in the session when I reviewed the major themes we had discussed earlier did I come back to the unfinished content issue. But, again, it was done in the context of the personal meaning the recurrence risk had for the counselees.

The occurrence of a genetic disorder often generates resentment and anger toward the spouse, the child, and, not infrequently, the physician. Frequently, feelings of guilt are expressed as anger. Also, anger may be used as a defense against making guilt feelings conscious. The genetic counselor can play an important role in providing an accepting milieu in which these feelings can be openly expressed. By being defensive of his/her reputation and expertise, or that of a colleague, the counselor may thwart the expression not only of angry feelings, but of any feelings at all.

Considerable data are available concerning the factors which promote or inhibit effective counseling [19, 20]. Carkhuff and Berenson [20] write,

> There is an extensive body of evidence suggesting that all human interactions designated by society as "more knowing" and "less knowing" may have facilitative or retarding effects upon the less known. *Thus, in significant counseling relationships, the consequences may be constructive or deteriorative on intellective as well as psychological indexes.* * In addition, there is extensive evidence to indicate that, to a large degree, the facilitative or retarding effects can be accounted for by a core of dimensions which are shared by all human processes. . . . These core dimensions . . . [involve] . . . emphathetic understanding, positive regard, genuineness, and concreteness or specificity of expression, offered by those persons designated as more knowing.

Effective counseling, measured on a variety of indices, occurs when the counselor provides high levels of these factors. Conversely, deteriorative consequences occur when low levels of these dimensions are provided. These findings suggest that if genetic counseling is a meaningful human encounter (as I believe it is), then it has the potential for both positive and negative consequences. From the psychotherapist's viewpoint, the provision of genetic information in the absence of a growth-promoting, therapeutic relationship would likely have harmful consequences for the counselees and for the persons around them. When cognitive and affective growth does occur, it may be obtained despite, not primarily because of, the information being transmitted by the counselor.

DECISION-MAKING

Under most circumstances, counselees should make their own decisions regarding abortion, reproduction, etc. Decisions made by the counselor for another person are not experienced as being one's own and, like other alien thoughts and feelings, tend not to be integrated well into the cognitive and affective aspects of one's functioning [21]. In the short run, the counselees may be pleased to have

*Sentence italicized by author.

a decision taken out of their hands. In the long run, however, it is self-defeating for it reinforces their sense of inadequacy, incompetence, and helplessness.

One of the frequent difficulties in genetic counseling is for the counselor to push for closure on issues too quickly. I suspect that often, when a counselee asks what the counselor would do or decide in his/her place, the counselee may be responding to a perceived pressure to reach a decision before he/she is ready to do so. The genetic counselor needs to be especially attentive to the counselees' metamessages, as well as his/her own anxiety at this point, and to be ready to back off if he/she is indeed applying pressure for a decision.

An important task for the counselor is to assist the counselees in obtaining a better understanding of the factors that impede or facilitate their decision-making process. This might require that he/she be able to help them develop relatively more effective patterns of responses to one another, to their children, etc. Knowledge of crisis intervention and family therapy skills would be invaluable in this regard. Frequently, important life decisions evoke approach-withdrawal responses, ie ambivalence. The counselor might point this out to the counselees and help them explore the personal meanings of both sides of the ambivalence, as well as the function that the ambivalence plays in impeding their reaching a decision.

The counselor's interventions should always be aimed at helping the counselees become involved in the counseling and in actively finding their own answers and solutions. In the context of psychotherapy, Angyal [21] writes that the atmosphere most conducive to a successful exploration of the decisions that the counselees need to make ". . . is that of a common enterprise, the counselees and the counselor looking at the facts together in as open-minded a way as they can and trying to make sense of them. The spirit in which the counselor conducts this enterprise affects not only the development of insight but also the counselees' confidence in their ability to get at the truth. . . . If the counselor gives interpretations dogmatically, with an air of superior wisdom, the counselees' weak confidence in their own experience is further undermined." (I have changed the wording so that it is more relevant to counseling.) In past relationships with medical professionals, many persons have been placed or have placed themselves into a relatively passive role. This role has major psychologic consequences [22], some of which are antithetic to feeling that one is a master of one's fate. One of the principal therapeutic functions that the genetic counselor can perform is helping the counselees move from a relatively passive to an active psychologic place. By communicating his faith in their wisdom and in their ability to manage their lives and by facilitating rather than directing, he can assist the counselees to become aware of the truths and answers that reside in themselves.

BENEFITS OF A PSYCHOLOGICALLY-ORIENTED APPROACH

I see four major benefits of a psychologically-oriented approach to genetic counseling. First, this approach provides a realistic foundation for understanding the processes of interpersonal communication and decision-making, as well as the other behavioral processes that comprise the subject matter of genetic counseling. This approach places the focus on the dynamics and principles of human behavior, without which little else in genetic counseling makes much sense.

Second, it provides a basis for understanding the counseling process, the nature of the counselor-counselee relationship and the goals of counseling. This approach unifies the principles and practices of genetic counseling with those of other areas of personal counseling. By doing so, it opens the way for geneticists to draw upon the experiences and experimental wealth of colleagues in these allied fields.

Third, it provides a holistic approach to the counselees and their concerns. The problems posed by a genetic disorder and the responses of the counselees to these challenges are placed into the perspective of their overall personality structure and interpersonal functioning. This approach provides an opportunity to help the counselees make important changes in their affective, cognitive, and intellectual functioning. The occurrence of genetic disorders are crises which shake up personal and family modes of functioning and which impose demands for new ways of functioning. These are precisely the moments during the life cycle of the individual and family in which psychotherapeutic intervention is known to be the most effective in changing attitudes, beliefs, and behavior [23].

Fourth, this approach helps define the role of the counselor as a guide or facilitator, involved with the counselees in a common enterprise, participating as a whole person — fallible, feeling, experiencing, and growing — rather than as an uninvolved professional, a technician, or an omniscient answer-man or woman. Of the approaches to genetic counseling, the psychologically-oriented one is probably the most demanding of the counselor. Not only must he/she be proficient in genetics and skilled as a counselor, he/she must also be constantly reaching for greater self-awareness and understanding. To the extent that the counselor can achieve such awareness, he/she can help others achieve it as well.

REFERENCES

1. Harper RA: "Psychoanalysis and Psychotherapy: 36 Systems." Englewood Cliffs: Prentice-Hall, 1959.

2. Bruch H: "Learning Psychotherapy." Cambridge: Harvard University Press, 1974.
3. Patterson CH: "Theories of Counseling and Psychotherapy." New York: Harper & Row, 1966.
4. Haley J: "Strategies of Psychotherapy." New York: Grune & Stratton, 1963.
5. Sorenson JR: Counselors: Self-portrait. Genet Counseling 1:31, 1973.
6. Watzlawick P, Beavin JH, Jackson DD: "An Anthology of Human Communication." Palo Alto: Science & Behavior Books, 1963.
7. Satir V: "Conjoint Family Therapy." Palo Alto: Science & Behavior Books, 1964.
8. Gillum RF, Borsky AJ: Diagnosis and management of patient noncompliance. JAMA 228:1563–1567, 1974.
9. Sorenson JR: Genetic counseling: Some psychological considerations. In Lipkin M Jr, Rowley PT (eds): "Genetic Responsibility." New York: Plenum Press, 1974, pp 61–67.
10. Fraser FC: Genetic counselling and the physician. Can Med Assoc J 99:927–934, 1968.
11. Glick ID, Kessler DR: "Marital and Family Therapy." New York: Grune & Stratton, 1974.
12. White RW: Strategies of adaptation: An attempt at systematic description. In Coelho GV, Hamburg DA, Adams JE (eds): "Coping and Adaption." New York: Basic Books, 1974, pp 47–68.
13. Hamburg DA, Adams JE: A perspective on coping behavior: Seeking and utilizing information in major transitions. Arch Gen Psychiatry 17:277–284, 1967.
14. Freud A: "The Ego and The Mechanisms of Defense." New York: International Universities Press, 1946.
15. Brenner C: "An Elementary Textbook of Psychoanalysis." New York: International Universities Press, 1973.
16. Kessler S: "Genetic Counseling: Psychological Dimensions." New York: Academic Press, 1978.
17. Anthony EJ, Benedek T: Parental aggression in fantasy, actuality and obsession. In Anthony EJ, Benedek T (eds): "Parenthood: Its Psychology and Psychopathology." Boston: Little, Brown & Co, 1970, pp 421–425.
18. Lazarus RS, Averill JR, Opton EM Jr: The psychology of coping: Issues of research and assessment. In Coelho GV, Hamburg DA, Adams IE (eds): "Coping and Adaption." New York: Basic Books, 1974, pp 47–68.
19. Truax CB, Carkhuff RR: "Introduction to Counseling and Psychotherapy: Training and Practice." Chicago: Aldine, 1966.
20. Carkhuff RR, Berenson BG: "Beyond Counseling and Psychotherapy." New York: Holt, Reinhart & Winston, 1967.
21. Angyal A: "Neurosis and Treatment. A Holistic Theory." New York: John Wiley & Sons, 1965.
22. Szasz TS, Hollender MH: A contribution to the philosophy of medicine: The basic models of the doctor-patient relationship. Arch Intern Med 97:585–592, 1956.
23. Sanford N: Notes toward a general theory of personality development – At eighty or any old age. Presented at the 81st annual convention of the American Psychological Association, Montreal, August 27, 1973.

13. The Genetic Counselor as Moral Advisor

Sumner B. Twiss, PhD

It is often asserted that, as a professional act, the offering of genetic counsel is morally neutral — intentionally so. One is confronted by a welter of claims that the aim of genetic counseling is to inform, to educate, to convey value-free facts and probabilities about genetic conditions, perhaps even to deal with psychologic problems, but never to advise and counsel about the moral aspects of mate selection and reproductive decision-making. In this stereotypic view, the ideal genetic counselor seldom (if ever) recommends courses of action to clients, tries always to be nondirective, and only gives explicit practical advice — especially about moral concerns — at his or her own peril.

Genetic counselors who hold this view, frequently as a matter of policy, are deceiving themselves. Whether they are aware of it or not, want to recognize it or not, morality is and should continue to be a professional issue in genetic counseling. Moral concerns lie at the core of genetic counseling. The genetic counselor will almost by necessity be a moral advisor to his or her clients; thus, the moral advisory component of counseling is inescapable.

On their face, these claims appear to revert to and endorse the themes of paternalism and arrogation of moral authority commonly associated with outmoded conceptions of the physician/patient relationship. However, far from being reactionary, these claims can be justified by sound, forward-looking, rational arguments. They should not be quickly assimilated to old paradigms and summarily dismissed.

SOCIAL ROLE OF GENETIC COUNSELOR

One may begin to see the genetic counselor as moral advisor by examining the social role of the genetic counselor, which is pertinent because counselors appeal to this role when they want to understand and defend themselves as acting responsibly in relation to their clients. Counselors invoke this role when they

Birth Defects: Original Article Series, Volume XV, Number 2, pages 201–212
© 1979 The National Foundation

speak of acting in a certain limited capacity, of being constrained by their position, or of standing in a specific relationship with their clients.

To act in a social role involves taking the point of view of the role and operating within its normative context. This context refers both to evaluative aims, ends, or goals, and to presciptive, regulative, or constraining rules. Evaluative aims comprise a spectrum, ranging from specific tasks and institutional functions, all the way to background social and moral norms. Prescriptive rules include constraints on reasoning (eg within the priorities of the role's aims) and constraints on action (ie duties specified by the role) [1].

The role of genetic counselor is established within the social and institutional context of health care. As such it is oriented toward health care goals, and it incorporates certain rules, in the form of duties, by which counselors regulate dealings with clients. To act in the role of genetic counselor involves engaging in more or less distinctive activities defined by certain aims and duties with clients who have genetic problems and concerns. Precisely what these aims and duties are, or should be, is one of the questions at issue, but this much can be said: they constitute points of entry for the moral aspects of the genetic counselor's role, and the main problem is to determine their character in order to identify their moral implications.

The practice of genetic counseling — the role of the genetic counselor — exists to achieve certain evaluative aims within the context of health care delivery. Prescriptions within the role serve to regulate (constrain) the conduct of the counselor in trying to attain these ends. Various types of aims shape the normative context of the genetic counseling role. The most immediate and least abstract type of aim refers to the specific tasks undertaken by genetic counselors, eg imparting genetic information to the client. A second type of aim is connected with the role's function in the larger social and institutional context of health care, eg the reduction or prevention of genetic disease. Clearly, these latter aims are designed to serve the broader goals of health care. A third type of aim embraces background sociomoral norms, eg basic moral principles of nonmaleficence, mutual respect, fairness, and basic moral rights of self-determination, personal inviolability, and liberty. These background norms serve as a groundwork to justify, criticize, and even humanize the tasks and institutional aims of genetic counseling.

Prescribed rules of various types also shape the normative context of the genetic counseling role. Two kinds of rules warrant special attention: constraints on deliberation and constraints on action. The first class of rules sets limitations on what count as acceptable reasons for undertaking activity in the counseling role. Such limitations help to structure the role so that its aims can be achieved and the client can be well served. For example, the counselor knows that certain considerations must always be taken into account (eg client's knowledge and attitudes, genetic facts and risks, reproductive options), other factors may or may not be considered relevant (eg eugenic projections), and yet other factors are almost always not relevant (eg client's social status). In the complex role of genetic counseling, limitations on deliberation depend logically on the priorities assigned to aspects of the role's aims. For example, if institutional aims regarding public health were heavily weighted, then perhaps eugenic factors would move into the category of considerations that must always be taken into account.

Prescribed rules relating to action within the counselor's role refer simply to the other-regarding duties constitutive of the role. Examples include the duty to inform the client as fully as possible about relevant genetic facts and available technology, the duty to alleviate psychologic anxieties associated with genetic counsel, and the duty to maintain confidentiality of genetic information. Such duties help insure that the aims of the role will be achieved, and specify what sorts of actions are justifiable within the role. And they check the counselor's exercise of power by setting limits on what can be done to achieve the aims of the role; for instance, the prohibition of eugenic sterilization. In general, these duties are of a relatively complex, extensive, and diffuse character, establishing a sphere of responsibility requiring the careful exercise of discretionary judgment and action.

These, then, are the sorts of elements that make up the normative context of the role of genetic counselor: a set of aims of increasing generality, ranging from specific tasks to the recognition of basic moral norms, and a set of prescriptions, including both constraints on deliberation and duties to perform certain actions. In order to make these aims and prescriptions more concrete and to identify certain moral issues, it is necessary to explore the role of the genetic counselor in its historical, systematic, and normative dimensions.

It is not possible here to undertake a thorough examination of the historical dimension of the genetic counseling role. However, a few comments about the role's origins and historical precedents are in order. The role of the genetic counselor descended from the early eugenics movement. For example, during the first three decades of the 20th century, the Eugenics Record Office at Cold Spring Harbor offered heredity counseling to individuals and couples at the premarital, preconception, and postconception stages of their life-development. Shaped by the moral crusading concern of the eugenics ideology, this early counseling aimed to advance the cause of positive and negative eugenics by proffering highly directive advice about mating and reproductive behavior. Individuals and couples were advised on eugenic grounds whether or not to marry and whether or not to reproduce.

The excesses of the eugenics movement were repudiated in the 1930s, but it has also been pointed out that the practice of genetic counseling is a survival of the heredity counseling associated with the eugenics movement. Further, it has been observed that as human genetics became incorporated into clinical medicine it encouraged the development of practices with eugenic overtones, however muted. It is not uncommon to see genetic counseling represented as a form of eugenic preventive medicine. Indeed, in 1960, Curt Stern openly stated that the social implications of specific advice in genetic counseling situations were not to be disregarded by the counselor [2]. And as recently as 1973, James Neel characterized the practice of genetic counseling as part of the new eugenics movement [3].

The point of these historical remarks is twofold. First, the role of genetic counselor was and still is shaped in part by eugenic objectives, which, regardless of their controversial nature, impart a paradigmatic social and moral dimension to the normative context of the role. Second, insofar as this is the case, the category of moral advice offered on behalf of the public welfare, is prima facie appropriate to the role of genetic counselor. Following from this historical understanding of the role, the genetic counselor seems duty-bound to point out the sociomoral and eugenic significance of the genetic problems, concerns, and decisions of clients. Whether these implications of the historical reference of the genetic counseling role can stand up to critical scrutiny will be addressed shortly.

Several human geneticists have proposed a new systematic dimension for the role of genetic counselor which attempts to define and systematize the role de novo, without reference to historical precedents. Review of representative agreements reached by groups of human geneticists and medical professionals on the role's definition would help to clarify this new role definition. As Sorenson and Culbert point out in Chapter 6 of this volume, most of these recent definitions agree on including the elements of provision of genetic information, exploration of reproductive-parenting options, and assistance in helping clients select a course of action appropriate to their situation. This new systematic dimension, then, appears to emphasize immediate task aims in relation to the broader institutional aim of helping clients to realize their personal life-plans in pursuit of what they perceive to be a good and happy life. Further, the counselor's duties to provide information, to educate, and to give psychosocial support for whatever decisions clients may make are singled out for attention. In this widely accepted new view, eugenic considerations and the giving of sociomoral advice about genetic concerns are systematically excluded from the role.

The apparent moral neutrality of the systematic dimension, however, is belied by sociologic evidence indicating that practicing genetic counselors do consider other institutional aims to be relevant to their role. [See "counseling outcomes" in Table 3 of Chapter 6.] Moreover, sociologic data indicate that genetic counselors consider it right to give advice, for instance, by informing clients about what most other people in their situation have decided, or by providing guidance about those factors which the counselor feels will lead clients toward an "appropriate" decision. No doubt many counselors would distinguish this providing of information from directly advising clients as to what the counselors really think the clients ought to do. Consequently, they would draw a sharp line between such information provision, on the one hand, and moral advising, on the other. As will be seen, these distinctions are disingenuous and misleading.

In examining the role of genetic counselor, the normative dimension deserves particular attention. This dimension involves argued judgments about what the role should be in order to establish propositions about what it is. The chapters in this section of the present volume represent just such argumentative appeals, eg information giver, decision maker, psychotherapist, and, of course, moral advisor. The point to be made here is that in spite of historical precedents and systematic agreements, controversy over the nature of the genetic counseling role persists. In the final analysis, any determination about the nature of this role — particularly about its moral aspects — depends on the cogency of the argument supporting that determination.

The normative dimension, then, suggests that it is appropriate to clarify the nature of the genetic counseling role by determining the aims of the role in relation to the institutions of health care and society generally. Thus, one important line to pursue is to determine how institutional and background aims give moral shape and direction to the role of genetic counselor. The task aims and prescribed duties of the role's normative context derive from and are justified by these more general aims. The primary aims of health care are to maintain the integrity of the person, with special reference to the physical substratum of that integrity, and to preserve life-capacities that underlie the realization of life plans in pursuit of the good and happy life. These aims imply two broad sorts of duties to act in the interest of maintaining good health.

First, there are duties to serve the welfare of the individual client. These duties constitute the personal medical care model, involving medical interventions which minister to bodily integrity; and they are constrained by basic moral rights. Second, there are duties to serve the welfare of the community — the collective patient. These duties involve medical and social interventions that attempt to optimize, or at least protect, the health aspects of the life-environment of the population. These duties constitute the public health model, and while they are constrained by basic moral rights, the state may determine that in some cases these duties override such rights in the interest of the public welfare.

An important question, from the standpoint of genetic counseling, is whether or not these two models in health care suggest or, more strongly, imply any priorities for the normative context of the role of genetic counselor. At least two observations appear to bear on this question, though neither is conclusive. The first is a logical point. The personal medical care model may be given logical and moral primacy over the public health model, since in fact it provides the rationale for public health measures. Public health agencies are concerned with community welfare, precisely because protecting or optimizing the health aspects of the environment in the final analysis benefits the health and bodily integrity of each individual member of the community. Even geneticists who emphasize the cause of genetically informed environmental hygiene say at the same time that the principal target of human genetics is the alleviation of individual distress, and that applied human genetics should be constrained by the patient-oriented values of the medical profession.

The second observation is empirical and tends to countervail the first point. It is not at all uncommon for geneticists to claim that medicine is dysgenic. The point of this claim is to suggest that the concerns of public health via genetics ought to shape the aims of medical genetics and, by implication, the normative context of the role of genetic counselor.

Such remarks and arguments about the normative dimension of the genetic counseling role result in a dilemma. Should this role conform to the requirements of personal medical care in the physician/patient relationship, or should it be construed along the lines of public health agency? Or should the role be conceived as internally complex, involving a dual responsibility to client (client advocate) and to society (public advocate)? This dilemma is not to be confused with the controversy over whether the role orientation in genetic counseling is more properly conceived as doctor/client than doctor/patient, for this controversy already assumes the legitimacy of something like the medical care model and simply argues over whether the task aims of the genetic counselor ought to include a psychosocial component. By contrast, the dilemma of medical care model versus public health model runs deeper than the more limited controversy of client versus patient.

A prima facie case can be made for conceiving of the genetic counseling role to involve a dual responsibility to clients and to the population as a whole. First, the historical dimension of the role provides precedents for this conception. Second, the sociologic data introduced in connection with the role's systematic dimension gives empirical support to this view. Third, the many claims made by reflective medical geneticists, genetic counselors, and medical sociologists that medical genetics is a form of eugenic engineering, that genetic counseling is basically a type of eugenic preventive medicine, and that genetic counseling is a kind of planned parenthood, lend support to this dual conception of the role of the genetic counselor as both client advocate and public health professional. Of course, appeals such as these are far from conclusive; historical remarks, empirical data, and speculative assertions scarcely amount to a cogent normative argument.

More important, perhaps, are considerations relating to the characterization of genetic disease as a public health problem and the interest of the state in the genetic quality of its citizens. As medical science and human genetics progress, more and more diseases are found to have a genetic etiology. As much as 25% of total morbidity in the population may be attributable to genetic factors, and 5% related to specific genetic defects [4]. Genetic diseases are growing in relative health importance. Indeed, much of the current discussion about genetic conditions and the role of genetic counseling programs seems to assume that genetic diseases constitute a public health problem.

Whether the state has a justifiable interest in reducing the incidence of genetic disease by shaping the role of genetic counselor turns in large part on the validity of the analogy between the public health problems posed by contagious disease on the one hand and genetic disease on the other. The validity of the analogy is debatable. Certainly genetic conditions do not present a public health hazard in the same sense as infectious diseases might, but communicability of infectious and genetic diseases is a point in common, even though the means and degree of transmissability are different in each case.

The question of state interest in genetic disease and, by implication, in genetic counseling does not rest solely on this analogy. Society takes a substantial interest in both the quantity and quality of children born within the community. This interest is clearly evidenced by publicly supported family planning programs, provision of contraceptive services, national commissions on population policy, legal requirements concerning mandatory education, court decisions ordering medical care for children against parental wishes, and laws in the area of child abuse. In these and other ways, the state expresses societal interest in the quantity and quality of its citizens' progeny. This interest is bound up with the social utilitarian aims of maximizing the number of socially useful people and minimizing the number of socially burdensome people. In terms of health, these aims materialize in a state interest in insuring that future citizens are healthy and in avoiding costs involved in caring for defective persons. Public policy has encouraged and sanctioned the use of the state's police power to minimize illness in the population, eg mass screening for tuberculosis, compulsory vaccination, mandatory premarital blood tests, and, most recently, mandatory genetic screening.

There are other clear signs that the state is concerned with the genetic quality of its citizens and, more specifically, in reducing the incidence of genetic disease. A small number of genetic diseases are thought to be prevalent enough to warrant a public health concern. Moreover, genetic diseases do affect the public interest through the allocation of public funds and medical resources for researching therapies, providing institutional care, and supporting genetic screening and counseling programs.

Consequently, there is a prima facie case for holding that the state has a legitimate interest in reducing the impact of genetic disease on the population. Although not conclusive, this case and its supporting considerations are sufficiently cogent to be taken to affect the moral shape of the genetic counseling role. Thus, although the primary responsibility of the genetic counselor may be to minister to the client's genetic problems and concerns, the counselor is also a health professional who bears some degree of responsibility for the genetic health of the community.

This secondary responsibility at least suggests, if it does not imply, the propriety (duty) of engaging in moral advising on behalf of the public interest in "genetic health," in addition to giving clients moral advice about personal and familial problems and concerns. At this point it becomes necessary to focus on the moral advisory aspects of the genetic counseling role and to delineate these in more precise terms.

ADVICE IN GENETIC COUNSELING

In order to locate the place of moral advice in the role of genetic counselor, it must be recognized that the practice of genetic counseling falls under the general category of advising. So much stress is laid on the task aims and duties of informing and educating clients that this fundamental fact is often ignored. Yet it is noteworthy that genetic counsel is characteristically sought by clients who have practical concerns and problems relating to mate selection and reproductive behavior. That is, confronted with practical problems about possible genetic consequences of their behavior, clients seek advice from genetic counselors because they expect counselors to be of some assistance in solving their practical problems. This almost trivial observation suggests that the main purpose of genetic counseling is advisory in nature, to assist clients confronted with a certain range of practical problems, and to help them in determining what to do. This suggestion, in turn, implies that the normative context of the role of genetic counselor is very much shaped by the logic of advice; that is, the role's aims and duties are advisory in character. Thus, along with the notion of social role, the category of advice confers another distinctive vantage point on the practice of genetic counseling.

The point of view of the clients becomes important when considering the genetic counseling role under the aspect of advice. In giving genetic counsel, the counselor is ordinarily expected to try to understand and reason from the clients' practical basis, their perspective, their standpoint about their problem: this follows from the very logic of advice [5]. On its face, genetic counsel may involve providing genetic information relevant to the mating and reproductive concerns of clients, and it may involve making suggestions or even recommendations pertinent to their concerns. Neither type of activity is excluded prima facie by the logic of advice. In supplying genetic information to clients, the counselor thereby enables them to draw their own practical conclusions from this advice and from other considerations that may not be known to the counselor. In suggesting or recommending courses of action to clients, the counselor leaves it up to the clients whether they will adopt such suggestions or recommendations.

What seems clearly inappropriate to genetic counseling conceived under the category of advice is for the counselor to substitute or impose his or her own personal practical basis — eg personal views about mating or reproduction — in giving advice to clients. Unless the counselor's personal views are consonant with those of the clients, nothing follows from these personal views about what the clients must do in order to resolve their practical problems. This caveat, however, does not necessarily imply that the normative context of the genetic counseling role is irrelevant to genetic counsel conceived under the category of advice. This caveat and its negative implication require clarification.

In principle there are at least two ways in which the aims of the genetic counselor (ie the institutional aims of the genetic counseling role) may enter into or shape the advice (genetic counsel) given to clients. The counselor may reason not only in terms of the clients' problems, but also in terms of the aims of the role to a practical conclusion about what the clients ought to do. Now whether a genetic counselor is entitled, or should be permitted, to do this is a question that needs to be carefully addressed. Under certain conditions such advisory activity may be permissible or even required, under other conditions it may not. This question will be taken up shortly. The aims of the genetic counselor may enter into or shape the advice in another, slightly less controversial way. To determine what the clients should do, the counselor may consider what he or she would do in the clients' situation from their point of view. Here the counselor supposes that his or her grounds for decision and action are similar to those of the clients. The main problem with this type of advisory activity is that it is exceedingly difficult to come to know on short acquaintance the practical basis and point of view of clients. In other words, the counselor's supposition about the consonance between the aims of the genetic counseling role and the point of view of the clients would rarely, if ever, be justified.

Aside from the controversial issue just raised, it seems that the general considerations adduced about genetic counseling qua advice-giving imply that an important premise underlies the practice. The premise is that mating and reproductive concerns are essentially private in character. Consequently, genetic counselors are entitled or permitted to advise clients on such matters only because the clients request this advice, ie genetic counsel. The vantage point for accepting this premise involves affirming the moral autonomy of clients in making decisions about their lives. Interestingly, this affirmation simply entails serious acceptance of the background aims of the role of genetic counselor: basic moral rights of self-determination as these relate to the integrity of the person and the family. These rights demarcate a sphere of individual privacy and moral autonomy in mating and reproductive matters. Authority for making decisions in these matters rests with the clients, who are properly viewed as autonomous moral agents responsible for their life-development. It appears, therefore, that the background sociomoral norms of the genetic counseling role place significant constraints on how the counselor is permitted to reason and to act.

GENETIC COUNSELOR AS MORAL ADVISOR

Given these implications of the logic of advice for the practice of genetic counseling, how is it possible to construe a moral advisory capacity within the role of genetic counselor? There are "weak" and "strong" answers to this question. The weak but not insignificant response runs as follows. Genetic counsel is sought by clients who, as parents and prospective parents, are trying to be morally responsible in their reproductive decision-making and behavior. Thus, much genetic counsel in the form of advice is sought as a result of practical moral concern that clients have about the genetic consequences of their decision-making and behavior, eg in terms of adverse impact on the welfare of their prospective progeny, their families, and even the society in which they live. As a consequence of their moral concern, clients may request and thereby entitle the genetic counselor to assist them in their decision-making. With this request or entitlement in hand, it seems that the genetic counselor's task and institutional aims and other-regarding duties obligate the counselor to assist clients in identifying morally relevant factors in their situation. For example, by discussing the financial burdens of raising an affected child, possible deleterious effects of a genetic disorder on family life, possible economic and/or eugenic burdens of a genetic disorder on society, and the like, the genetic counselor, by virtue of the normative context of the role, is helping clients to see the nature and range of the moral issues at stake in their future decisions and behavior. To label this sort of discussion as simply "information provision" is misleading, for the genetic counselor *is* morally advising clients in their practical situation, even though he or she may not be explicitly examining the whole range of the clients' moral beliefs and views on life. Rather, the counselor is exploring how certain considerations, of a kind which the clients view as morally significant, are relevant (or not) to their practical moral concerns about genetic disease. On request of the clients and following the personal medical care model, the genetic counselor has the duty to engage in such moral advisory activity by virtue of the genetic counseling role.

The strong answer to the question of a moral advisory capacity within the role of genetic counselor follows from the consideration of that role in its historical, systematic, and normative dimensions. On this view, a genetic counselor may well be concerned and duty-bound to urge the admission of morally relevant factors to the practical basis or point of view of clients. In this case, rather than waiting on a request and then reasoning from the clients' practical basis, the genetic counselor actively seeks to promote what he or she considers to be moral action in the clients' situation. Here the counselor claims to see the moral problem confronting the clients, regardless of whether they see that problem. For example, even if the clients fail to raise eugenic issues, or issues of fulfilling extant obligations to family members, or issues of economic burdens on society, etc, the genetic counselor initiates discussion about these issues and urges the clients to consider them. The counselor does this because of institutional aims and duties regarding public health that are part of the role's dual responsibility to clients on the one hand and to society at large on the other.

This strong understanding of moral advice in the role of genetic counselor may appear to contravene the very logic of advice and the implied notion of the moral autonomy of clients. Many would reject the strong view on precisely this basis. But, in fact, this objection is far from being conclusive. First, it may be argued that as mature moral agents the clients would (or should) want to know if they were inadvertently or negligently avoiding a moral problem relevant to their behavior. Second, it may be observed that by their very nature moral problems are not purely private and personal, since they involve situations in which the interests and welfare of others are affected. The public character, so to speak, of moral problems undermines the contention that the genetic counselor can speak to moral issues only if and when requested or given entitlement by clients.

In moral matters criticisms of title are frequently, if not always, inapplicable; that is, it is never morally wrong (and it may always be morally right) to give unsolicited moral advice, because the welfare of others is at stake. These two lines of rebuttal suggest that the genetic counselor may indeed be acting appropriately within the role if in counseling he or she actively indicates to clients moral considerations about certain courses of action, eg in taking a high risk in conceiving a seriously defective fetus, in bearing a child with a serious genetic disorder, in failing to inform relatives that they may be at-risk for having a genetic disease or carrying a deleterious trait. To act in this way — to proffer moral advice — in the role of genetic counselor may be justified by the normative context of the role, especially its institutional aims (eg reduction of the incidence of genetic disease), its duties (eg relating to public health), and even its background aims (eg moral principle of nonmaleficence).

Counter-arguments to building either the weak or strong sense of moral advice into the role of genetic counselor would no doubt refer to the limits of the counselor's professional competence and authority. Opponents might claim that genetic counselors have neither moral competence nor authority in relation to their clients. This claim has some force, but it is overstated. Surely genetic counselors have the competence to make moral decisions based on the evaluative aims and prescribed rules built into the role whatever its specifics. However, counselors have no moral authority to impose these decisions on their clients. But this claim is somewhat trivial, for nowhere has it been argued that genetic counselors have any authority to impose decisions, moral or otherwise, on their clients. What has been argued is that *if* clients request (entitle) genetic counselors to advise them on moral issues, then counselors may do so, and they may well have the duty to so advise. Furthermore, whenever genetic counselors observe that clients are ignoring relevant moral considerations, then counselors may raise these considerations with their clients, and they may well have the duty to do so, by virtue of the normative context of the genetic counseling role and by virtue of the nature of morality itself.

Now with regard to the strong sense of moral advice the poignant question arises: In a morally pluralistic society, would not genetic counselors overstep their role if they indicated to clients some moral considerations relevant, for example, to choosing between reproductive and parenting options? The answer is by no means plainly in the negative, for the counselors' authorization, so to speak, for raising such considerations derives from duties logically based on institutional and background aims shared with clients. If this is the case, whence comes the violation of the role? Note finally that even the dual conception of the genetic counseling role does not dispute the moral right of clients to make their own decisions. It only proposes that on behalf of the public welfare the genetic counselor is permitted, and perhaps has the duty, to initiate moral discussion with mature moral agents. It is not self-evident that the exercise of this duty implies paternalism, arrogation of moral authority, or overstepping the bounds of technical expertise.

The charge of paternalism is rebutted by noting that in the end the final decision-making authority of clients is upheld. Against the charge of arrogation of moral authority, it must be reiterated that the counselor is not playing the role of being a moral authority, only a role-agent with certain aims and duties. And against the charge of overstepping the bounds of expertise, it needs to be said that genetic counseling is not just an applied science but an interpersonal role-relationship defined in large part by social and moral norms which are often shared by both counselor and clients.

REFERENCES

1. Kadish MR, Kadish SH: "Discretion to Disobey." Stanford, CA: Stanford University Press, 1973, pp 15–26.
2. Ludmerer KM: "Genetics and American Society." Baltimore: Johns Hopkins University Press, 1972, pp 174–193. Curt Stern cited on p 178.
3. Neel JV: Social and scientific priorities in the use of genetic knowledge. In Hilton B et al (eds): "Ethical Issues in Human Genetics." New York: Plenum Press, 1973, pp 353–355.
4. Lederberg J: Biomedical frontiers: Genetics. In Kunz RM, Fehr H (eds): "The Challenge of Life." Basel: Berkhauser Verlag, 1972, p 234.
5. Gauthier DP: "Practical Reasoning." Oxford: Clarendon Press, 1963, pp 53–57.

III. Moral, Social, and Legal Problems in Genetic Counseling: Introduction

It may be that to point out now that medicine has ramifications far beyond its surface preoccupations has achieved the status of comfortable platitude. Ten years ago, that was, if not a new idea, at least a controversial one. Today, however, it is increasingly the case that attention is paid to the other implications of the work of medicine. The journal article on an ethical or legal issue is no longer a rare event, and often even in professional gatherings otherwise devoted to technical concerns a session is set aside for "ethics."

Unfortunately, all the nontechnical concerns tend often to be lumped together, resulting in, say, muddling a private moral concern (if I am over 35, should I undergo prenatal diagnosis?) with a public policy issue (should the government subsidize prenatal diagnosis programs for women over 35?) and/or a legal one (can a woman over 35 successfully sue her obstetrician if he fails to suggest prenatal diagnosis and she bears a child with Down syndrome?). That muddling is partly due to the novelty of these still unfamiliar concerns. It is also due to the perfectly accurate perception that it is often very difficult (and perhaps not even desirable) to draw precise demarcations between those subjects. They are not only related to each other; they often really cannot be successfully handled without reference to each other.

Therefore, the concluding section of this volume succumbs to the temptation to consider these concerns together, though it also divides the papers here into three groups of two, each group concentrating chiefly on moral, policy or legal questions.

In the first paper in this section, psychologist Sidney Callahan provides an ethical analysis of the idea of responsible parenthood. This is an idea, she points out, which seems somewhat novel because there has been very little ethical analysis of the relationship between the family and the rest of society, an analysis which she sees as central to discussing the kinds of responsibilities parents have for the genetic inheritance and potential of their children. Acknow-

Birth Defects: Original Article Series, Volume XV, Number 2, **pages 213–215**

ledging what we all would acknowledge, that parents have important basic obligations to their children, Callahan nonetheless points out that the formulation of such duties may not be as simple as it sounds. At what point does this parental obligation come into being: at birth, during pregnancy, at conception, or perhaps long before? How much control should we exert over our own reproduction? How much risk-taking is ethically acceptable in order to achieve parenthood? Ethicist John Fletcher then brings a policy dimension to that kind of analysis by discussing the development of a moral framework that will balance the ethical status of the developing fetus against the needs of family and society. He argues the need to push a technique like prenatal diagnosis further, until it becomes possible to administer in utero therapy, which he sees as a goal morally far superior to the current "treatment" following prenatal diagnosis, selective abortion.

Under the heading "The Public Interest in Reproductive Behavior," ethicist Sumner Twiss applies principles of social justice to certain policy issues in medical genetics, chiefly eugenics policy. Priorities in the allocation of scarce resources — bluntly put, how do we decide how much of the public dollar should be spent on genetics? — is also taken up in his article. In the following article, some public policy issues in genetic counseling are explored jointly by ethicist James Childress and lawyer Kenneth Casebeer. That collaboration produces a simultaneous moral and legal analysis of whether and how public policy toward genetic counseling should be made. Since they view our society as favoring, at bottom, procreational freedom, they pay particular attention to proposed policies that might circumscribe freedom and privacy, two issues where ethics and the law strongly mesh.

Two other lawyers take up the thread in the last group of two articles, devoted specifically to legal issues in genetics. The first, by Philip Reilly, tackles a very concrete and controversial issue in medical genetics, the question of accreditation. The necessity for setting professional standards seems more and more pressing as clinical genetics grows and changes, as more and more women seek prenatal diagnosis, as genetic counseling expands its services and employs more (and new kinds of) people on the counseling team. After looking at the experience with licensure in other professions, Reilly concludes that medical genetics would do well to avoid that route, and indeed, to maintain for as long as possible its current flexible, heterogeneous approach. Other classic legal issues are assessed by Alexander Capron: professional responsibility and liability (that is, the usual concerns in malpractice cases), but also issues of professional responsibility with regard to confidentiality, a difficult problem in clinical genetics, where a counselor may feel a moral duty to disclose information to relatives, though his legal obligation may be to remain silent.

The fact that we have grouped all these subjects in a separate section means that we do see them, in some important sense, as nontechnical and related to each other. It is not, however, intended to obscure the fact that we also see them as very much akin to, and growing out of, the other sections of this volume. If people have become more sensitive to the moral—social side of medicine in the last few years, nowhere is that sensitivity more important than in genetic medicine, whose ministrations touch not just the individual patient, or his immediate family, or even his relatives and the rest of society, but all the future generations of human beings that will follow our own.

TMP

14. An Ethical Analysis of Responsible Parenthood

Sidney Callahan, MA

INTRODUCTION: WHAT IS RESPONSIBLE PARENTHOOD?

How does the growing knowledge of genetics and medical technology affect parental responsibilities? The concept of responsible parenthood includes many questions relating to procreation, the control of reproduction, child-rearing, and the role of the family in the larger community. At the moment all of these issues are in a state of flux from an ethical, legal, and social point of view. It is as though the rapid expansion of medical technology had caught a whole society unprepared. We do not know how to deal with specific genetic issues because there has been so little ethical analysis of the role of parents and the family in relationship to the rest of society. There has been even less analysis of the responsibilities of parents in relationship to their genetic inheritance and potential [1, 2].

To begin to cope with the question, it should be recognized that the term "responsible parenthood" is used in two different ways. In one usage, responsible parenthood refers to parents who care for their existing children in a careful, dedicated manner, meeting all of their parental obligations. They are responsible or able to respond to their children. The other usage of responsible parenthood refers to wise decisions that people make or actions they take in becoming a parent either for the first time, or to add to a family already begun. Here the use of "responsible" is that of initiating or causing some outcome, or being held accountable for the action [3]. Obviously the two meanings of responsible parenthood are interrelated, since ideas about what parents are and how they should respond to their children will affect decisions and attitudes towards becoming a parent.

A potential parent may view questions of mate selection, contraception, selective abortion, and the promotion of genetic health in the light of his or her

Birth Defects: Original Article Series, Volume XV, Number 2, pages 217–238
© 1979 The National Foundation

view of parental functions and obligations. Another aspect of responsible parent-hood, of course, is that usually two people are involved. If a mate is present, there are the added complications ensuing from shared responsibility and joint decision-making. Before getting to the complex questions of responsible de-cisions about becoming a parent, a review is in order of what responsible parents do.

I think that in "doing ethics" and in considering morality, ethical questions can never be separated from a consideration and analysis of what seems to be the case. Of course, inevitably, the perceptions of some facts and conditions are fil-tered through personal values, but it still seems better to organize an ethical in-quiry with a preliminary account of what is happening or what has happened in the past.

What is expected of parents, and what is the role of the family?

THE ROLE OF PARENTS AND THE FAMILY

At the most elementary biologic level, parents must insure the health and sur-vival of their offspring by diligent care. Basic nurturing consists of feeding, groom-ing, sheltering, and protecting the young from harmful aspects of the environ-ment. Parents must be active and aggressive at times in defense of their offspring and be the buffers between the outside environment and their young. All of the above could be true of many species, but in the case of human parents, physical protection and providing for biologic survival is not enough. While caring for the needs of a child, parents also effect the necessary socialization of a child by instruction, discipline, play, contact-comfort, and emotional attachment [4]. Love, respect, and affection between parents and children promote the inter-nalization of moral and social norms [5]. Parents provide a primary partner relation-ship in the learning of language and all the other social aspects of living. At the same time, a parent is the child's advocate in the world. It is also the case that the more competent and better equipped the adult parent partners are, the more advantaged the children [6].

In the beginning of a parent–child relationship, the parent who is more powerful than the child must exercise initiative and judgment. While infants have now been found to be much more active and effective than had been thought previously [7, 8], still the parents must be dominant and even coercive in order to protect. But as the normal child grows and matures, the unequal power relationship changes slowly into one of more and more equality. Inde-pendence training is an important part of parental functioning. A gradual separa-tion and mutual weaning takes place, which culminates in adolescence and the social launching of young adults into the larger society. If all goes well, and a child is normally healthy and competent, parents work themselves out of a job: In ecologic terms, good parenting is biodegradable. New adults are produced, able to love, work and found families on their own.

Such a process of active helping and parental care, when done adequately, takes enormous amounts of time, effort, and emotional energy. It also requires an increasing amount of material resources to feed, clothe, and educate each child. In other societies and in different historical periods, parental functions and the economic burdens and expenses of child care have been distributed in different ways than our own. Either extended family systems or developed systems of public child care, health care, and education have eased the parental load [9]. In America, immigration and mobility have eroded economic and social supports to parents from extended families while at the same time public support is minimal. Even the traditionally provided public systems of school and scholarship funds are being reduced. Good public daycare and child heath care also are unavailable generally.

Most public and community help offered to parents is accompanied by stringent means tests and some stigmatization. Ironically, the withdrawal of social support for parents has been accompanied by an increase in economic and emotional expectations and pressures on the family. Among other things, more and more single parents are doing the job alone. Several experts have traced the decline of IQ and achievement scores and the rise of juvenile disturbances to the reduction of parent-child relationships [10]. Perhaps there has never been such a society anywhere that demands so much from individual parents and yet provides so little help from others. Even in the realm of moral teaching and the transmission of culture, the traditional supports of church, school and neighborhood have been lessened. Nuclear families can be quite isolated in smaller and smaller units, all the while being pressured with more and more demands to provide their children with present and future economic, emotional, and moral well-being.

The increasing pressures of raising a new generation for the future has meant for most Americans less family energy and resources available for old parents and other aging relatives. When new adults have been raised, launched, and become independent, there is some question in our society as to just how much they owe to their parents. Social security, pension funds and medicare have done much to alleviate the economic burdens of older parents, but no one would claim that the social situation of the aging in America is satisfactory. The family has always been the institution to cope with human dependency in the beginning and end of life, but in other times and places there also has been much more group and community support for the family in its function. The ascribed status of the family, or that relationship which is involuntary and irreversible, has in other more family-centered social systems been as important as an achieved status of work, education, and productivity [11]. When an ideology of individualism, independence, achievement, mobility, and self-fulfillment become dominant in a society, then family ties and status suffer [12].

Links between the generations, and the provision of mutual aid and family support, depend upon an ideology of community group cooperation and interdependence. Dependency at the beginning and end of life need not be considered unfortunate, but simply a natural part of life. While most persons in America would not welcome a return to older European concepts of the extended family system which so often suppressed individual rights and initiative, still some re-dressing of the balance may be hoped for. More and more it is realized that children and older persons are helped by participation in a network of ascribed kinship relationships which do not depend upon productivity and achieved status. If an extended family can be psychologically supportive and ready to aid when necessary, individual parenthood is made easier. Public social measures which provide substitutes for family aid may also increasingly be adopted if the political demands for them increase [13].

BECOMING A PARENT: PSYCHOLOGIC AND ETHICAL CONSIDERATIONS OF PARENTAL MOTIVATIONS

One of the difficulties of analyzing responsible parenthood from an ethical point of view is that so little attention has been given to parental motivation. Why do people have children? Why do people want children [14]? Mostly, it has been considered either too private or too controversial a matter and a com-plicated, confused question it appears to be. One interesting dimension of the picture is that of conscious compared to unconscious parental motivation. Do people want children because they are responding to an unconscious biologic drive or program to reproduce, as in many lower species? Arguments from a socio-biologic perspective would see an animal's drive for dominance, or the effort to get more of one's genes into a population as an unconscious motivating force [15]. Parental competition, protective-aggression, territoriality, and "care" could be seen as general socio-biologic imperatives working in the human species like any other. Parental altruism, self-sacrifice, and caretaking would be seen as more biologically programmed than other activities. Parent behavior has been asserted to be basically built into the adult repetoire of each member of the primate species, only waiting to be stimulated by the presence of the young of the species [16]. In this view, there may be an inherent attraction to infants in primate groups which binds the groups together and insures altruism and survival.

Another approach to the motivation of parents comes from the psycho-analytic school of thought [17, 18]. Here both conscious and deep unconscious factors are thought to be operating with early family relationship predominating. A complicated development of sexual and reproductive motivations is postu-lated, which includes hostility, love, identification processes, and efforts to com-pensate for childish inferiority. Positive desires and defenses may both be operating semiconsciously. Some depth analysis would also propose that an un-conscious force may be at work in human beings, urging them to reproduce in order to overcome death [19]. The desire for immortality is translated into a desire for children who will live on after one's death. There is a deep felt need to become one's own father and mother, give a child to a beloved mate and live out an urge for "generativity" and completeness [20]. Only those who are convinced of immortality or whose ego development is deeply involved in other generative functions can easily sublimate procreative functions.

By contrast, in a social learning theory approach to parent motivation, it would be the modeling of a child's parents and the learned social conditioning of society that would impel persons to want to produce children [21]. In western society the transmission of culture from one generation to another takes place primarily in the family unit, so that each new entrant into society inevitably learns that the normal adult role involves being a parent. Women in particular have been given few alternatives to the maternal role [22]. But in a learning theory approach it is always possible for other satisfactions and models to be learned and substituted for the parental role. It is only a question of society and social change reinforcing and rewarding other modes of living. The reason that parental motivations may appear to be universal, unconscious, and instinctual is simply that heretofore, in a less crowded world, it has been highly adaptive for populations to reward and condition a desire to reproduce. At least this would be true in agricultural societies.

Moreover, few other alternatives or other motivations have been accessible or available to be learned by the majority of people other than planning, sustaining, and enjoying family life in a cycle of generations. The way our social life is currently organized, much love, affective, and leisure time are organized around family and kinship ties. Generally, few substitutes have been found for the institution of the family, and this may be because the limited information processing and emotional makeup of children and adults predispose to life in small groups. It may be psychologically difficult to become deeply involved and continuously stay in touch with more than six to eight people in a household, the size of the usual family group [23, 24]. Human interest in a variety of both ages and sexes, and the need to organize life in long periods of time, may make it "natural" to desire children to complete generational cycles. If there is an economic advantage or social advantage to having children to increase the size of a clan or family work force then the learned motivation to produce children will be even more strong.

In some cultures, including our own, there has also been a strong religious component to parental motivation [25]. In the Judeo–Christian religious tradition, a good creator God has given mankind a mandate "to increase and multiply," to have dominion over the earth and the animals. Having children is thought of as a service to the creator of all good things. In imitation of God's creativity, man and woman, through their love of one another, create new children for the greater glory of God. Care of children by loving adults is modeled on God's loving care of mankind. The responsibility and joyful duty of most human beings is to raise up sons and daughters, training them, disciplining them, loving them and being rewarded by seeing one's children's children. Occasionally in the past, this responsibility to procreate was interpreted as a way of paying for the sensual pleasures of sex, but generally the tradition of serving God through procreation was thought of as a blessing [26]. Procreation is seen as one of man's highest forms of stewardship over creation.

Occasionally too, this service of God was seen as a way of populating heaven rather than as an exercise of stewardship over earth. Also at times the desire to produce more believers in the households of the saints than in the households of the unbelievers may have been mingled with a religious motivation. Similar group-oriented "front mentalities" or pronatalist motivations have been held by national and ethnic groups who are threatened in some way. To defend against extinction or produce defenders of a way of life has also been an ideologic motivation which influences individual parental motivations.

Other defensive personal parent motivations for having children have also been described: to prove fertility, sexual prowess, or maturity; to obtain an inheritance or some other economic advantage; to gain revenge or secure a mate; to work out pathologic neurotic needs for power; or to obtain a scapegoat; to satisfy curiosity or provide a novel experience; to have a toy or compete with others; to prevent some other occurrence such as draft selection; to dominate another or to placate.

Obviously, none of the parental motivations described above need be exclusive of the others. Individuals may have very mixed motivations in becoming parents. And as we see in some theories the motivations may not all be conscious. An ethical analysis of these responses, however, can still be made on some general principles. Surely the relationship between a person and his or her child-to-be should not be less subject to ethical standards, than an intimate personal relationship between adults. It is generally accepted that the "alien dignity" of each person should be recognized as a means of keeping each person free from exploitation and validating human dignity [27]. The child as a person is not an extension of the parent, must also possess an "alien dignity" and does not exist to fulfill a parent's needs and desires. There is also a morally accepted standard that the more in need and dependent another person is, particularly in one's own family, the more valid is his claim to be helped. This is surely a minimal standard for any relationship between parent and child as well.

The only difference between parent–child and other intimate personal human relationships would be the greater demand upon the parent's altruism, helping behavior, and recognition of a child's right not to be exploited. The unequal power relationship between parent and child and the disparity in ages takes away any justification for demanding an equal giving of goods or satisfactions in furthering the relationship. If there is symmetry in the relationship, it can only be expected when there is more equality, ie when the child becomes an adult. Even then the general "repayment" of parental care is usually invested in a third generation of grandchildren.

Therefore a motivation for parenthood could be assessed ethically by how much the potential child's inalienable separate human dignity was recognized, along with its right to dependent care. The more egocentric the parental attitude, the more exploitative and less acceptable it would be. Obviously all the pathologic desires for a child in order to gain a chance for sadism, power, or revenge would be deemed immoral and unethical. A less obvious exploitation would be the trivializing of the parent-child-to-be relationship through wanting a child as a plaything or curiosity. Desiring a child of a particular sex or with certain special characteristics which the parent wants would also be less than acceptable, since the parent's satisfaction would be seen as more important than the child's own welfare and alien dignity as a separate unique person.

Wanting to have a child to fulfill some ideologic group motivation, such as nationalism, ethnicity, or religious motivation might be either positive or negative. If the ideologic motivation created an appreciation of the child as a unique child, with its own intrinsic value and dignity, it would be positive. If the individual child's welfare was being submerged or ignored for the sake of the greater cause, or even willingly sacrificed to the cause, the parental motivation could be judged as unethical and immoral. Wanting and having a child in order to consciously experiment with a new child-rearing regime, or to indoctrinate it with an ideology, would be exploitative if the child's own welfare, point of view and intrinsic rights were not being considered.

The unconscious motivations for parenthood posited by biologists and depth psychologists bring up the question of how one could possibly ethically judge unconscious motivations. Do motivations have to be conscious and rational to be thought positively good? Certainly in a case of self-judgment a motivation has to be accessible and conscious. But since we know so very little about the human unconscious that is not speculation and theory, it seems far too premature to assert anything about its moral effects. We do not really know whether there is a deep unconscious desire to conquer death by providing one's immortality in one's children; we do not really know whether the sociobiologists' analysis of parental care and the urge for dominance by placing one's genes in the next generation is operating with human beings. Personally, I think cultural conditioning and social learning are much more potent than any unconscious life force [28].

The socially learned motivations for parenthood, such as reproducing one's own family, or taking an adult role in the organization of society, can be ethically and morally judged on the same principles of nonexploitation of another. If becoming a parent is seen as engagement with another person in a giving, nonegocentric relationship that will benefit the child, it would be seen as a good and acceptable motivation.

In other words, the most ethically acceptable parental motivation involves the most conscious commitment to giving a unique child what the child needs for its fulfillment. People who want to be parents should want to be parents in order to give, not get. It is immoral and unethical to knowingly want a child to satisfy needs or desires which take no account of the child as a human person with intrinsic rights to dignity and nurturance. While many have claimed that parental giving, protecting, and advocacy of one's children within the family framework produces one of the greatest of life's satisfactions and joys, still the ethical essence of the parental role is altruism and unselfish nurturance of another.

While many would agree with the above assessment of parental motivation, there would be more disagreement and conflict over the amount of control and intervention parents should use when engaging in the parental enterprise.

DIFFERENT CONCEPTS OF PARENTAL INTERVENTION AND CONTROL

The argument over the extent of intervention and control parents can and should exercise in genetic and reproductive questions is a subset of general arguments over control and intervention in natural processes. There are, of course, certain limits beyond which it is still humanly impossible to do anything about life, death, or the control of nature. Human beings have no choice in these situations and simply must accept the course of events. But at the same time it is clearly the case that human life also consists of some control and intervention in nature; the human species depends upon initiative, control, planned activity, and technology in order to exist. No human child can survive to adulthood without its caretakers massively controlling the environment in order to protect the immature life. Adaptive human life consists of both acceptance of certain limits in the environment and active control of life processes. The ethical and value questions that concern us here are the questions of how much parental control of reproductive processes is good, and for what ends?

These questions are more pressing today because it is the first time man has had the medical technology and knowledge to intervene so extensively in his own life processes. More choices are now available to many. But also troubling to contemplate are the appearances of destructive side-effects and unforseen ecologic consequences of medical and psychologic interventions which were seen at the time as unalloyed cases of progress. When does the active control and technology necessary for adaptive human life become destructive? When does the receptivity, interdependency, and passivity necessary for adaptive human life become destructive? In particular in the case of genetic controls and interventions, when does the parent–child relationship become damaged, and/or the society in which parents and children live?

In evaluating the ethics of control over the reproductive process, particular disagreements usually arise from very deep differences about the nature of the universe and man's role therein. The different approaches are also seen as having profoundly different effects upon relationships between parents and children and other human relationships. One could loosely group these approaches to human control and intervention as those advocating minimal human control, maximal human control and an in-between mixed approach. At one extreme there are people who feel that in reproduction, human intervention and controls should be minimal. All interventions of technology and control in reproduction and parenting are resisted except perhaps for a minimum of medical intervention in furthering fertility, birth, and the physical welfare of newborns and children. If in a "natural" course of events a conception or pregnancy occurs, it is a positive "natural" event to be accepted as a given. Human beings should personally control the exercise of their sexual capabilities, but without medical technology of an artificial, intrusive type.

In terms of a perceived "locus of control" for reproduction, this minimal view sees an external rather than an internal locus of control [29, 30]. External forces of nature, over which an individual can have no control and should have no control, determine new life. Human beings have the role of receptively co-operating with these forces when they are seen as benign, or submitting to these external forces when they are evil. Usually this view springs from a religious view of the world as created and ruled by a good God or good fate or nature, which in the end will make all things work together for good, either in this world or the next. Death and suffering are not meaningless or the end of the story; human life in all its manifestations is sacred and not under any mere human being's authority.

In an extreme minimal view of justified human control (which implies, of course, a maximal trust in the order of the universe), it would be unacceptable to engage in genetic screening, genetic mate selection, contraception, amniocentesis, abortion, or infanticide. Nor would eugenics or the promotion of genetic health be seen as the business of human beings. God or Nature or a combination of both will take care of life. A defective child should be received like any other, no matter how severely damaged or with what suffering, as providential.

While most of those who share this minimal view of intervention, with its external locus of control, would not argue from the utilitarian consequences of their principles [31], some such arguments can be made. Even though parents may be committed to nonintervention because they believe it is the right-principled and trusting thing to do, regardless of consequences, some positive outcomes can be seen. Every child conceived can see himself and be seen by others who care for him as a part of a meaningful divine plan, not just a random event of no moment. The significance and validation of each human life does not arise from other people's recognition, but from the essential nature of the universe. Such an acceptance of events and a basic trust in the processes of human life and reproduction are very adaptive for much of the parenting role. Erik Erikson, among others, has noted the need for parental trust and belief in the universe in order to be able to give basic trust to a newborn child [32].

Seeing a child as a unique other, who is distinct and separate from all definitions, desires and standards set up by his parents helps a parent—child relationship. The inalienable dignity of a child who is an individual apart from his parents' wants and desires is safeguarded by the idea of the child as providentially sent rather than as a product of parental efforts. It is also easier for parents to let go and let a child grow up and away in his or her own direction if the child is seen as coming to them from far beyond an exercise of human will. Any lack of perfection or real inadequacies in a child are not seen as inferiorities produced by parental action, but as a part of a reality beyond the control of human beings. Moreover, the sacrifices and frustrations of child care can be seen as meaningful and unavoidable, part of the providential plan which should be accepted with good grace. Parental responsibility is seen as primarily the ability to respond to what comes. Parental guilt is allayed in this world view, for forces beyond human control are seen to have determined so much of every parent—child situation.

At the opposite pole are those who espouse a world view in which human beings should have as much an internal locus of control as possible. The more a person can shape the environment and himself, the more he lives up to human responsibility. Here responsibility is seen in its meaning of active initiation and control of outcomes. Perhaps the ultimate statement of this view in respect to human reproduction could be seen in Fletcher's statement:

"A 'test tube' baby made artificially by deliberate and careful contrivance, would be more human than one resulting from sexual roulette — the reproductive mode of the sub-human species" [33].

The implication here in this view is that the more initiative and control that parents can exercise over the processes of human conception and birth, the better. All the techniques of genetic and medical technology which can remove human life from the undependable forces of chance operating in the universe should be employed. Genetic screening, eugenic mate selection, contraception, artificial insemination, amniocentesis, fetology, abortion, and in some cases, infanticide, would be seen as a proper exercise of human responsibility and initiative.

The argument here is usually a utilitarian one describing the good consequences that will occur if human beings make active decisions to control their destiny, including their own reproduction and evolution as a species [34]. Processes of nature are considered to be neutral or negative, only awaiting human intervention for human purposes. Quality of life is considered more important than any idea of the sacredness of life in itself. The greatest good for the greatest number is sought in the employment of medical technology and knowledge. The parents' planned intention, decision, and desire to have a child is considered the most important justification of a child's conception and birth. In cases of conflict or doubtful outcomes, the mother's decision is considered most important. Also it is considered that parents have a right to have a healthy, normal child, only when and if they choose. If a fetus or newborn is suspected or found to be defective, then human responsibility can be exercised and abortion and infanticide sanctioned in the interests of a replacement, or future child who can be healthy [35].

In this world view, the parental role is seen as consciously, voluntarily chosen and contracted. Up through the neonatal state, the parents and especially the mother have the right to withdraw or cancel, if they do not wish to enter into the parent—child relationship at this particular time, or with this particular child. Proponents of this exercise of parental control see this right and freedom as furthering the good of all concerned. Neither individual parents nor society has to be burdened with the enormous care, suffering, and cost of defective children. No family has to be burdened beyond its capacities so that sibs have to suffer. When the parent—child relationship is a voluntarily entered free relationship, each child who is alive will know that he or she was chosen and voluntarily accepted. Each child will be a wanted child. When parents realize that they can choose to be parents, they can accept full responsibility of their fully voluntary decision, thereby being better parents in all ways. Active in the child's conception, they will be more active and take more initiative to protect and care for their children. Parent—child relationships are bettered by active parents who control the environment and the fate of themselves and their dependent children.

As usual, between these two extremes of advocating a complete internal locus of control and intervention versus an acceptance of an external locus of a control, there is an ambiguous middle position advocating a mixed approach which most people, including myself, hold. In this world view, intervention and an internal locus of control is demanded and necessary, but there are also limits which must not be trespassed, both on grounds of principle and pragmatic consequences for human life. Lines have to be drawn and reasons given for each action and limitation. In parent—child relationships and reproductive decisions, this view would see the need for both an initiating of control and an accepting of events and situations which come. In other words, both an internal and external locus of control would be needed when deemed appropriate.

In this mixed view, parental functions are seen as being helped by both control and acceptance, since dangers arise from too great a degree of either. Too much control and the child easily becomes an extension or manufactured product of the parent to be exploited or rejected at will in name of parental standards and requirements. On principle there has to be acceptance of the inalienable dignity of the child as a person who is different and unique and cannot be defined or ordered as some form of consumer product which must please its parents. Seeing a human life as having its existence depend upon the private desires and standards of others, especially when that life is helpless and powerless, goes against the fundamental principles of western civilization and law. Human beings have fundamental inalienable rights which are not to be subjected to private decisions by the more powerful of two parties in a conflict of interest. An infant is not to be exempted from the principles protecting other human life. Children, like women and slaves before them, cannot be seen as the private property of their parents. Infanticide is based upon an unacceptable concept of the infant as a subhuman form of private property.

Furthermore, if parents are to exercise control unto death over the lives of their children, it can be seen to corrupt family existence. Each child will fear its parents who can do away with new sibs of inferior condition and resent the fact that the parent holds such power and can demand to be satisfied. When parents can reject a new life at will because of genetic defects or anything else, it destroys that sense of trusting secure acceptance so necessary for a child's development. The contradiction of the child's primary protector and advocate harming his or her own child is upsetting logically and emotionally. On the parent's side, the realization that they could have once rejected a child can produce insidious resentments and a demand that children measure up. The family becomes one more achieved relationship rather than maintaining its ascribed status. All imperfections, inadequacies, and frustrations are not tolerated when a parent feels he has a right to the optimal baby. The rise of child abuse, child murder, and the abandonment of children all might seem a logical outcome of changing the parent—child bond from an absolute, irreversible, binding and accepted part of the natural processes of life to an arena of parental controls, personal desires, and voluntary contract.

On the other hand, the dangers of too little control are also obvious. Unlimited fertility without reliable contraception produces burdens on families and individuals. If women cannot control the number of their pregnancies, they are made subject to many grievous penalties, as are their children. The suffering of families who get no public help with handicapped children can be overwhelming. Adults must be able to take initiative and have control over their reproductive destiny, or else they cannot be expected to take initiative and act on behalf of their children. Making judgments about the future and matching one's obligations to one's capabilities are distinctively human characteristics. Fundamental human rights and the good of all family members require a measure of reproductive freedom, preventive measures, discretion, self-reliance, and self-control. Planning and hard decisions are part of the human condition and an exemplary aspect of parenthood. A passive acceptance of everything that comes would be the end of active parental protectiveness.

Most people taking a mixed view, advocating limited controls and appropriate acceptance of natural processes, are quite sure of the outer boundaries of both. They draw one line at infanticide; killing infants is inadmissable no matter how utilitarian the reasons proposed. A new human life, however defective, should be accepted and cared for just as would the most powerful, wealthy and influential adult in need of therapeutic care. (Neither adult or infant might be kept alive by extraordinary measures if they were in intractable physical pain with no hope of future remission, but the decision should be the same for the most powerful and the most powerless human being.) At the same time, when no helpless human life is at stake, a mixed view would advocate the controls and preventive interventions involved in voluntary genetic screening, contraceptive family planning, and efforts to avoid serious genetic defects through reproductive counseling. In other words, holders of this view would all say yes to contraceptive family planning but no to infanticide.

But it is in the question of whether to intervene with selective abortions that disagreements appear. The arguments over the morality of abortion, and particularly selective abortion for severe genetic defects, are between those who see abortion as basically more a form of early infanticide and those who see abortion as basically more a form of late contraception and family planning [36]. The former resist its use on principle, and the latter accept it with all the attendant pragmatic arguments described above.

Others would see the intervention of amniocentesis, followed by selective abortion, as justified by serious enough reasons; parental discretion would be allowed up until some designated cut-off point, say viability, when abortion would change its moral status from that of contraception to that of infanticide. But in any case, at some point, by birth at least, medical intervention to sustain a human life, or considerations for withdrawing support systems, could no longer depend solely upon parental discretion and decision.

Our society's principles about guarding human life and the professional ethics of physicians and others involved should, I would argue, take precedence over parental decision-making and desires once a human life is in existence. The beginning of human life is as entitled to fundamental human rights granted without discrimination as any other age or stage. Parents become parents at the birth of a child (at least), and, whether intentionally procreating or not, become subject to the same strictures against child abuse and child murder as operate with older children. If a child is mistreated or abandoned by its parents, then it becomes the responsibility of others in the society to step in, protect, and perhaps take over its care [37]. One may abandon or refuse the parental role, but not by killing one's child.

Since there is so much controversy and difference of opinion between those holding different world views with different concepts of justified medical intervention, it becomes difficult to protect the integrity, conscience, and freedom of all of the individuals involved. In a disputed moral matter which is mostly undefined by law, it becomes a delicate and stressful endeavor for parents, genetic counselors, attending physicians, and others who confront a situation to treat each other with respect and agree or disagree on very difficult courses of action. Another particular aspect of taking a practical course of action which causes controversy is making decisions about taking risks before a crisis.

THE ETHICS OF RISK-TAKING IN REPRODUCTION

The question of risk-taking is a primary one for a parent-to-be no matter how much intervention and control of reproduction is advocated theoretically in their world view. All humans alive risk an unknown future, but having a child intensifies the leap into the unknowable. Not only are all the possible genetic combinations of any new child unknown, but all the environmental factors which can begin to have an effect immediately after conception are unknown. Science has only begun to penetrate the mysteries of human development. Furthermore, no parent-to-be can guarantee that he or she will live to carry out the parenting function or that the larger social situation will be favorable for his or her child. War, economic disasters, epidemics, disease, and other larger forces may come despite all personal effort. How do you assess which risks one ought to take?

Generally, in taking risks one might hold to a principle of proportionality. The safer the risk, and the more one is able and willing to personally pay the price of the failure of some gamble or risk, the more morally justified it is to take it. But in the case of most parents, it is a joint risk, in that two people are facing the unknown together. When two people enter any venture together, their internal relationship becomes of paramount importance, and of course this is intensified in childbearing and child-rearing, where the marriage relationship is so crucial. Mutual trust between reproductive partners and their ability to communicate and support each other will change the nature of the risk-taking. Two persons may take more or fewer risks than one alone. A great deal of research has been done to ascertain when and under what conditions people will make a "risky shift" or be willing to take more chances [38, 39]. Much will depend, I would argue, on their world view of cause and effects and their past experience [40]. But if there is mutual agreement and commitment between a couple, then there is that much more human support to meet reproductive obligations entailed. If, in addition, other resources are available, such as economic power, extended family ties, education and high intelligence, health, youth, etc., the more justified the risks.

It is also the case that, in human affairs, psychologic factors such as self-confidence, hope, and emotional attitudes are very influential. Might not one see an interesting process at work in parental risk-taking? Those parents and potential parents who see themselves as strong, able, eager, confident, and are full of optimistic trusting views of themselves and the future, quite often take risks and create the conditions which fulfill their hopes. Hopeful confidence in the future often begets extra effort, just as the despair that leads to giving up can also create self-fulfilling prophecies. The psychologic factors of attitude and emotional outlook invariably interact with events and situations in the environment, especially where parenthood is concerned.

Thus different persons can view an objective probability and a risk to be taken in very different ways. A one-in-a-hundred chance of some future happening may be perceived very differently by different persons. It also may make a difference whether the uncertain future happening is positive or negative [41]. Subjective probability and objective probability are almost always discrepant and differentiated according to individual differences in personality and attitude. Attitudes may also change after experiencing certain events.

The experience of previous outcomes makes a difference in subjective assessments of probability, but not always in a strictly logical way [42]. Parents who have experienced some negative outcome with a previous child may view the probability of a similar event occurring again with quite different subjective assessments. Some parents would become far more conservative in ever taking such a risk again, while others might be more positive in future risk-taking. Those who were more positive might be reasoning under the faulty gambler's fallacy which hopes each event in an independent series is not independent, ie that after a number of boys in a family one is more likely to get a girl. Or those parents who are more positive in taking a second time risk that would be unacceptable to others, may have found by their previous experience that the supposedly negative outcome was not so dreadful after all.

Perhaps the most important ethical principle involved in reproductive risk-taking is to have a concern for the potential third party who may be involved. No potential parent or parents can judge risks simply upon their own ability and willingness to sacrifice for the consequences. Will an innocent third party, ie one's own child, have to bear the burden or suffer from parental risk-taking in reproduction in a disproportionate way? The term "disproportionate" is very important, since each new human life that comes into the world will inevitably have to suffer pain, frustration and death. Moreover, imperfections, flaws and limitations are inevitably part of every person's genetic heritage. The relevant question is: when does the potential suffering of a new life become an immoral imposition of the parents who brought it into being while knowing the risks involved? (Lack of knowledge creates an ethically different situation, of course.)

One might say that one standard would be whether a potential child would suffer far beyond and inevitably more than another child in his or her generation. Not that the parents would suffer, or that society would have to expend costs, but that the child from its own conscious perception would suffer intensely no matter how much effort might be expended in compensatory care. By this standard a retarded child, or a handicapped child not in pain and well cared for, would not suffer as much as a child of high intelligence subject to an incurable, painful, anxiety-producing condition or disease that had no known therapy available. To risk an action in which another almost certainly will suffer grievously no matter how much buffering can be provided by parents or society's resources seems immoral.

The usual risk-taking decisions of potential parents facing some genetic problem, however, will be even more complicated. Many factors will have to be weighed simultaneously: known objective probabilities interacting with subjective assessments, available family resources, available society resources, effects on sibs and marital relations, commitments to values and world view, and finally how these would all work together in affecting the welfare of a future child. Since so much of this assessment process is deeply personal, private, and intimately involved with individual differences, prudence has dictated that these decisions be left to the individuals involved. Since in our social system outside help for parents has been minimal, in the normal course of events, reproductive decisions have remained private. Society has also left unanswered the question of whether potential parents have an obligation to find out any possible known risks. This may be due partly to different world views in regard to control of life [43] and partly to the unavailability of genetic education and counseling until after some crisis event. What will be the future role of preventive measures such as mate selection?

MATE SELECTION AND RESPONSIBLE PARENTHOOD

Should a person obtain genetic information about one's reproductive potential and perhaps the genetic potential of some potential mate, in the interest of responsible parenthood? The answer to this question depends upon the current state of the science of genetics and its ability to predict future genetic outcomes [44]. It also depends upon whether a future marriage is seen as necessarily including biologic reproduction. If a marriage without children is acceptable, or adoptive parenting would be an equal alternative to biologic reproduction, then the genetic potential of a future mate would not affect a marital choice. In the same way, if the technologic intervention of amniocentesis and selective abortion for genetic defects were completely acceptable, effective, and available, knowledge of the genetic potential of a future mate would be less important in making a choice. Any genetic problems could be controlled. At the opposite extreme any genetic knowledge would be irrelevant if persons were possessed by an extremely passive external locus of control attitude toward the world and felt that they should accept whatever came to pass.

Genetic considerations in mate selection would be most crucial for those individuals who felt they should take active initiatives in controlling reproduction but could not in conscience employ amniocentesis and selective abortion. To obtain forewarning and use contraception would be necessary in order to avoid possible genetic harm to children which might be incurred by mate selection. Such persons would want to know beforehand of any genetic risks to reproduction in a possible marriage in order to make informed decisions about marriage, reproduction, and contraception. If even contraception were considered unacceptable while biologic reproduction in marriage was considered an imperative, then the genetic condition of a possible mate would be vital. It would be the only acceptable way of exercising any initiative and control of the genetic welfare of future children.

I think it can be argued that genetic information about one's self and a potential mate would always be helpful in mate selection and marriage. It would be one more consideration in making decisions about marriage and life goals. As marriage and reproductive decisions become less routine and more deliberate, under the social pressures of the changing roles of women, changing sexual mores, and population concerns, knowledge of their genetic potential could help an individual or a couple assess alternatives for a future marriage. Already some informal genetic considerations often operate in mate selection, and in a matter as serious as marriage and potential reproduction, the more informed the decisions, the better. In my estimation, taking an action with some foreknowledge of the possibilities involved helps avoid later recriminations and furthers parental responsibility.

If genetic screening and genetic consultation were offered as a service to all young persons and all newly married couples, it would probably soon become a matter of course. Chest xrays, cancer examinations and eye examinations are not considered stigmatizing, and neither would the obtaining of pertinent genetic information once it is more widely understood. Since genetic information helps a person make decisions which might affect the welfare of a potential child, and involves a potential parent—child relationship, one of the most intense and altruistic of human bonds, such information will be sought and welcomed. The reluctance to learn that one may be carrying deleterious genes would, I think, be a minor factor compared to the ability to avoid producing a child suffering from a genetic condition.

Information is not passive but an active ingredient of human interrelationships. Genetic information about an individual derives from the individual's participation and very existence in a specific human family of the human species. To withhold relevant genetic information from a mate with whom one is jointly going to create a continuation of families would seem to be inadmissable, no matter what conflicts might be envisioned. So too, everyone in an extended family whose future course of life might be affected by certain genetic information should be able to know. To withhold any information from anyone when it might affect their serious life decisions even more when involving the welfare of potential children, would be seen as morally unacceptable. Only if genetic information truly affects only one person's future could it be seen as truly private and privileged. Of course this general view will entail many cases of conflicts of interest which would have to be argued in much more detail in an effort to be just to all parties.

CONFLICTS AND TENSIONS BETWEEN INDIVIDUALS AND SOCIETY

Ethical considerations of responsible parenthood from the point of view of the individuals involved does not begin to take on the questions of larger individual—society conflicts. What happens when an individual's actions in regard to reproductive decisions are seen as unacceptable to others either for moral reasons or on allocation of available resource grounds? Do these others, along with the various legal authorities, have the right to make laws, set policies, intervene, of coerce? This is a huge question involving fundamental questions of the role of law, the extent of civil liberty and the nature of justice in a pluralistic democracy, areas beyond the scope of this paper [45]. But a few thoughts are unavoidable.

Reproductive decisions and parental actions have in no social system ever been completely private actions, probably because the survival of human groups has depended upon an adequately socialized new generation. Social regulations about mating and family life have always had either social or legal force, often both, as in the prohibition against incest in our society. Today, each parent or parent-to-be is also a social person, participating in many subgroupings and institutions of society. Parents are three-way agents in a way: Responsible to and for themselves, to and for society, and to and for their child. In their child-producing and child-rearing, parents have a temporary mandate or temporary proxy control over a child who as a future adult citizen must be adequately socialized. Parents have to be given enough authority and rights in order to carry out their increasingly difficult role.

But parents cannot be given total control and authority, for it is often the case that society has to protect children from their parents. The increase in reported child abuse and child murder has forced child abuse legislation, which in emergencies can remove a child from a parent who is failing to protect and socialize adquately [46]. At the same time, professionals and representatives of the society can also fail children, and many a parent has had to struggle against outside professionals, authorities, and so-called protective institutions in order to protect their children. In cases of conflict between parents and others, it is always difficult to discern the truth, much less the best interests of all concerned in either the short or the long run. Therefore, except in very extreme situations, great caution and hesitation have been very rightly exercised by society's various representatives when any question arises of coercing parents. Instead, voluntary cooperation has always been sought through education, persuasion, and incentives.

Such an educational voluntary approach seems even more appropriate in setting up programs and goals involved with genetic issues, where so little is yet known and there is so much controversy. Programs can be offered, persuasive educational measures can be taken by various institutions and groups, but coercion, intervention, and legal measures are a most serious step in any pluralistic and free society. The bitter ongoing controversy over abortion legislation is an example of deep divisions which exist in the society. How could any legal coercion and intervention in parental reproductive decisions be justified in the promotion of genetic health? One may argue persuasively for the immorality or irresponsibility of certain individual reproductive actions, but it is another matter to create a coercive law or family penalties which will probably mostly affect innocent children. It is especially a problem, since reproductive behavior is so personal, private, and involves unknown future events. What would you need for enforcement? Some reproductive preventive detection? Compulsory sterilizations and abortions? And decided by whom? The idea is ethically repugnant and politically impossible.

CONCLUSION

Parents will be exercising reproductive responsibility mostly apart from any legal restrictions or coercion. They will be influenced by their responses to the many interrelated factors discussed in this paper: the social role of the family; parental motivations; concepts of intervention and control; attitudes toward risk-taking and mate selection; and available education about genetic issues. When searching for an ethical perspective the distinction has to be made between exercising responsibility *as* a parent and responsibility in *becoming* a parent. A parent is primarily responsible for his or her child or children. The special relationship involved in this unique dependency situation implies a primary obligation to parental altruism and unselfishness. In any conflict of needs the child's interest almost without exception over that of the parent. To be a parent is to be protector, caretaker, buffer, advocate, and initiator—educator with obligations to fulfill this role toward one's own dependent child before others. If there is a conflict of interest between the good of one's child and the good of a social institution or some other person, then the parent takes the side of his child. In other words, it seems right that the parent protect and be the child's protector—advocate, first and foremost, before other personal obligations as a member of any other group. The responsibility to one's child comes first, then to self and society.

Of course the parent is also engaged in socializing the child and preparing him or her for gradual emancipation and adult group membership. Sometimes this will involve withdrawing some parental protection strategically, but only in the best interests of the child. In general the parent should as parent challenge, if need be, every professional, every institution, every authority, any other person in order to protect and provide for his or her child. As long as the society has not forcibly removed a child and the parent has not legally relinquished the parental role, then the parent's primary role is protection, advocacy, and a prejudiced biased championing of their own. Who else is there if parents fail? Protection necessarily means putting the protectee's interest ahead of one's own (unless in a conflict one's own interest will serve the protectee better). The parental role is one in which altruism is demanded once one is a parent.

But it is more complicated to think ethically about the process of becoming a parent or assuming the parental role. Before becoming a parent there is as yet no dependent child to whom one owes protection and advocacy. The would-be parent's obligations to themselves, their existing family, to society at large could be far more compelling than that to a potential child-to-be. Many, many cases can be imagined in which an individual or couple's prior obligations, or the needs of others, would override the individual's justifications for procreating potential children. There would be a continuum of cases, ranging from the very ordinary situation of already having as many children as one can care for to the extraordinary crisis situation of living during a famine or in a concentration camp.

Those who stress the problems of earth's overpopulation argue for limiting births from the analogy of the famine situation, and/or the obligation to future generations not to make the earth unlivable.

In other words the would-be parent may take into account obligations to himself, the society now and in the future with a different set of priorities, than the parent who now has a child. Questions about the would-be-child's nature and the nature of the parent's motivations, capabilities, and potential genetic risks can be asked which become beside the point once embarked upon the parental enterprise. But the primary guiding ethical principle of decision-making seems as inevitable as in considerations of parental motivation, parental control and parental risk-taking. What will be best from the potential child's point of view? Any parents contemplating entry into the basically altruistic role of parenting can hardly justify putting their own motivations, desires, or even ideologies ahead of their child's welfare.

Granted the primacy of obligatory parental altruism and commitment to his or her own child, several crucial moral and ethical questions remain. At what point in the course of a developing human life, from conception to birth, does one become a parent with parental obligations of altruistic protection and primary advocacy? To what extent is it ethically justifiable to control human reproduction, given a range of options from nonintervention to infanticide? And, finally, what is ethically acceptable in parental risk-taking? The answers to these questions basically determine the different approaches to the ethics of responsible parenthood discussed above. Since different individuals in this society radically disagree over these basic questions and do not succeed in persuading each other, we will all be living for many years to come with serious and unresolved social and ethical dilemmas. Two final quotes, which are both true, suggest the essential problem:

Human reason needs only to will more strongly than fate and she is fate.
Thomas Mann

One may well want to reconsider the relationship between the will to master totally, in any form, and the will to destroy.
Erik Erikson, in "Young Man Luther"

REFERENCES

1. Fletcher J: The Parent-Child Bond. Theological Studies Vol. 33, No. 3, 1972.
2. Twiss SB: Ethical issues in genetic screening. "Ethical, Social and Legal Dimensions of Screening for Human Genetic Disease." Edited by D Bergsma, M Lappe, RO Roblin, JM Gustafson. New York: Stratton Intercontinental Medical Book, 1974.
3. Gustafson JM, Laney JT: "On Being Responsible: Issues in Personal Ethics." New York: Harper & Row, 1968.

4. McCandless BR: "Childhood Socialization, The Handbook of Socialization Theory and Research." Edited by DA Goslin. Chicago: Rand McNally College Publishing, 1969, pp 791–819.

5. Wright D: "The Psychology of Moral Behavior." Baltimore: Penguin Books, 1971.

6. Baumrind D: Current patterns of parental authority. Developmental Psychology Monographs, 1971.

7. Rheingold HL: "The Social and Socializing Infant, Handbook of Socialization Theory and Research." Edited by DA Goslin. Chicago: Rand McNally College Publishing, 1969.

8. Bell RQ: Stimulus control of parent or caretaker behavior by offspring. Develop Psych 4:63–72, 1971.

9. Bronfenbrenner U: Two Worlds of Childhood: U.S. and U.S.S.R. New York: Russell Sage Foundation, 1970.

10. Zajonc RB: Family configuration and intelligence. Science 16, April 1976.

11. Parsons T, Bales RF: "Family Socialization and Interaction Process." New York: The Free Press, 1955.

12. Goode WJ: "World Revolution and Family Patterns." New York: The Free Press, 1970.

13. Steinfels M O'B: "Who's Minding the Children: The History and Politics of Daycare in America." New York: Simon and Schuster, 1973.

14. Berelson B: The value of children: A taxonomical assay. "Raising Children in Modern America." Vol. I: Problems and Prospective Solutions. Edited by MB Talbot. Boston: Little Brown, 1976.

15. Wilson EO: "Sociobiology." Cambridge, Mass: Harvard University Press, 1975.

16. Wilson EO: Ibid. Money J, Ehrhardt A: "Man & Woman: Boy and Girl." Baltimore: The John Hopkins University Press, 1972.

17. Flugel JC: "The Psycho-Analytic Study of the Family." London: Hogarth Press, 1929.

18. Freud A: "The Concept of the Rejecting Mother, Parenthood: Its Psychology and Pyschopathology." Boston: Little Brown, 1970, pp 376–387.

19. Benedek T: "The Psychological Approach to Parenthood: Its Psychology and Psychopathology." Boston: Little Brown, 1970, pp 109–185.

20. Erikson E: "Childhood and Society," 2nd Ed. New York: WW Norton, 1963.

21. Bandura A: Social-learning theory of identificatory process. "Handbook of Socialization Theory and Research." Edited by DA Goslin. Chicago: Rand-McNally College Publishing, 1969.

22. Blake J: Population policy for Americans: Is the government being misled? Science 164: 522, 2 May, 1969.

23. Bettelheim B: "A Home for the Heart." New York: Knopf, 1974, p 149.

24. James J: A preliminary study of the size determinant in small group interaction. Am Sociol Rev, LV: 6 May, 1950, pp 474–477.

25. Fagley R: Doctrines and attitudes of major religions in regard to fertility. Proceedings of World Population Conference 1965. New York: United Nations, 1967.

26. Noonan JT: "Contraception." Cambridge: Massachusetts, Harvard University Press, 1966.

27. Thielicke H: The Ethics of Sex. New York: Harper & Row, 1964.

28. Callahan S: Are parents born or made? "Parenting: Principles and Politics of Parenthood." New York: Doubleday, 1973, pp 137–169.

29. Ratter JB: Generalized expectancies for internal versus external control of reinforcement. Psychol Monographs 80:1, 1966.

30. Weiner B, Frieze I, Kukla A et al: Perceiving the causes of success and failure. "Attribution in Social Interaction in Social Interaction: Perceiving the Causes of Behavior." Edited by E Jones, DE Karause, HH Kelley, RE Nisbett, S Valins, B Weiner. Morristown, New Jersey: General Learning Press, 1971, pp 1–27.

31. Frankena WK: "Ethics." Englewood Cliffs, New Jersey: Prentice-Hall, 1973.
32. Erikson E: "Childhood and Society," 2nd Ed. New York: WW Norton, 1963.
33. Fletcher J: Ethical aspects of genetic controls. N Engl J Med, September 30, 1971, pp 5–6.
34. Hardin G: "The Moral Threat of Personal Medicine, Genetic Responsibility of Choosing Our Children's Genes." Edited by M Lipkin, Jr, and PT Rawley. New York: Plenum Press, 1974.
35. Tooley M: Abortion and infanticide. Philosophy and Public Affairs 2:37–65, 1972.
36. Callahan D: "Abortion: Law, Choice and Morality." New York: Macmillan, 1970.
37. Katz SM: "When Parents Fail: The Law's Response to Family Breakdown." Boston: Beacon Press, 1971.
38. Rettig S: Ethical risk-taking in group and individual conditions. Journal of Personal Soc Psychol 4:6, pp 648–654.
39. Pearn JH: Patients' subjective interpretation of risks offered in genetic counselling. J Med Genet 1:129, 1973.
40. Kelley H: Attribution in social interaction. "Attribution: Perceiving the Causes of Behavior." Edited by E Jones, DE Karause, HH Kelley, RE Nisbett, S Valins, B Weiner. Morristown, New Jersey: General Learning Press, 1971, pp 1–27.
41. Karause DE, Hanson LR: Negativity in evaluations. Ibid.
42. Langer EJ: The illusion of control. J Personal Soc Psychol 32:2, 311–328, 1975.
43. Gustafson JM: Genetic screening and human values: An analysis. "Ethical Social, and Legal Dimensions of Screening." Edited by D Bergsma et al. New York: Stratton Intercontinental Medical Book, 1974, pp 201–223.
44. Sorenson JR: Some social and psychologic issues in genetic screening. Public and professional adaptation to biomedical innovation. Ibid, pp 165–184.
45. Green HP, Capron AM: Issues of law and public policy in genetic screening. Ibid, pp 57–84.
46. Gil DC: "Violence Against Children: Physical Child Abuse in the United States." Cambridge, Mass: Harvard University Press, 1970.

15. Prenatal Diagnosis, Selective Abortion, and the Ethics of Withholding Treatment From the Defective Newborn

John Fletcher, PhD

INTRODUCTION TO ETHICAL ISSUES IN PRENATAL DIAGNOSIS

There are several intensely debated moral problems concerning the use of prenatal diagnosis with selective abortion. Questions of risk to fetus and mother, abortion itself, indications for prenatal diagnosis, and the development of social policy on prenatal diagnosis have each occasioned sharp differences. The major purpose of this chapter is to analyze one further debate about the ethics of prenatal diagnosis, namely, the question as to the relationship between abortion of the defective fetus and decisions about treatment of the infant born with the same degree of impairment. A brief description of the other four issues will provide the reader with an introductory review of the spectrum of ethical arguments on prenatal diagnosis so that the subject of this chapter can be seen against the background of available discussion.

Risks of Amniocentesis

According to safety studies conducted by the National Registry for Amniocentesis Study Group [1] and a collaborative study in Canada [2], amniocentesis does not adversely affect mother or fetus, with the exception of cases where more than one needle insertion was made during a single occasion to obtain fluid. There is always a theoretic risk of infection, spontaneous abortion, or injury to the fetus, but these two studies of more than 1,000 cases in each country show that amniocentesis is a safe procedure when done by a trained physician. In the early literature on prenatal diagnosis, there was discussion of risk factors, but it is of interest that risk was emphasized more by advocates of selective abortion than by its critics. Fuchs and Littlefield [3, 4] held that

Birth Defects: Original Article Series, Volume XV, Number 2, pages 239—254
© 1979 The National Foundation

women unwilling to accept abortion should be refused amniocentesis because accepting the (then) unknown risks could only be justified by abortion when necessary. Since the general safety of amniocentesis has been demonstrated, risk can be separated from the issue of abortion and that central problem discussed on its own merits.

Accuracy of diagnosis is a source of greater concern than safety. There were six cases in the U.S. study and seven cases in the Canadian study incorrectly diagnosed due to human error. Two infants thought to be normal were born with Down syndrome and two with neural tube defects. These tragedies raise moral problems that will be addressed in the main body of the paper.

Selective Abortion

The critics of prenatal diagnosis do not attack the procedure on questions of safety or accuracy but because abortion is used as the major response to early detection of defects. Their ethical arguments proceed largely from the principle of equality of the right to life as applied to the fetus. Lejeune, a physician, and ethicists Ramsey, Dyck, and Lebacqz [5—8], define the basic purpose of medicine as the saving of life, and they oppose selective abortion because it 1) undercuts the role of the physician as an advocate for the life of the fetus, 2) transforms the conscientious physician into a mere technical agent of the parents, 3) gives unwarranted power to physicians to decide who shall live or die, 4) exploits the innocent fetus that cannot consent, and 5) mistakenly makes the desires of parents legitimate objects of medical care.

Ethicists or physicians who argue for the justification of selective abortion usually reason from evidence of good consequences to be attained as opposed to the bad consequences of not aborting. Physicians such as Milunsky and Hirschhorn, and ethicists such as Aiken and Joseph Fletcher [9—12] understand the purpose of medicine as the reduction and prevention of suffering and that selective abortion serves this goal. Milunsky and Macintyre [9, 13] stress that prenatal diagnosis saves more fetal lives than those lost through selective abortion, because prenatal diagnosis more frequently dispels fears of defects and leads parents to decide to keep the fetus. Within the literature supporting selective abortion, there is a wide range of opinion about the restrictions that should be placed on abortion. Joseph Fletcher understands any unwanted pregnancy as a "disease" and advocates abortion with no sense of regret or guilt [12]. Hirschhorn takes a pragmatic position with respect to selective abortion but notes that abortion decisions must be made in the light of "individual rights" [10]. The present author attempted to create a wider latitude of choice, including protection from economic or social pressure against those who conscientiously object to abortion [14].

Indications for Prenatal Diagnosis

Should physicians admit persons for prenatal diagnosis who are severely anxious about fetal abnormality but lack any substantial family history of a genetic problem? Should parents be admitted when identification of fetal sex is the only motivation? The major argument against admission is that the physician ought not to use prenatal diagnosis to "treat the desires" of parents and become a mere technician for their wishes [8]. The major argument for respecting anxiety as one criterion for admission is that the probabilty is high that a life will be saved since diagnosis is overwhelmingly negative, and since the overall risk of having a chromosomally defective child is 1:200, there is a basis for admission [9]. There are no attempts in medical-ethical literature to justify abortion for reasons of sex preference, but Hirschhorn stated that if parents threaten abortion in the face of the physician's resistance to comply with their request, the physician should admit them in the hope of saving a life.

Social Policy for Prenatal Diagnosis

The rapid proliferation of prenatal tests will offer opportunities to governmental and medical bodies for mass programs of genetic screening, prenatal testing, and selective abortion. Three kinds of ethical issues are involved in program policy formation: 1) the degree of need to justify mounting a mass program beyond private clinics, 2) the concepts of health, especially genetic health, that undergird the program, and 3) the degree of voluntarism about abortion permitted in the program. Murray and Callahan have debated the role of cultural factors in concepts of genetic disease [15], a force that would operate in any mass program.

SELECTIVE ABORTION AND THE CARE OF DEFECTIVE NEWBORNS

A case can be composed from the National Registry of Amniocentesis Study that will frame the issue of human error in prenatal diagnosis [16]:

> Of 1,040 diagnoses made, 6 were wrong. Two babies were born with Down's syndrome even though prenatal diagnosis indicated they would be normal. The errors were . . . the result of human error as far as can be determined. It is possible that samples of amniotic fluid were mislabeled . . . and that the investigators were looking at maternal rather than fetal cells but did not realize it.

Does the moral reasoning that applies to the prenatal situation bear any relation to decision-making after the birth of a viable infant? This general question is made more poignant by the facts in a case of false—negative diagnosis. If the parents would have chosen to abort the fetus at 20—22 weeks of gestation for Down syndrome, do they and the physician have an obligation to care for the infant that slipped through the screen due to human error? One can imagine the feelings of sorrow and rage in the parents and physicians. How should they act in such a situation? Does the situation warrant euthanasia if the parents would have chosen abortion?

A second example of a moral problem stems from the following case of false—negative medical advice for prenatal diagnosis:

> Mrs. C is a 41-year-old mother of 2 children, who are 14 and 9 years of age. She accidentally conceives and consults the obstetrician-gynecologist who delivered her on both occasions. She inquired as to whether she should have prenatal diagnosis and he advised against it because he believes that "it will just upset you and there is not a good reason in your case." Seven and one-half months later, a baby with Down syndrome was delivered. The infant required surgery for esophageal atresia. Mrs. C refused to give consent for the surgery and asked that the infant not be supported. She acknowledged her anger against her physician and her pain at having missed the opportunity to diagnose the chromosomal disorder earlier and have an abortion. (Personal communication, David Abramson, MD, Georgetown University Hospital.)

Was the obstetrician-gynecologist negligent in his first recommendation? Does Mrs. C have any moral justification for her position in regard to the required surgery? How should physicians and parents now understand their obligation to care for the defective neonate in the light of arguments for abortion after amniocentesis?

The debate in ethics about such cases is presently polarized between a right-to-life argument that tends to equate genetically indicated abortion with infanticide [17, 18] and a quality-of-life argument that tends towards positive arguments for the morality of abortion and selective euthanasia of the defective neonate [19, 20]. A third view, based upon a developmental argument, distinguishes between the two situations — accepts the morality of abortion in cases with severe handicaps, but disapproves of euthanasia of the defective newborn based on the prior commitment to abortion [21].

Paul Ramsey, a leading exponent of the first view, fundamentally questions abortion decisions based upon prenatal diagnosis, because he holds that the reasoning that leads to abortion could be used to justify deliberately bringing about the death of an infant [22]. He holds that there are no clear differences between the decision-making in the two situations. He asks if there is an argument for abortion that will not also be an argument for infanticide [22]. Ramsey's concern in raising this question is not based upon a sociologic prediction that we will begin to commit infanticide because we do abortions to prevent genetic diseases. He is saying that if we have moral reasons not to commit infanticide, then we should not do the abortions. In short, there are means that are intrinsically wrong in themselves regardless of the good ends that may be desired through the means. If the argument for abortion could bring about infanticide, then there must be a fatal moral flaw in the argument.

Joseph Fletcher's position, leading the second view in the debate, not only supports prenatal diagnosis and abortion of defective fetuses, but also tends towards setting aside restraints against euthanasia for defective neonates [20]. He also holds that there is no significant moral difference between the two situations, and that if we would see a moral justification for abortion based on genetic defects, then there would surely be a legitimate argument for euthanasia, painlessly putting an end to the life of an infant born with the same serious impairment. To do less would be hypocritical and morally disingenuous.

Consequentialist reasoning supports his position, for which "only the end (a proportionate good) makes sense of what we do (the means)" [12]. He does not say that any end justifies any means, but that the ends of prevention of human harm and relief of suffering by abortion and euthanasia clearly justify these actions in cases where there is clear medical evidence.

These rival views, though polarized in their practical recommendations, are united in a commitment to consistency when each compares the moral and legal status of the fetus with the newborn. Each ethicist, in his own terms, understands the fetus on the same level of value and dignity as the infant. To Ramsey, the status of the fetus as a fellow human being begins at implantation, and the status is given from God, an unconditional source of irreducible dignity [23]. For Joseph Fletcher, the bestowal of humanhood is a human choice that ought to be based upon the needs of the adults making the decision about humanhood. We ought, therefore, to work out "indicators for humanhood" that cause us to delay conferral of human status to the infant until qualitative and quantitative measures can be made [24].

A common strength in both arguments is consistency. We yearn to be able to do the fitting and right thing in similar situations. We need to account for our actions in patterns that are not susceptible to too many contradictions, whether we use deontologic or consequentialist forms of reasoning. The particular strengths and relevance of each argument to the two cases will be evaluated.

The Right-to-Life Argument

The strongest feature of the right-to-life argument is the clarity that derives from the objective reality of the fetus. There is human life present. All of the genetic information is present that will interact with the environment to produce the child that will be. Furthermore, the fact that the fetus is the result of the procreation of two human beings is a de facto case for claiming that a human life has begun that deserves equal protection with each and every other human life.

If the fetus is a fellow human being, any medical procedure should be done with a guarantee to do no harm to the fetus. Whether the argument is grounded in biology, theology, or equal human rights, the effect is to take the issue of the conferral of humanhood out of human control. The effect of being transcended by sources of meaning and dignity beyond oneself is profoundly reassuring and adds to the clarity of the basic premise. Clarity in moral reasoning supports consistency and is very effective in ordering the priorities in decision-making. The first move in the argument is always in the direction of respecting the objective reality of the fetus.

If one applied the right-to-life argument to the two cases presented, the following two possibilities would result in each case, but with the same moral outcome:

1) Human error in prenatal diagnosis. a) Since prenatal diagnosis is in practice associated with selective abortion, which is inherently immoral except in a situation required to save the mother's physical life, one ought not to have entered into it in the first place. One ought to protect the life of the infant with the same degree of loyalty that is required to protect the life of the conceptus. Therefore, even if one has made the moral error of entering prenatal diagnosis, one must not commit another wrong by questioning the right of the defective infant to life. Every possible step must be taken to preserve the life of the infant born after a false—negative prenatal diagnosis.

b) Since prenatal diagnosis is medically safe, however morally dangerous, one can seek the knowledge that it provides as long as one intends not to act upon it to seek abortion. The only exception to the rule against abortion is when the disease of the infant threatens the life of the mother. The primary reason for obtaining a diagnosis is to prepare for the birth of the infant with every known resource that modern science can provide to concerned parents. We should seek prenatal diagnosis to be more prepared to care. In case of an error that results in a false—negative diagnosis, one ought to remain faithful to the original commitment to bring a new human life into the world without prejudice about his or her right to life, however badly the infant might be damaged by heredity or accidents of birth.

2) False—negative medical advice for prenatal diagnosis. a) The obstetrician-gynecologist is not culpable in any sense since he ought originally to have expressed his opposition to prenatal diagnosis due to its link to selective abortion which is inherently immoral. The mother is wrong to base any reason for passive euthanasia on the faulty premise of a missed opportunity for abortion. She should consent to the surgery in order to save the life of the infant, and if she can recover her lost commitment to the sanctity of human life, she should commit herself to the loving care of a child with the potential to love and respond to parental care, despite the mental and physical problems associated with Down syndrome.

b) The obstetrician-gynecologist ought to have originally recommended prenatal diagnosis, because of the known risks of mental retardation in children born to mothers of advanced age. But his recommendation should have been coupled with an argument against abortion, if he were going to continue to act as the woman's physician. A physician who respects human life can separate prenatal diagnosis from abortion and should help parents seek as much information as they can to be fully prepared for the birth of a child. If he had acted in accordance with his best medical knowledge and his conscience, he would have obtained the mother's consent to go through with the pregnancy even if a positive diagnosis were made for Down syndrome. Then they could have prepared for and faced the birth together, been prepared for the likelihood of surgery, worked through the disappointment at an earlier stage, and devoted every precious minute to the saving of the life of the infant. It would not be morally or legally reasonable for the woman to sue the physician for failing to give accurate medical advice, because the presumption of such a suit would be the missed opportunity of the abortion of the fetus.

The right-to-life argument will accomplish what it sets out to do: equal protection of the fetus and the infant. That is an additional strength, in that congruity between consequences and intentions lends weight to moral argumentation.

What the right-to-life argument does not do is satisfactorily involve and resolve another set of interests and values which, by virtue of the basic promise of the argument, are not admitted into the realm of moral discourse:

Will the physical and mental problems of this infant be an overall detriment to the personal life of the mother, the well being of her family, and the resources of the society in question?

Will the public health be well served by allowing this child to live?

If the pregnancy was originally unwanted, do not the needs of the mother count in moral terms?

Does this mode of reasoning do justice to the possibility that allowing the infant to live will do greater injury to it than allowing it to die?

Is death for this particular infant better than continued existence?

The Quality-of-Life Argument

The basic strength of the quality-of-life argument rests in its link to the power of authentic human responsibility. In reality, *only* human beings decide about what is truly human, even if they do so in the power of the belief that humanhood is derived from God, biology, or natural law. If only human beings make these decisions, the argument proceeds, we must not shirk the implications of the responsibility to distinguish personal life from biologic life. Biologic facts do not in themselves provide the values that enhance personal human existence. To turn over any part of our responsibility to decide to forces outside human control is an abdication of the imperative to act in every way to increase the realm of human control and its quality. To act as though we could not control more of the consequences of inborn errors is bad faith and a denial of our own dignity. Therefore, we ought to promote a climate in which decisions about the fetus and the neonate are made in the light of the *needs* of the living adults making the decisions and the *social consequences* of the decisions, rather than in response to the imagined "rights" of beings who are so damaged that they will never be able to claim a right.

If one applied the quality-of-life argument to the cases under discussion the following results would ensue:

1) Human error in prenatal diagnosis. The very occurrence of human error in prenatal diagnosis should serve to illustrate the justification for a policy of delaying decisions about humanhood until after birth. Women who need prenatal diagnosis should be fully informed about the minimal risk of error, and the counselor should open all of the implications of error and argue for a consistent position on abortion and euthanasia. The investigators who mislabeled or misread fetal cells should not be punished or should they be liable for suit for malpractice, even if the parents and physicians decide to support the unwelcome infant, because the latter have abdicated their medical and moral responsibility by allowing the infant to live. The payment of damages to the parents presumes that the continued existence of the infant is of sufficient value to require compensation, and such is not the case. The pain and suffering relieved by a decision not to support the infant (or in a more responsible society by procedures for euthanasia) would be a greater good than the possible psychologic compensation to the parents of the continued existence of the infant. There should be a policy for error in prenatal diagnosis consonant with the personal freedom of adults to decide for themselves what constitutes acceptable human life. If the parents would have aborted a defective fetus for Down syndrome in order to protect themselves, society, and the infant from the mental and physical consequences of that disorder, then they are surely justified in acting upon the same intentions at the birth of the infant. Birth does not change the real situation as defined earlier; the only significant factor is the passage of time and that is hardly a deterrent to a responsible decision.

2) False—negative medical advice for prenatal diagnosis. The obstetrician-gynecologist should definitely be liable for malpractice and the mother should be able to recover for damages to her mental and psychologic health from the results of misadvice. If the physician was covering up his opposition to prenatal diagnosis on the basis of his beliefs about abortion, he should have been open and honest with the woman. He could have distinguished between the benefits of the test and the dangers of abortion (in his eyes), but he should have logically withdrawn from the case if she intended to act by abortion on a positive diagnosis. His personal beliefs about abortion should not have influenced a recommendation for a test that is definitely safe and will provide the person with information for action.

The attending physicians at birth should accede to the mother's desire not to perform surgery on an infant that would have been aborted at an earlier time for Down syndrome. The atresia is an added problem that could not have been detected in utero but should not be the basic justification for nonsupport. Down syndrome is in and of itself a defect sufficient to warrant nonsupport because of the lack of therapy, the lifetime of special care and protection needed for the affected person, the lack of a potential approaching real quality of life, and the extraordinary demands such a person places on the family. The physicians and parents should not be liable to prosecution for a decision of nonsupport, and existing laws should be changed to protect the freedom of individuals to make these decisions according to their own needs. We should always allow persons in this situation to exercise their responsibility rather than to pass it to someone else. The expense and conflict of a medical decision to disagree with the mother, to proceed with a court order for surgery, and to place the infant in an institution as a ward of the state would be greatly outweighed by a decision consistent with an earlier commitment to therapeutic abortion.

Like the right-to-life argument, the argument from quality brings results consonant with its original intention: protection of the responsibility of adults to decide for themselves to control the consequences of reproduction. Within the major premise of the argument, the rights of the infant are excluded in order to serve a higher social good, increase the sphere of freedom of the adults directly concerned, and create new alternatives to try for a healthy child or accept the limits of the present family.

Questions remain, however, not addressed by the argument, that are excluded from the debate by force of the premise of responsibility:

What is the relevance of biologic development to a moral position on the status of the fetus or neonate? (The quality-of-life argument can so completely separate biologic from human freedom as to rest its case entirely on the latter.)

Does society owe a protection to the newborn that overrides the self-interests of parents and physicians?

If we are free to define what is human based upon needs and social consequences, does not this mean that the taking of life in other contexts (terminal illness, senility, coma) could be justified on the grounds of social good?

Will a human being with this disorder inevitably be unhappy and unfulfilled? Is there not a potential for such a person that is within a reasonable attainment, given the right attention?

Does not the quality of life argument ignore the fact that people regard the newborn as a real individual and build up loyalty steadily during pregnancy to the expected child? Will not the extension of the quality of life argument postpone the development of the essential trust required between parents and the newborn?

Might not some parents meet a real need to love and care for a handicapped child?

Clarity and consistency are not the only tests for the adequacy of bio-ethical arguments [25] . Several other tests must be applied. Our theory of moral responsibility should be able to examine the widest range of biologic, social, and other kinds of evidence to support or deny a proposed action. Both views that we have examined are exclusionary on this first count: the right-to-life argument counts heavily on biologic facts but excludes data on socioeconomic need or the severity of the defect from consideration; the quality-of-life argument does not need to refer to biologic facts at least until after birth to establish its major point. Second, the moral perspective should be able to include many contending values, conflicts, and tensions that come into play in biomedical decisions. Both positions exclude important interests and values from the debate. Third, an argument should not furnish principles for guidance in one situation (abortion) that could be used to destructive ends in another situation (euthanasia of neonates or terminally ill persons). The quality-of-life argument is especially vulnerable to this test. Finally, because our society is pluralistic and no one's moral development is complete, our modes of reflection should show an openness to multiple sources of criticism. In short, one should show how he can learn from the basic strengths of the arguments of the other, rather than set out to demolish those arguments.

I have indicated that I favor a third line of reasoning that offers a greater balance between the two polar positions in the debate, assists us in making hard decisions in both prenatal and neonatal situations, and allows for more ethical pluralism than the two views previously considered.

A Developmental View

A developmental view begins with the observation that there is a *process* of interaction between the genetic program of fetus and its environment that is normative both for biologic and moral understanding. Those geneticists or philosophers who hold this view are by no means agreed on a single theory of development [25] . Thinkers choose different stages in the developmental process to assign the status of human life or personhood deserving of protection. The presence of all of the organ systems, the beginning of brain waves, completion of the brain structure, viability, and birth are only some of the stages that have been singled out. All of the views on development, however, agree that life is present from fertilization forward in the sense that all of the genetic information is present and as the process of development continues this life will interact and grow towards the stage in which human life of personhood is a fitting description.

In addition to a developmental view of the growth of the fetus, the medical literature amply describes pregnancy as a crisis bringing about in the parents, especially in the mother, behavioral changes that prepare them for caring for the infant [26—29] . We should expect loyalty to the developing life to grow, change, and increase during the whole course of pregnancy. Taking the developmental view, one would argue that there ought to be care and regard for the fetus that are appropriate to its development. This proportionate care should be understood in the total context of reproduction.

For example, since every pregnancy should be a wanted, planned, and caring experience, one ought to begin to care for the nascent life by ordering priorities before conception. Care must be taken to avoid the drugs, pollutants, or exposure to hazards that may harm the crucial first stages of fetal development. The last statement assumes that one desires to be a parent, has conceived willingly, and is competent to make the changes in life-style and self-understanding to make a good beginning as a parent. In the world in which we live, however, there are coerced or unwanted pregnancies. Many persons can adjust to an unplanned pregnancy so that it can become wanted. Not many can adjust to an unwanted pregnancy. Medically regulated abortion should be available as early as possible as a remedy to unwanted or coerced pregnancy, but no woman should be coerced into making an abortion decision. The norm for the care of the beginning of life should be consonant with planned conception.

As part of planning for parenthood, couples should have at least familiarized themselves with the genetic histories of their own families. Public education about birth defects and genetics will continue to raise the consciousness of young parents about defects in the fetus due to no human intentionality. Prenatal diagnosis should not be presented as the "answer" to genetic ignorance, but as a tool that increasingly well-informed and educated persons employ to learn the truth about an at-risk pregnancy. Seeking prenatal diagnosis can be a caring act in a series of caring acts during pregnancy, assuming that there are proper indications.

An earlier section presented my position on criteria for abortion in the event of a positive diagnosis. That view attempts to balance the value of the developing life of the fetus with the individual and social interests of the parents. The right-to-life argument correctly observes that prenatal diagnosis and abortion are separable, but incorrectly argues that abortion is morally wrong except to save the mother's life. The quality-of-life argument would tend heavily towards encouraging abortion as prevention for the birth of each detected at-risk fetus for which there was no therapy. My own view accepts the morality of abortion for the reasons stated, because I do not hold that the fetus prior to viability is yet a fellow human being to whom wider social protection is due beyond the kind of educated care on the part of parents and physicians described above. Thus, if a severe defect is detected at this stage of development, one is morally justified to abort even though there will be much more emotional involvement in the second trimester since the fetus has been felt to move [30]. Parents who choose to abort at this stage act out of a desire to protect themselves, their family, and society from harm. They do not incur any moral guilt because all of the conditions for humanhood are not present and the defect is weighed against a stage of development in which the fetus is still totally dependent upon the mother. Parents who choose not to abort after a positive diagnosis, because of conscientious objection to abortion, should not be penalized or pressured in any way and should be helped to prepare for the alternatives that birth will present.

There is one major difference between the prenatal and neonatal situations that has direct moral relevance. Following viability, the separate physicial existence of the infant apart from the mother confronts parents, physicians, and legal institutions with independent moral claims for care and support. Pediatricians may consider the "fetal-maternal unit" as a patient prior to viability, but after viability, the infant is clearly a patient. The movement of the fetus prepares the parents emotionally for the acceptance of the infant as a separate individual, but before extrauterine viability the fetus should not be considered independently from the mother's condition. McCormick has questioned how one would delineate the strength of the moral claim of the fetus before and after viability [31]. The right-to-life argument holds that the claim is so strong prior to viability that only life-saving interventions (eg ectopic pregnancies or their equivalent) are allowed. The quality of life position would hold that the developing fetus had no more moral claim than the adults concerned with it would allow, and that its moral claim would depend entirely on their wishes, needs, or plans. The first view overestimates the moral claim of the previable fetus, and the second view underestimates it.

The moral claim of the previable fetus should be understood as proportionate to its stage of development, what is known about that stage, and what ought to be done within that stage to assure maximal fetal development. The previable fetus does have a moral claim for care upon parents, especially the mother, and those who assist her in developing her parenthood. There are two sources of the moral claim: 1) the value of the developing life and 2) the human potential of the developing life. We ought to regard the developing life with a value for us that increases with each discernible stage of growth. The more we learn about fetal development, the more informed our valuing becomes. There is a more powerful "lure" in the potential of the person over his or her lifelong development and growth in value for self and others. The future of the fetus is a far greater source of its value than its past. If one understands the value of the fetus as totally "given," then one must accord the same rights that adults deserve. If one understands that the fetus has no value until after adults assign personhood at some point following birth, then rights must be withheld. Neither of these static views are sufficiently informed by the dynamic process in which increasing value accompanies increasing growth and interaction. The real question here is how much human experience counts in a theory of moral behavior.

The strength of the previable fetus' moral claim is weaker than that of the viable fetus because the life of the former is totally dependent upon the mother, whose needs and rights may conflict with the developing life of the fetus, especially if a serious defect is discovered. Prior to viability the fetal claim to protection can only be responded to through the mother, whose needs and rights in a situation of serious conflict should predominate when the bodily life of a defective fetus with little or no potential threatens her more developed personal life. Following viability, when the life of the fetus is not dependent upon the mother and the infant can live apart from her, the fact that physicians and others can respond directly to the body and life of the fetus without any bodily conflict with the mother is only the beginning of the independent existence of the infant, but it is a sufficient beginning to warrant wider protection.

A fetus without a severe defect, or with a defect for which there is a therapy, has a stronger moral claim on the mother and those who assist her than a fetus with a severe and nontreatable defect, because the former can more probably respond to the promise of becoming a person in a community of persons and assuming the rights and privileges that the future holds. The detection of a severe defect and the known suffering that will be incurred further weaken an already dependent moral claim to existence and allow the parents sufficient reason to make an abortion decision if they so choose. When the future potential of a fetus is disclosed and found to be minimal or nonexistent, the larger pull of the future is vastly diminished or lost. The independent moral claims to life and protection of a viable infant are to be valued more highly than the previable fetus because as soon as the fetus actualizes its potential viability it can play a full social role and be recognized as a person [32]. The basic moral principle involved in judging between the strength of the two claims is that of the justice that is due to the mother over the previable fetus prior to viability and to the viable infant itself after it is supportable apart from the mother. The difference between claims of justice when the body of the mother is the vehicle through which remedies must be sought and when we could respond directly to the body of the infant should be obvious. It is simply not fair to the mother to accord the previable fetus an equal or external status to her condition, since she will endure the consequences of any decision made while still carrying the fetus.

There are two additional differences that help to distinguish between the fetal and neonatal states, although these reasons are more descriptive of the two states rather than constitutive in the moral sense. First, after birth the disease in the infant is more available to physicians for palliation, or partial therapy that will not involve the mother. The hope of many researchers is to be able to treat fetal disease in utero, as in the case of erythroblastosis fetalis (Rh disease). For the present, however, the real situation for parents and physicians is that they must wait until birth to respond to a disease in the newborn with decisions to treat or not to treat. The basic presupposition of neonatology is that the neonate is a patient and should be treated where there is a reasonable hope of intervention.

Second, I have referred to the change in parental loyalty and acceptance of the infant as a real person at birth, compared to the same sense of loyalty in the earlier stages of pregnancy. An example of the depth of parental loyalty can be seen when parents of a defective newborn "mourn" the loss of the expected healthy child and reconsider acceptance of the child with a defect.

The effect of the moral difference of viability, combined with the additional two descriptive differences establish the newborn infant, even with a serious defect, as a fellow human being who deserves protection on both a legal and an ethical basis, and the force of these differences contributes to an argument against euthanasia based on any earlier commitment to abortion.

We are now in a position to see how this perspective would consider the two cases under discussion:

1) Human error in prenatal diagnosis. There is no inherent reason why a parental commitment to abortion in the case of a positive prenatal diagnosis for Down syndrome would carry over to the situation of a false—negative diagnosis and warrant active euthanasia or nonsupportive management. The options open to parents and physicians include 1) vigorous support and surgery if required to enable the parents better to accept and serve the infant as their own, 2) the same regimen to allow for optimal placement of the infant in the event that the parents choose to dissolve their parental rights and give the infant for adoption, or institutionalization, or 3) a program of intensive care and hospitalization in order to monitor the infant for additional problems than were presented at birth. Part of the informed consent procedure of prenatal diagnosis should include facts about the possibility of human error and the commitment of the physicians to the viable infant in case technical error occurs. If these facts are explained clearly, the physicians responsible for the error should not be held liable, but rather they should do everything in their power to ease the problems of the parents. There should be compensatory measures designed to help the economic situation of parents in this particular situation, paid for out of special liability insurance funded by centers that specialize in prenatal diagnosis. Extended counseling and support should be provided by the physicians to strengthen the parents for their initially unhappy role.

If the third option were followed and further complications developed that were not present at birth, the physicians and parents may have to face decisions to intervene that would promise only minimal hope of satisfactory recovery. In this situation, extraordinary care needs to be taken that every reasonable medical intervention had been made or evaluated negatively.

2) False—negative medical advice for prenatal diagnosis. The obstetrician-gynecologist should definitely be liable for malpractice because he did not explain the risks of mental retardation or the options open to his patient. His malpractice insurance should pay for the support of the infant while under medical care and in addition pay damages to the mother for the mental anguish she suffered due to his mistake.

The decision about surgery should not be made in the light of the missed opportunity for prenatal diagnosis, but solely in the perspective of the infant's medical picture and its potential within the limits of Down syndrome and any additional complications that have developed after birth. The same options are open in this case as are open in the former case. Again, there should be no necessary relation between a lost opportunity for abortion and a program of nonsupport that is not warranted by additional complications.

CONCLUSION

The thrust of my argument is that prenatal diagnosis and its relation to neonatal care should be conducted within an ethic that balances the growing right to life of the developing fetus with the needs and interests of the parents and society. As success grows in the efficacy of prenatal diagnosis, those who administer it must not accept selective abortion too easily as a final solution for genetic disease. If we enter the neonatal event with a too-easy conscience about what we allow in abortion, the ambience of caring which is so necessary to the beginning of human life might be seriously harmed. Parents and physicians are free to be inconsistent with the reasoning that justifies selective abortion and to choose to do everything reasonable to support the life of a neonate that slips through the screen of prenatal diagnosis by human error, injustice of the distribution of resources, or parental commitment to the right to life. The conduct of genetic counseling should be done in a climate of caring for human life, even though abortion is an unhappy solution to severe defects, and only an interim solution prior to genetic therapy. Underlying my final remark is an assumption that human genetics will someday be more completely understood and that knowledge will lead to possibilities for genetic therapy and permanent prevention of genetic disease. Between today and that future, geneticists, their patients, and their nonscientific colleagues must negotiate their way through the cultural and ethical complexities of the application of technical insights to genetic problems without sacrificing the humanity which justifies the scientific quest itself.

REFERENCES

1. NICHD National Registry for Amniocentesis Study Group: Mid Trimester Amniocentesis for Prenatal Diagnosis: Safety and Accuracy. JAMA 236:1471–1476, 1976.
2. Simpson N, Dallaire L, Miller J et al: Prenatal diagnosis of genetic disease in Canada: Report of a collaborative group. Can Med Assoc J 115:739–748, 1976.
3. Fuchs F: Amniocentesis: Techniques and complications. In Harris M (ed): "Early Diagnosis of Human Genetic Defects." Washington DC: US Government Printing Office, 1972, pp 11–16.
4. Littlefield JW: The pregnancy at risk for a genetic disorder. N Engl J Med 282:627–628, 1970.

5. Lejeune J: On the nature of man. Am J Hum Genet 22:121–128, 1970.
6. Ramsey P: Screening: An ethicist's view. In Hilton B, Callahan D, Harris M (eds): "Ethical Issues in Human Genetics." New York: Plenum Press, 1973, pp 147–160.
7. Dyck AJ: Ethical issues in community and research medicine. N Engl J Med 284: 725–726, 1971.
8. Lebacqz KA: Prenatal diagnosis and selective abortion. Linacre Quart 22:109–127, 1970.
9. Milunsky A: "The Prenatal Diagnosis of Hereditary Disorders." Springfield: Charles C Thomas, 1973.
10. Hirschhorn K: Practical and ethical problems in human genetics. In Bergsma D (ed): "Advances in Human Genetics and Their Impact on Society." White Plains: The National Foundation–March of Dimes, BD:OAS VIII(4):17–30, 1972.
11. Aiken HD: Life and the right to life. In Hilton B, Callahan D, Harris M (eds): "Ethical Issues in Human Genetics." New York: Plenum Press, 1973, pp 173–183.
12. Fletcher Jos: "The Ethics of Genetic Control." Garden City/New York: Anchor Press/ Doubleday, 1974.
13. Macintyre NM: Professional responsibility in prenatal genetic evaluation. In "Advances in Human Genetics and Their Impact on Society." Op cit, pp 31–35.
14. Fletcher JC: Moral and ethical problems of prenatal diagnosis. Clin Genet 8:251–257, 1975.
15. Murray RF, Callahan D: Genetic disease and human health. Hastings Cent Rep 4:4–6, 1974.
16. Culliton BJ: Amniocentesis: HEW backs test for prenatal diagnosis of disease. Science 190:537–540, 1975.
17. Ramsey P: Feticide/infanticide on request. Religion in Life 39:170–186, 1970.
18. Dyck AJ: Perplexities of the would-be liberal in abortion. J Reprod Med 8:351–354, 1972.
19. Tooley M: Abortion and infanticide. Phil Public Affairs 2:37–65, 1972.
20. Fletcher Jos: Ethics and euthanasia. Am J Nurs 73:670–675, 1973.
21. Fletcher JC: Abortion, euthanasia, and care of defective newborns. N Engl J Med 292: 75–78, 1975.
22. Ramsey P: Abortion. Thomist 37:174–226, 1973.
23. Ramsey P: "The Morality of Abortion. Life or Death," Labby DH (ed). Seattle: University of Washington Press, 1963, p 73.
24. Fletcher Jos: Indicators of humanhood: A tentative profile of man. Hastings Cent Rep 2(5):1–4, 1972.
25. Callahan D: "Abortion: Law, Choice, and Morality." New York: Macmillan, 1970, pp 395–396.
26. Kennell JH, Klaus MH: Care of the mother of the high risk infant. Clin Obstet Gynecol 14:926–954, 1971.
27. Bibring GL: Some considerations of the psychological processes in pregnancy. Psychoanal Study Child 14:113–121, 1959.
28. Caplan G: "Emotional Implication of Pregnancy and Influence on Family Relationships in the Healthy Child." Cambridge: Harvard University Press, 1960.
29. Nadelson D: Normal and special: Aspects of pregnancy. Obstet Gynecol 41:611–620, 1973.
30. Solnit AJ, Stark MH: Mourning and the birth of a defective child. Psychoanal Study Child 16:523–537, 1961.
31. McCormick RA: Life-saving and life-taking. A comment. Linacre Quart 22:110–115, 1975.
32. Englehardt HT: Viability, abortion, and the difference between a fetus and an infant. Am J Obstet Gynecol 116:429–434, 1972.

16. Problems of Social Justice in Applied Human Genetics

Sumner B. Twiss, PhD

This chapter explores the judgments and criteria of social justice that pertain to applied human genetics. There are two principal occasions for discussing social (or comparative) justice in applied human genetics: 1) legislation and public policy regarding the social uses of human genetics; and 2) allocation of scarce resources for the research and development of genetic technologies. The first occasion raises problems about the implementation of human genetics in medical, public health, and more broadly, social programs. These problems include, for instance, the dilemmas of eugenic policy. The second occasion raises problems about the setting of priorities and the distribution of funds for advancing the techniques of applied human genetics. These problems often involve issues about the most appropriate ways to allocate resources equitably. Although they are not entirely unrelated, these circumstances raise distinct conceptual and moral issues that require separate attention.

SOCIAL JUSTICE IN APPLIED HUMAN GENETICS: EUGENICS

In attributing human worth to everyone we may be ascribing no property or set of qualities, but rather expressing an attitude — the attitude of respect — toward the humanity in each man's person. That attitude follows naturally from regarding everyone from the "human point of view," but it is not grounded on anything more ultimate than itself, and it is not demonstrably justifiable. It can be argued further against skeptics that a world with equal human rights is a *more just* world, a way of organizing society for which we

Birth Defects: Original Article Series, Volume *X V, Number 2,* pages 255—277

would all opt if we were designing our institutions afresh in ignorance
of the roles we might one day have to play in them. It is also a *less
dangerous* world generally, and one with a more elevated and civi-
lized tone. [1].

Eugenic Survivals and Revivals

In spite of the repudiation of the eugenics movement in the 1930s, there
has been a renewed interest in eugenic problems, especially since the Second
World War. As Ludmerer has shown, this resurgence of interest in eugenics can
be attributed to a number of factors [2]. First, in the late 1930s and early
1940s, certain individuals like Osborn attempted to formulate a new eugenics
ideology, firmly based in the sciences and in the conception of a democratic
political framework: a new, revamped eugenics creed was advanced [3]. Second,
the advent of the atomic age stimulated scientific and public concern over the
genetic hazards of radiation exposure. This concern highlighted the problem of
the genetic load of the population and thereby revitalized the eugenic theme of
genetic deterioration of the human species [4]. Third, as human genetics became
incorporated into medicine, it encouraged the development of practices having
eugenic overtones, however muted. In fact, it has been argued that the practice
of genetic counseling, for example, is a survival of the original eugenics movement, which offered hereditary counseling services as a form of eugenic preventive medicine [5].

Contemporary advances in applied human genetics could readily lead to a
new eugenics movement. Indeed, in discussing the uses of genetic knowledge at
a 1971 conference on genetic counseling, Neel stated openly, "What we are
really discussing is the new eugenics, where I define eugenics simply as a collec-
tion of policies designed to improve the genetic well-being of our species." And
he continued, "All of the value judgments and ethical issues that previously
made eugenics so thorny an issue are still there, albeit with some added precision" [6]. In the last twenty years, extraordinary progress has been made in
the basic understanding of human genetics and in the development of new
genetic technologies. The following developments could be used for programs
of "negative eugenics," aimed at reducing the frequency of deleterious genes or
at least the incidence of genetic disease: genetic screening and counseling, techniques of prenatal diagnosis and selective abortion, and new sterilization procedures.

Other technological advances could lend themselves to programs of "positive eugenics," aimed at improving the genetic quality of the population: artificial insemination, cloning of selected human genotypes, and gene therapy. In
fact, experiments in negative eugenics may have already gotten underway in the
guise of legally mandated, compulsory mass genetic screening programs. Certainly, these developments and prospects in applied human genetics have led to

a resurgence of eugenics proposals from a number of geneticists, ranging from H.J. Muller and J. Huxley in the 1940s and 1950s, to B. Glass and J. Lederberg in the 1960s and 1970s. Most recently, there has been an increasing amount of talk about eugenic sterilization for dominant genetic disorders, the right of every child to be born with a sound genotype, and the desirability to make genetic screening, counseling, and even prenatal diagnosis compulsory for certain high risk groups in the population.

In the light of these developments and proposals, it is not unreasonable to suggest that a new eugenics ideology is beginning to take shape, particularly around decisions made as to the genetic worth of prospective human beings. It has even been predicted that as this new eugenics ideology grows, new technological developments will be simply plugged into the eugenics arsenal as medical advances without so much as a second thought [7].

The major controversy surrounding the "new eugenics" is one of the social ethics of ends and means, just as in the case of the earlier eugenics movement. The ethical dilemmas and motifs have not changed much, nor has their urgency abated. Even if effective, how precisely would proposed eugenic measures affect the genetic composition of the population or the species? What constitutes a so-called desirable (undesirable) gene or trait, and how can these value judgments be defended? And most important, what are the human consequences ("from the human point of view") of implementing a eugenic policy, and are these acceptable from the vantage point of social justice and human rights to liberty and equality?

There are three ethical dilemmas endemic to eugenics, whether "old" or "new." The first involves the identification and appraisal of eugenic objectives. The second concerns the specification and justification of criteria for implementing eugenic policies. And the third involves the moral evaluation of the cases for positive and negative eugenics.

Genetic Pollution vs Genetic Variability

Eugenic objectives are articulated, explicitly or implicitly, against the background of varying conceptions of the genetic status quo of the population [8]. These conceptions fall into two main classes that may be conveniently labeled "genetic deterioration" (or "genetic pollution") on the one hand, and "genetic variability" on the other. These two types of conceptions reveal a century-long debate over a question of fact central to eugenics.

According to many eugenic thinkers, from the time of Darwin to the present, eugenics was and is a necessary response to an assumed or projected deterioration of the genetic quality of the species. The basis for this response is that there has been, or will be, such a severe increase in the frequency of deleterious genes of traits in the population that the species is, or will be, threatened by a genetic apocalypse. For example, in 1960, Huxley warned: "If we don't do something about controlling our genetic inheritance, we are going to degenerate. . . . Most mutations are deleterious, but we now keep many of them going that would otherwise have died out. If this continues indefinitely . . . then the whole genetic capacity of man will be much weakened" [9]. In 1961, Theodosius Dobzhansky queried: "We are then faced with a dilemma — if we enable the weak and the deformed to live and to propagate their kind, we face the prospect of a genetic twilight; but if we let them die or suffer when we can save them, we face the certainty of a moral twilight. How to escape this dilemma?" [10] And more recently, in 1972, Sang concluded that "we may now be starting a phase of 'genetic pollution' roughly equivalent to the beginnings of environmental pollution a generation ago" [11]. Given, this "factual" premise, eugenicists have proposed remedial measures in the form of genetic interventions via applied human genetics.

On the other side of the controversy, there are scientists who view the vision of a genetic apocalypse as myopic and unwarranted. In the last few years conceptions of the genetic status quo have swung away from negative views of genetic deterioration to positive characterizations of the genetic diversity of the population. Optimistic proponents of genetic diversity argue that such diversity represents evolutionary capability and therefore should be regarded as "capital for investment in future adaptations" [12]. More moderate proponents simply predict that medical and environmental correction of genetic defects will far outrun the effects of any presumed genetic load [13]. One consequence of conceptions of genetic diversity is the recommendation that eugenic measures be avoided.

Thus, there are two polarized views of the genetic status of the population. One paints a negative picture of actual or imminent genetic pollution; the other a more positive picture of genetic variability. Both of these views have divergent policy implications vis-à-vis eugenic objectives. Which view is more accurate? The truth of the matter appears to lie between these polarized views, though it may be wise to admit a healthy degree of ignorance at this time. On the one hand, it does appear that certain social developments, including advances in medicine, contribute to the genetic load of the population by permitting individuals with genetic disorders to survive and reproduce. But at the same time it should be pointed out that medicine, for example, it not generating a large number of invalids. As Lappé has aptly summed it up, "The consensus of the best medical and genetic opinion is that whatever genetic deterioration is occurring as a result of decreased natural selection is so slow as to be insignificant when contrasted to 'environmental' changes" [14]. It may even be that far from being deleterious to the population, the so-called genetic load represents genetic diversity and contributes to the evolutionary adaptability of the population. Although the evolutionary significance of genetic diversity is not well characterized, the weight of genetic knowledge and opinion at this time encourages a positive acceptance of genetic diversity.

In identifying and evaluating eugenic objectives against the background of the genetic status quo, two questions must be raised and answered. First, is the objective feasible and scientifically warranted? Second, is the objective ethically justifiable? Answering these questions requires exploring the conceptual and valuational elements of an objective, along with its social policy implications. The objectives proposed for the use of genetic knowledge comprise a wide spectrum, ranging from treatment of the genetic ills of the individual to enhancement of the quality of the human gene pool [15]. From among these objectives, the leading contenders in eugenics are: improvement in the quality of the gene pool, maintenance of the quality of the gene pool by preventing genetic deterioration, and reduction of the incidence of genetic disease in the population. These are not the only candidates for eugenic objectives, but they are representative and invoked with a fair degree of frequency.

Improving the Species

The eugenic objective of enhancing or improving the quality of the human gene pool is historically important. It is premised on the view that eugenics is necessary for human progress. The argument for this eugenic objective consisted in appealing to man's ascendent place in the order of nature: a traditional natural law appeal restated in evolutionary terms [16]. Recently, in 1974, Sperry resuscitated this argument for the objective by stating, "Social values are necessarily built in large part around inherent traits in human nature written into the species by evolution." He concludes: "The upward thrust of evolution . . . becomes something to preserve and revere. This would imply a commitment to progress and improvement . . . in terms of furthering the advancement of the evolutionary trend towards greater complexity, diversity, and improvement in the quality and dimension of life" [17].

This position has been criticized and rejected by contemporary biologists and philosophers. For example, Simpson has argued that "there is no innate tendency toward evolutionary progress and no one, overall sort of such progress" [18]. In short, eugenic objectives cannot be read off the facts of human evolution. Speaking philosophically, the bête noire of this eugenic objective and its rationale is the naturalistic fallacy. Moreover, the very concepts of enhancement and improvement in this context elude analysis, both scientific and ethical. The criteria for their meaning are simply unavailable.

Survival of the Species

The eugenic objective of maintaining the quality of the gene pool by preventing genetic deterioration has long been in vogue, from the Social Darwinism of the early eugenics movement up to the present. It is premised on a certain view of species survival which shapes a fundamental concern of eugenics. And it presupposes a view of the genetic status quo which is still subject to intense controversy among the experts: the condition of genetic deterioration. Even conceding some degree of truth to this conception of the genetic status quo, the appropriate eugenic course of action is not self-evident. For it is not obvious what threat is posed to the survival of the species, nor whether that threat is imminent or remote. That is, it is not at all clear that the species will not survive if eugenic measures are not now undertaken [19].

The rationale for this eugenic objective is that there is a duty to promote the survival of the human species. If there is such a duty, it follows that there is a duty to implement eugenics controls to prevent the genetic deterioration of the species. This argument raises a number of issues, some factual, others normative. First, it is not clear that the species will deteriorate to the point of nonsurvival if eugenic controls are not implemented. The controversy over genetic deterioration versus genetic diversity is pertinent here. The consensus in favor of genetic diversity or some middle ground argues against adopting this eugenic objective. Second, it is difficult to see what is good about species survival as such. For example, even granting that the species is seriously threatened by genetic deterioration, it is possible that survival under conditions of strict eugenic control may not be worth the price, if eugenic measures were to seriously infringe fundamental human rights of social justice (see below). This point suggests that what is at stake may not be sheer species survival, but rather the survival of a way of life, eg, an unjust class society governed by the principles of Social Darwinism. Third, the source of the duties underlying this objective is not clear. For example, is the duty to promote species survival an obligation to promote what is good for future generations? If so, what is the moral status of this obligation, and what precisely does it entail for present generations?

The question of the meaning of genetic deterioration raises technical matters that belong to the provinces of evolutionary biology and population genetics. However, there is justification for exploring this issue in a less technical way, for the concept of genetic deterioration shapes beliefs about the problem of eugenics, its gravity, and its urgency. Moreover, the concept is not solely a technical genetic notion when it is used to justify eugenic measures. Rather, the concept turns out to be quasi-evaluative, and its employment by eugenicists suggests that some evil must be remedied. As it is used in eugenic discussions regarding applied human genetics, the concept is negatively value-laden. There are a number of problems associated with its use in policy discussions of genetic interventions.

The first problem is that historically its use often involved a logical fallacy — the fallacy of affirming the consequent. Many eugenicists began with the assumption that genetic deterioration was an established fact; and since this state of affairs implied a condition of disvalue, many disvalues were then taken to establish the situation of deterioration whose existence was already assumed. The eugenics movement was replete with assertions of the "hereditary" basis for disvalued human traits, eg feeblemindedness, pauperism, vagrancy, epilepsy, alcoholism, insanity, criminality. The movement was also replete with examples of fallacious reasoning. If there was genetic deterioration, there were these disvalues; there were these disvalues, therefore there was genetic deterioration. This was precisely the sort of fallacious reasoning used by eugenicists in support of the passage of the Immigration Restriction Act of 1924 [20]. This fallacy was easy to slip into, and it led to the tendency to connect all sorts of social evils with the condition of genetic deterioration.

Although this fallacy is not characteristic of eugenic thinking now, its historical use resulted in a second problem connected with the concept of genetic deterioration. Since it proved difficult to demonstrate a causal connection between genetic deterioration and the social problems and traits mentioned, eugenicists simply came to define genetic deterioration in terms of these problems and traits. The consequent envalued concept is still employed in eugenic discussions. From a policy perspective, continued use of the concept sets up false dilemmas in eugenic arguments, eg either counteract the condition of genetic deterioration by eugenic means or fail to deal with the problems and traits now in question (recessive and dominant genetic disorders, chromosomal abnormalities). This line of argument misdirects and conceals other policy alternatives, for it ignores the possibility of noneugenic, environmental solutions.

Yet a third problem connected with the notion of genetic deterioration is its conceptual opacity, inasmuch as it is defined in terms of so-called undesirable genes and traits. The main issue is that to speak of defective, deleterious, and undesirable genes and traits is to employ environmentally relative terms. Judgments about what count as undesirable genes and traits are relative to a given population. An example often cited is the sickle cell trait, which is judged beneficial in certain malaria-infested populations and not so beneficial in Western industrial societies. If such judgments about specific genes and traits are relative, then equally relative is the very concept of genetic deterioration of the population or the gene pool. These problems with the concept of genetic deterioration seriously undermine the cogency of the eugenic objective of maintaining the quality of the human gene pool.

Insofar as this eugenic objective appeals to the survival of the human species, it is appropriate to examine the nature of this appeal. It is by no means clear how sheer appeal to species survival can justify this objective (and policies associated with it). This is so for a number of reasons. First, the preceding criticism of the concept of genetic deterioration suggests that the postulated threat to species survival may well be specious. Second, what really seems to be at stake is survival of a way of life or type of social system (and an unjust one at that!). Third, even if species survival were at issue, it is quite possible that survival may not be worth the moral price of accepting repressive eugenic controls. Fourth, the duty to promote species survival is morally ambiguous. That is, assuming that the duty may be logically derived from accepted moral principles which extend to future generations, its implications for eugenics are unclear.

On the one hand, this duty can be interpreted in such a way as to justify prima facie eugenic measures: the present generation owes to the future the possibility of life and survival and the amelioration of those conditions which lessen the possibilities for living a full human life. On the other hand, the duty can be interpreted somewhat differently, with different consequences: the present generation has an obligation to refrain from doing things that might be harmful to the future, especially those things which would be irrevocably harmful in the long run. Other things being equal, the first interpretation justifies adopting the eugenic objective in question. The second prohibits adopting the objective, particularly since so little is known about the long-range consequences of implementing eugenic measures. Consequently, the objective's justificatory appeal to species survival is not only conceptually but also morally ambiguous.

Combating Genetic Disease

The reduction of the incidence of genetic disease in the population is a more concrete eugenic objective than the other two candidates. It has a fair degree of currency among geneticists in the fields of medicine and public health. Two primary concerns underlie this objective: increased mutation rates exacerbated by drugs, food additives, environmental pollutants, artificial radiation, and increased morbidity attributable to genetic factors. The genetic technologies associated with this objective include genetic screening and counseling programs, prenatal diagnosis and selective abortion, population policies, and genetically informed legislation. The basic aim of this objective and its associated technologies can be characterized in terms of public health, where genetic (medical and social) interventions are intended to optimize, or at least protect, the health aspects of the life environment of the populace. This eugenic objective raises two distinctive issues. First, is genetic disease properly characterized as a public health problem, threat, or hazard? Second, does the state have a justifiable interest in reducing the incidence of genetic disease in the population? Although these issues cannot be fully examined here, a few observations are in order.

As medical science and human genetics progress, more and more diseases are found to have a genetic etiology. As much as 25% of the total morbidity in the population may be attributable to genetic factors, and 5% related to specific genetic defects [21]. Thus, genetic diseases are growing in relative health importance. Much of the current discussion about genetic conditions and the role of genetic screening and counseling programs seems to assume that genetic diseases constitute a public health problem or even a public health hazard. This assumption is invidious, for it encourages premature state intervention into parenthood and reproductive behavior — a sphere of privacy and autonomy demarcated by basic human rights — on genetic (ie eugenic) grounds. Although vaccination against contagious diseases and premarital blood tests are sometimes made mandatory to protect the public health, there is currently no public health justification for mandatory screening for the prevention of genetic disease, to take just one example. The conditions being tested for in the screening programs are neither contagious nor, for the most part, susceptible to treatment at the present time [22] . To think otherwise is to apply without justification the idea of Typhoid Mary to genetic conditions and to accept uncritically the principle that those who are genetically diseased or even just carriers ought to be quarantined (eg by eugenic sterilization). As Hull says, this is to slide into social policies which ought to be squarely faced, debated, and adopted or rejected with full knowledge of the price paid in the currency of human rights and social justice [23] .

Whether the state has a justifiable interest in imposing eugenic controls to reduce the incidence of genetic disease turns in large part on the validity of the analogy between the public health threats posed by contagious disease, on the one hand, and genetic disease, on the other. The validity of the analogy is tenuous: means of disease transmission, etiology, communicability, and means of disease control are quite different for these disease categories. Conceptually, therefore, the case is weak. Empirically, also, the case is weak, for genetic diseases do not spread like a contagion, nor do they lead to hazardous epidemics of gross proportions. And it is worth pointing out that there would be an enormous time lag between the implementation of a eugenic policy and its effects (if any) on either a recessive or dominant genetic disorder, a time lag on the order of many decades and centuries to affect the frequency of deleterious genes.

The question of state interest in this eugenic objective does not rest solely on this analogy, however. There are other considerations. To begin with, civil society takes a substantial interest in both the quantity and quality of children born within the community. This interest is clearly evidenced by publicly supported family planning programs, provision of contraceptive services, national commissions on population policy and control, and by legal requirements concerning mandatory education, court decisions ordering medical care for children against parental wishes, laws in the area of child abuse. In these and other ways, the state is expressing societal interest in the quantity and quality of its citizens' progeny. This interest is bound up with the social utilitarian aims of maximizing the number of socially useful people and minimizing the number of socially burdensome people. In terms of health, these aims materialize in a state interest in insuring that future citizens are healthy and in avoiding costs involved in caring for defective persons. Public policy has encouraged and sanctioned the use of the state's police power to minimize illness in the population, eg mass screening for tuberculosis, compulsory vaccination, fluoridation of water, mandatory premarital blood tests, and, most recently, mandatory genetic screening [24].

There are clear signs that the state is concerned with the genetic quality of its citizens and, more specifically, in reducing the incidence of genetic disease. A small number of genetic diseases are thought to be prevalent enough to warrant a public health concern. Moreover, genetic diseases do affect the public interest through the allocation of public funds and medical resources for researching therapies and providing institutional care. Consequently, there is a prima facie case for holding that the state has a legitimate interest in reducing the impact of genetic disease on the population. Yet this case is not conclusive. It does beg the issue of whether genetic disease is properly characterized as a public health concern. And it tends to elide public health issues, on the one hand, with the health costs incurred to society as a result of genetic disease, on the other. This tendency results in confusion over the grounds for making social policy in the area of applied human genetics. On balance, however, in contrast with the eugenic objectives of enhancing or maintaining the quality of the human gene pool, the eugenic aim of reducing the incidence of genetic disease is by far the most feasible and most cogent of the three.

Obligation to Future Generations

The issue of articulating criteria for the moral appraisal of eugenic policies can be approached along two dimensions. The first involves norms and obligations entailed by the notion of intergenerational responsibility, ie obligations to future generations. The second involves those ethical values and norms which specify a conception of a just society. The first approach holds that future generations have moral claims against present generations, because both present and future constitute a common moral community [25]. Obligations to future generations based on these claims include, on the one hand, prohibitions against harming future generations, undermining the possibility of their planning for themselves, and jeopardizing the possibility of their exercising fundamental human rights, and, on the other hand, injunctions to provide for the possibility of life and survival of future generations, to produce the conditions necessary for insuring their survival, and to ameliorate those conditions which lessen the possibilities for living a full human life.

These obligations fail to supply unambiguous moral criteria for assessing eugenic policies. For example, the positive injunctions appear to sanction eugenic measures associated with any one of the three eugenic objectives introduced above, particularly those of maintaining the quality of the gene pool and of reducing the incidence of genetic disease. By contrast, the negative prohibitions appear to rule out eugenic measures altogether, regardless of objectives. The obligations are morally ambiguous on two other counts. First, it is paradoxical to have obligations only to some potential members of future generations and not others, eg discriminating against those who might have certain genetic defects. It does not make moral sense to claim that present generations have an obligation to some potential members of future generations to see to it that other equally potential members are not born. Second, it needs to be indicated that just because some future generations at some future time might have to adopt eugenic objectives and controls, it does not follow that in ignorance of appropriate goals and their consequences the present generations must now adopt such eugenic measures. Such a course of action would fail to make not only moral sense but also logical sense as well.

Social Justice and Individual Rights

The second approach to identifying criteria for the appraisal of eugenic policies is predicated on the view that there is a set of moral principles enjoining nonmaleficence, mutual respect, equal treatment, and fairness which comprise the core of what it means to be just. These principles specify a conception of the good life in a just society which involves basic individual (or human) rights, eg personal inviolability, liberty, equality, and the recognition of basic life-setting needs, eg primary material goods, physical and mental well-being, security. This notion of justice may be conceived on analogy with a game [26]. There are rules of the game that define its inherent end and what it means to be a player in the game. These constitutive rules are analogous to the set of moral principles. Closely related to these rules are those that define the positions of the players, not only in what they should do, but also in how they stand vis-à-vis others in the game. These positional rules are analogous to the rights of the individual. Then, of course, there are the moves and strategies that happen within the game according to its rules. These gaming elements are analogous to the basic needs recognized, pursued, and satisfied in the just life.

Clearly, this notion of social justice puts a premium on individual human rights and their preservation. As a consequence, the baseline for moral reasoning and action tends to emphasize the ethical constraints of rights when public policies are under consideration. Those public policies are to be preferred which accord primacy to human rights and their implications, eg the right to life with a self-determined destiny, the right to marry and found a family, the right to voluntary procreation. Further, if conditions require limiting these rights, then policies should be designed to minimize harmful consequences and to instantiate the norms of justice.

Summary rules applicable to proposed eugenic measures follow from this notion of justice and its consequences. For example, the right to free procreative behavior should be respected unless there are clearly demonstrable threats to the rights of others following from the exercise of this right, and even then, limitations should be proportional to the danger involved. In public health policies, direct encroachment on individual rights ought to be proportional to the public health dangers posed by the disease, and such encroachment is to be mitigated by the availability of therapy. In the case of eugenic measures, aimed, say, at the reduction of genetic disease, voluntary policies with few restrictions on the rights of individuals are preferable to compulsory policies, from the point of view of achieving social justice. Moreover, the acceptability of eugenic policies ought to depend on the degree to which restrictions on individuals are consonant with the needs to be satisfied by these same individuals. Further, the large time lag for the effects of eugenic policies indicates, from the point of view of justice, a greater responsibility to meet the basic needs of extant individuals rather than future generations. These summary considerations are best examined in the context of specific types of eugenic policies.

Types of Eugenic Policies

Eugenic policies raise the age-old problem of the relation between ends and means. Not every end justifies any means, particularly when the feasibility and the desirability of the end are in dispute, as is the case with eugenic objectives. Moreover, the acceptability of a means cannot be appraised solely in terms of its effectiveness in achieving an admittedly feasible and desirable end. For issues of basic human rights, freedoms, and social justice must be taken into account. This is especially true when considering eugenic policies, given the history of the eugenics movement and its social abuses. For convenience, eugenic policies may be classified into three major types, though these are neither mutually exclusive nor exhaustive: coercive eugenic policies, economic eugenic policies, and social eugenic policies [27].

Coercive eugenic policies that have been proposed include, for example, compulsory sterilization of the genetically affected and the behaviorally deviant, restriction on marriage and reproduction for carriers of undesirable traits, and even compulsory genetic screening, prenatal diagnosis, counseling, and abortion for women at high risk for bearing a defective child. Each of these proposed policies, among others, has its own particular problems, but they may be treated as a group. Clearly, such eugenic policies impinge on basic human rights and implied freedoms — eg personal inviolability as this pertains to childbearing and proprietary parenthood — and contravene the norms of social justice and the summary rules incorporating such notions as proportionate danger. It is important to underscore the fact that these policies have been seriously proposed and, in some cases, actually effected. For example, some compulsory sterilization laws enacted between 1911 and 1930 are still on the books in many states, and they are still being invoked [28]. For another example, in 1972, Glass recommended compulsory eugenic sterilization of persons suffering from genetic retinoblastoma, a dominant disorder [29].

In itself perhaps the use of coercion to restrict the exercise of a right is not all that problematic, since the possibility of coercion is implied in the protection of rights. One person's freedom is almost always limited when another person's right is protected. However, in deciding what to protect and what to restrict a crucial moral and social choice is made. For at the basis of this choice are the conceptions of the just life and the roles that human rights and freedoms play in this conception. It may be argued that interference with the human rights invested in voluntary procreation and proprietary parenthood can be counterbalanced only by a tremendous benefit to the person(s) affected, and that coercive restriction of these rights can only be justified as a "last resort" measure, if at all. Thus, the eugenic policy proposals under discussion only make sense and can only be justified (if at all) as "last resort" methods in situations where, eg human survival is at stake. But it is not clear that eugenic objectives incorporating appeals to species survival are cogent. And if human survival here really means survival of a certain social system, then it is far from clear that such survival is desirable from the point of view of justice. Consequently, these proposed eugenic policies, involving virtual penalization of purported "dysgenic behavior," lack moral justification.

Economic eugenic policies that have been proposed include, for example, incentive programs in the form of tax credits to encourage so-called superior couples to reproduce, withdrawal of welfare and tax benefits from high-risk couples who should decide to reproduce, financial inducements to carriers of deleterious traits not to mate or procreate, and even compensation for voluntary sterilization. Again, these policies may be treated as a group. On their face, positive incentives, inducements, and compensations seem noncoercive, ie they do not appear to diminish freedom, infringe rights, or produce injustice. Yet they may well be coercive and discriminatory in subtle and invidious ways, if in effect they leave no actual choice, remove a basic right or freedom (eg to procreate), or discriminate (eg against the childbearing of a certain group). Moreover, these policies may lead to undesirable personal and social consequences, the risk of which is not proportional to satisfying basic needs of the individuals involved, eg psychological problems resulting from sterilization, or social stigmatization resulting from being a member of a group targeted to have smaller than average families. Furthermore, negative incentives — withdrawal of maternity benefits and child allowances, reversal of tax benefits, etc — appear more directly coercive in depriving persons of free choice about procreation through the imposition of penalties. And it seems that these penalties would create a situation of social injustice for those who were being denied needed welfare and tax benefits. The justification for these eugenic policies is questionable, given the social and moral consequences of their implementation.

Social eugenic policies are intended to encourage rather than coerce individuals and couples to become genetically responsible. That is, they are designed to motivate people to think seriously about the genetic consequences of their mating and reproductive decisions and to provide opportunities for voluntary and informed genetic interventions. Examples of such eugenic policies include genetic screening and counseling programs, and the provision of prenatal diagnosis and selective abortion. These measures are conceived to be mechanisms that enhance responsible parenthood, while at the same time protecting fundamental human rights. The major ethical issue associated with these measures is that they assume a normative concept of genetic responsibility which has rarely been subjected to critical scrutiny [30]. Inasmuch as this concept is often used to refer to the right of every child to be born free of genetic defect and abnormality, or, alternatively, the right to be born with a sound mind and healthy body, it seems that these policies require (potential) parents to act responsibly by insuring, so far as possible, sound or normal genotypes for their progeny. Yet it is hard to know what counts as a "normal genotype"; and it is both biologically unrealistic and socially unfair to ask anyone to insure that a child be born with one. Further, the very notions of genetic health and genetic disease are rather elusive and arbitrary notions on which to base a eugenic policy, however voluntary that policy may seem to be.

To encourage eugenic thinking on the part of parents and prospective parents could have the effect of recasting the role of parenthood with undesirable and unjustifiable consequences. On the one hand, it may be argued that since decisions about prenatal diagnosis and selection abortion are individual decisions made in the context of genetic counseling, they are voluntary and informed and in no way lead to socially repressive eugenic controls. On the other hand, it seems that the case is not so simple and clear-cut, for decisions that have in fact been made to abort, for example, XYY fetuses are far from being informed and responsible, in light of present ignorance about the XYY chromosomal make-up. These decisions may well have been influenced by eugenic thinking of some sort, but the validity of this thinking and the decisions to which it led are problematic, not only scientifically but also morally. Injustice may have been done to both potential and extant XYY individuals. Thus, it appears that noncoercive social eugenic policies can have the effect of reshaping, on ambiguous grounds at best, the traditional values and human rights of parenthood. Acceptance of such a recasting of the parental role is not to be taken lightly. The social consequences of such a change in human relationships are unknown, and it seems unwise to alter prematurely the meaning and moral shape of parenthood and the family bond.

Positive and Negative Eugenics

From the standpoint of social justice, a few observations about both positive and negative eugenics are in order. To begin with, it needs to be said that a successful program of positive eugenics would most likely require the implementation of coercive eugenic measures. The early eugenicists recognized this point and despaired over it [31]. Later eugenicists, like H. J. Muller and J. Huxley in the 1950s and 1960s, attempted to talk only about voluntary programs [32]. But recent developments in coercive population controls in other societies belie the practicality of this voluntaristic emphasis. Indeed, American experiments in applied human genetics, past and present, also call into question voluntarism for successful eugenic control. If success in positive eugenics requires authoritarian measures, then the moral price for such success (if it can be had) may well be too high.

Turning to negative eugenics, it must be said that its programs are not only inefficient but also unjust. Most eugenicists admit the point about inefficiency. The major exception is the eugenic control of a dominant genetic disorder by means of compulsory sterilization. However, even this category of exceptions is disputable. For example, to reduce significantly the frequency of a rare dominant disorder like genetic retinoblastoma would take hundreds of generations, because it is thought to have a very high mutation rate. More important than inefficiency in this case is that for hundreds of generations basic human rights would have to be infringed, all for a small benefit of dubious worth to the individuals affected. On balance, the social justice of this course of action appears uncertain at best. And again the questions must be raised: Are programs of negative eugenics worth their moral cost?

SOCIAL JUSTICE IN APPLIED HUMAN GENETICS: MACROALLOCATION

The larger questions of medical and social priorities are almost, if not altogether, incorrigible to moral reasoning [33].

Pervasive Problems

For obvious reasons the problem of scarce resources has a direct bearing on setting priorities for the research and development of genetic technologies. Since many of the technologies will result from research in human genetics, macroallocational decisions about the distribution of funds to support this research represent a particularly exigent area of concern. These decisions will strongly influence the directions of genetic research and therefore will determine in large part whether certain genetic technologies will ever exist. Problems of social justice in this area involve identifying the proper distributive norms and showing how these norms are to be used. These problems are particularly germane to applied human genetics, since many hard questions are pressed in this area, not the least of which is whether expenditures for developing treatments or other modes of management for relatively rare diseases can be justified.

There are a number of considerations that indicate that issues of social justice in the research and development of genetic technologies have not yet been settled. First, it is not uncommon for reflective members of the biomedical community to apply to medical genetics G. B. Shaw's caustic observation that medical treatments are governed by fashion just as are clothes [34]. The same observation is also made from the standpoint of technology assessment: biomedical interests and available capital for these interests tend to run in tides. The present tide in the biomedical sciences is the biochemistry of inheritance; this has been called somewhat pejoratively as the "dominance of the almighty gene" [35]. Policy questions derived from such observations ask whether this interest in applied human genetics, especially the lure of sensational innovations in genetic technology, is simply a passing fad, and consequently whether large public investments should be made in this area.

Second, it appears that escalating public demands for biomedical innovations not only are making the economics of therapy difficult to manage but also are compelling certain areas of biomedical research and development to take a defensive posture. This point is applicable to applied human genetics. Again, it is not uncommon for reflective clinicians and researchers to assert that much research and development in applied human genetics have little, if any, bearing on the prevention of disease or the improvement of health or medical care for the public [36]. In this case a general point about diminishing returns from scientific research is applied with a vengeance to human genetics: in the course of scientific development, the easy problems are solved first and the more complex and intractable ones are put off to the future. The observation appears trivial until one puts it in the economic context of resource allocation and notes the import of later attempting to solve the shelved problems. Their solution requires a large resource investment subject to the classic law of diminishing returns: costs rise, the significance of results diminish on the average, and the waiting times for innovation breakthroughs increase dramatically [37]. When these implications are brought to bear on applied human genetics, the point is made that much policy-making about genetic technologies may well divert significant resources from the delivery of presently available modes of health care in other areas: the implicit judgment is that this macroallocation is unjust. A related point is that the benefits of research in applied human genetics may never redound to the welfare of the investing generation but only to their successors; this is judged to be unjust also.

Third, it is sometimes observed by reflective physicians and economists alike that the direction of biomedical research and technology is often controlled, so to speak, by the desires of the biomedical community. Hence, vested interest groups account for many patterns of resource allocation in this field. And there has been far too little rational planning by public policy-makers about the priorities and issues of macroallocation. These observations apply to research and development in applied human genetics.

All three of these considerations indicate the importance of clarifying the proper distributive norms for the macroallocation of scarce resources, particularly in the area of applied human genetics. In approaching this task, it is necessary to keep in mind the distinction between the theoretical and technical aspects of applied human genetics, since nuanced norms and procedures may be applicable to the phases of basic and applied research, on the one hand, and clinical developments and uses, on the other [38].

Efficiency and Justice

Three generic features of the macroallocation of scarce resources may help to specify the role of social justice in decisions about the research and development of genetic technologies. First, macroallocations can affect the welfare of an entire class of patients or potential patients and can virtually determine whether or not certain diseases or even broad categories of illnesses will receive attention and to what extent. Thus, at the macroallocational level it is possible to discriminate against certain classes of patients, certain diseases, and even categories of diseases. Second, at least in principle, macroallocations involve rational planning and deliberation; they are not made on an ad hoc basis. Thus, at the macroallocational level it is possible, and even required, to make decisions according to carefully formulated and rationally defensible norms. Third, by their very nature macroallocations are matters of public policy, and decision-makers at this level are accountable and liable to large constituencies, often at the state or national scene.

The important point that emerges from this brief characterization of macroallocation is that preeminent among the criteria or norms of distribution are those of efficiency and justice (equity). The intuitive idea is that there is a dialectical process at work here, between the constituency's claims of right to fair access to available resources for its medical needs, on the one hand, and the policy-maker's duty to create an allocation system that distributes resources efficiently and justly to meet these needs, on the other. The intuitive idea has to suffice, for this is hardly the place to articulate and defend a conception of an ideal society and a theory of justice.

To begin with, this view implies that the sole norm of pareto efficiency is not adequate for macroallocational decisions regarding the distribution of scarce resources for the research and development of biomedical technologies. This is so for two reasons. First, an allocation is pareto efficient when there is no other feasible allocation that will make everyone better off. According to this norm, it is acceptable to have a system which allocates a large share (even all) of the resources to a few, if there is no way of increasing the welfare of the many without at the same time harming the few. Moreover, this norm also sanctions an allocation system which benefits the majority at the expense of minorities, if there is no way of increasing the welfare of the minorities without detracting from the welfare of the majority. Clearly, the norm of pareto efficiency is a weak and unacceptable criterion from the standpoint of social justice [39]. A pareto efficient allocation need not be equitable. But social justice, along with the policy-maker's duty, requires that considerations of equity play a significant role in the macroallocation of resources to constituencies.

If this point is still unclear, then consider the following case. Suppose that it is pareto efficient to emphasize and allocate resources for the research and delivery of health care for only the major infectious and communicable diseases and cardiovascular diseases at the expense of avoiding research and medical care for genetic diseases. Ex hypothesi this resource allocation would be efficient. But would it be just and equitable? Is pareto efficiency the only relevant norm for macroallocation? Surely not.

A second reason for the inadequacy of the norm of pareto efficiency can be indicated by asking whether the standard method for the distribution of scarce resources — the price system, the equilibriated commercial market, aiming at pareto efficiency — is applicable to the research and development of bio-medical technologies, even on the economist's own terms. The answer is that it is not, for the reasons outlined by Arrow more than a decade ago [40]. The uncertainty involved in maintaining good health, combined with the premium put on health, undermines the very applicability of a price system in this area. The consequence is that macroallocations of scarce resources for the research and development of biomedical technologies cannot be governed solely by the norm of pareto efficiency. Rather, efficiency must be constrained by equity or justice.

The next problem is to specify a relevant norm of equity from the viewpoint of social justice and then relate it to macroallocation of scarce resources in the biomedical field. As stated before, it is not possible to provide a theory of justice here. So a proposal for a relevant norm of equity which appears both plausible and workable will be sketched. This norm of equity is cast in the form of justice-as-fairness, and may be articulated briefly as follows. In ideal economic conditions, the norm of equity requires the equal distribution of resources. As Feinberg says, "Strict equalitarianism, then, is a perfectly plausible material principle of distributive justice when confined to affluent societies and basic biological needs" [41]. In less than ideal economic conditions, such as those of scarcity, the norm of equity requires a decision procedure that insures equality of opportunity or equal access to the resources, and it tolerates inequalities in resource allocation only if these are arranged to benefit the least advantaged [42]. It is more than likely that macroallocational decisions regarding biomedical research and development will continue to be made under these less than ideal economic conditions. So the second formulation of the norm of equity appears applicable.

How, then, does this norm of equity apply to macroallocational decision-making in the biomedical field, particularly with regard to research and development in applied human genetics? It may be safely assumed that advances in medical and health care generally represent a high priority area for the macroallocation of scarce resources, since such care ranks high among the real or perceived needs of the constituency. This assumption is not open to serious debate. Indeed, at least one philosopher and social critic has gone so far as to claim that this assumption carries the weight of necessary truth [43]. Of course, the assumption and this sort of judgment hardly resolve the problems of macroallocation in the biomedical field. They say nothing about macroallocations for biomedical research versus preventive medicine, or less severe prevalent diseases versus severe rare diseases, and the like. It should be observed that the norm of efficiency might have much to say about such marcoallocational dilemmas, perhaps coming down on the side of preventive medicine and the treatment of the more prevalent diseases. With the tools of modern economic analysis, the norm of efficiency can churn out macroallocational decisions in short order. But at the level of public policy, efficiency is constrained by other considerations, not the least of which is social justice in the form of equity. Efficient unequal distribution must work to the benefit of the least advantaged. Assuming that the least advantaged can be specified in part by less prevalent severe diseases, then these must receive their fair share of resources. Or at least, "equal access" negates macroallocations that systematically discriminate against certain diseases in the population. It has been observed that "strict macroallocation logic" based on economic efficiency is "rarely the only, and sometimes not even the decisive, element in the decision" to allocate "funds for the operation of scarce life-saving cures" [44].

In the case of biomedical research, it appears that "efficiency constrained by equity" bears on the macroallocation of resources in the following ways. Recognizing that biomedical research must be diversified, these norms require the continued support of promising lines of research until a particular treatment has been proven to be effective. On the other hand, these norms also require a constant review of progress so that unproductive research does not continue unchecked. In the particular case of research in applied human genetics, the application of the norms of efficiency and equity have some additional consequences. Since research into genetic diseases cannot be systematically discriminated against, this research has a just claim on available resources. The degree of this claim cannot be measured precisely, but relevant decision-making factors certainly include the frequency of these disorders and their severity (ie mortality and morbidity).

Cost/Benefit Analysis

At the stage of clinical developments in applied human genetics, the norms of efficiency and equity take on a distinctive form. For example, the norm of efficiency often takes the form of cost/benefit analysis and cost/effectiveness studies. In particular, given a specific objective and two or more alternative modes of genetic intervention, the norm of efficiency requires the application of the optimal task thesis asking, "Which is the best or most efficient mode of intervention?" [45] When considering the macroallocation of scarce resources, this is an acceptable resolution procedure, all other things being equal: employing cost/benefit analysis is required by the macroallocational norm of efficiency. However, the ceterus paribus clause must not be overlooked. For when the costs involved in choosing between two alternative interventions refer to "social costs" (eg infringement of human rights, inequalities) and when other objectives may be at issue, then the resolution procedure moves beyond efficiency and requires more than cost/benefit analysis [46]. In many cases it is the norm of equity that identifies when the resolution procedure moves beyond efficiency and enters the arena of social justice.

Indeed, the norm of equity or social justice contravenes many of the claims made on behalf of cost/benefit analysis in applied human genetics. For example, contrary to some overly zealous claims about its ability to solve macroallocational problems, cost/benefit analysis does not solve issues of health policy in applied human genetics; it does not determine the social validity of programs of genetic intervention; and it does not provide proof of the social value of genetic screening and counseling programs [47]. Thus, it appears that cost/benefit analysis is of limited value in making macroallocational decisions in applied human genetics, except in the case where there are two potential resource-consuming genetic technologies aimed at precisely the same justifiable objective and involving no other moral or social policy considerations. As Tsukahara and Kadota so eloquently conclude in their cost/benefit study of genetic screening programs for Tay-Sachs disease, "It is important to recognize that none of the economic approaches suggested earlier addresses the difficult problem of equity . . . it must be remembered that efficient use of resources is not necessarily the supreme criteria for policy choices. . . . Ethical arguments are perhaps more persuasive than the slippery justification revealed by monetary assessment of program costs and benefits" [48].

Allocations for Future Generations

In the preceding analysis an observation was made to the following effect: the benefits of biomedical research, including genetic research, may only redound to the welfare of successive generations. This observation, among others, raises the poignant question: Do present policy-makers have any duty of justice to allocate funds to research and develop genetic technologies for the benefit of future generations? From the standpoint of social justice, does the norm of equity require such macroallocations for future generations?

Although there is a growing philosophical literature on obligations to future generations, most of it is irrelevant to the present question. For this question is concerned with an extended concept of social justice and whether that concept entails a duty of justice to future generations. Given the macroallocational context, it seems plausible to frame the question in terms of equity of justice between generations. Thus, one approach to tracking the issue is provided by Rawls' theory of justice. Obviously, this theory cannot be detailed here. Suffice it to say that within a theoretically powerful contract theory, Rawls develops a notion of justice which states in part that inequalities are to be arranged so that they are to the greatest benefit of the least advantaged. To this he adds the following assumptions: the long-term prospects of the least advantaged extend over future generations, and the parties to the contract represent family lines with ties of sentiment between successive generations. The result is the recognition of duties incumbent on each generation to preserve the gains of culture and civilization, with this savings coming in various forms, eg net investment in technology, education, etc [49].

The problem is to determine a just savings principle, a rate of savings. Though Rawls admits that it is not possible to define precise limits for this rate, he suggests that there are ethical constraints that permit limits to be determined by each generation. For example, one asks what is reasonable for members of adjacent generations to expect of one another, on analogy with parents balancing goods for their children against what they believed they were entitled to receive from their own parents. And one adopts the standpoint of the least advantaged in each generation and requires that their expectations be maximized, subject to the savings that they would acknowledge.

The upshot is that different generations have duties of justice to future generations seriatim. The implications of this position for the question about the extended concept of social justice on the part of policy-makers are obvious. First, they may well be duty-bound to allocate funds to research and to develop biomedical, including genetic, technologies for future generations, to the extent that this macroallocation sits well with the least advantaged group in the present generation. Second, this line of reasoning mitigates the negative force of the observation that such research may never redound to present investors but only to their successors; the point is that the performance of an extant duty of social justice on the part of policy-makers is at stake. Third, this line of reasoning seems to imply that an extended concept of social justice (norm of equity) is indeed applicable to the macroallocational context as this may apply to the research and development of genetic technologies. Further, on the grounds of social justice in the form of just savings, it may well be argued that technologies in applied human genetics represent an eminently suitable form of such savings.

REFERENCES

1. Feinberg J: "Social Philosophy." Englewood Cliffs, New Jersey: Prentice-Hall, 1973, p 94.
2. Ludmerer K: "Genetics and American Society." Baltimore: Johns Hopkins University Press, 1972, ch 8.
3. Ludmerer, ibid, pp 174–175.
4. Ludmerer, ibid, pp 193–201.
5. Ludmerer, ibid, pp 178, 187–188.
6. Neel JV: Social and scientific priorities in the use of genetic knowledge. In Hilton B, et al (eds): "Ethical Issues in Human Genetics." New York: Plenum, 1973, pp 353–355.
7. Beckwith J: Social and political uses of genetics in the United States: Past and present. Ann NY Acad Sci 265:54, January, 1976.
8. Lappé M: Can eugenic policy be just? In Milunsky A (ed): "The Prevention of Genetic Disease and Mental Retardation." Philadelphia: W.B. Saunders, 1975, p 460.
9. Huxley J: In Tax S, Callendar C (eds): "Evolution After Darwin 3." Chicago: University of Chicago Press, 1960, p 61. Cited in Golding MP: Ethical issues in biological engineering. UCLA Law Rev 15:453, February, 1968.
10. Dobzhansky T: Man and natural selection. Am Sci 49:285–299, 1961. Cited in Lappé, M: Moral obligations and the fallacies of 'genetic control.' Theol Studies 33:417, September, 1972.
11. Sang JH: Nature, nurture, and eugenics. Postgrad Med J 48:227, 1972. Cited in Lappé, 1975, p 460.
12. Lappé M, 1972, p 422–423.
13. Medawar PB: Do advances in medicine lead to genetic deterioration? Mayo Clinic Proc 40:33, 1965.
14. Lappé, 1972, p 421.
15. Lappé M: Allegiances of human geneticists: A preliminary typology. Hastings Center Studies 1, No. 2:65–74, 1973.
16. Lappé, 1975, p 466.
17. Sperry RW: Science and the problem of values. Zygon 9:7, 1974. Cited in Lappé, 1975, pp 466–467.
18. Simpson GG: The concept of progress in organic evolution. Soc Res 41:28, 1974. Cited in Lappé, 1975, p 467. Also see Flew, A: "Evolutionary Ethics." London: Macmillan, 1967.
19. Golding MP: UCLA Law Review 15:1968, op cit, pp 461–462.
20. Ludmerer K: "Genetics and American Society." op cit, pp 20–33.
21. Lederberg J: Biomedical frontiers: Genetics. In Kunz RM, Fehr H (eds): "Challenge of Life." Basel: Berkhauser Verlag, 1972, p 234.
22. Genetics Research Group: Ethical and social issues in screening for genetic disease. N Engl J Med 286:1131, May 1972.

23. Hull RT: Why 'genetic disease'? This volume, p 57–69.
24. Twiss SB: Ethical issues in genetic screening: Models of genetic responsibility. In Bergsma D, Lappe M, Roblin RO, Gustafson JM (eds): "Ethical, Social, and Legal Dimensions of Screening for Human Genetic Disease." New York: Stratton Intercontinental Medical Book, 1974, pp 239–240.
25. Callahan D: What obligations do we have to future generations? Am Ecclesiastical Rev 164:265–280, April, 1971. Golding MP: Obligations to future generations. Monist 56: 85–99, January 1972.
26. Fried C: "Medical Experimentation." Amsterdam: North-Holland, 1974, pp 92–93. Cf Twiss SB: Ethical issues in priority-setting for the utilization of genetic technologies. Ann N Y Acad Sci 265:24–25, January 1976.
27. Golding MP, Golding NH: Ethical and value issues in population limitation and distribution in the United States. Vanderbilt Law Rev 24:509–515, April 1971.
28. Beckwith J: Ann N Y Acad Sci 265:1976, op cit p 48.
29. Glass B: Human heredity and ethical problems. Persp Biol Med 241–245, Winter, 1972.
30. Twiss SB: "Ethical, Social and Legal Dimensions of Screening for Human Genetic Disease." op cit pp 225–261.
31. Haller MH: "Eugenics." New Brunswick, New Jersey: Rutgers University Press, 1963, pp 81, 141.
32. Golding MP: UCLA Law Review 15:1968, op cit pp 470–471.
33. Ramsey P: "The Patient as Person." New Haven: Yale University Press, 1970, p 240.
34. Zuckerman L: The doctor's dilemma. In Kunz RM, Fehr H (eds): "The Challenge of Life." Basel: Berkhauser Verlag, 1972.
35. Gordon TJ: The feedback between technology and values. In Baier K, Rescher N (eds): "Values and the Future." New York: Free Press, 1969, p 151.
36. Zuckerman L: "The Challenge of Life." op cit, p 430.
37. Rescher N: Ethical issues regarding the delivery of health-care services. Unpublished paper read at Conference on Ethical Issues in the Distribution of Health Services, Brown University, Providence, Rhode Island, April 15–16, 1975.
38. Twiss, 1976, p 23.
39. Varian HR: Distributive justice, welfare economics, and the theory of fairness." Philosophy and Public Affairs 4:223–247, Spring 1975.
40. Arrow K: Uncertainty and the welfare economics of medical care. Am Econ Rev 53:941–954, 1963.
41. Feinberg J: "Social Philosophy." op cit p 110.
42. Rawls J: "A Theory of Justice." Cambridge, Massachusetts: Harvard University Press, 1971, ch 2.
43. Williams BAO: The idea of equality. In Bedau HA (ed): "Justice and Equality." Englewood Cliffs, New Jersey: Prentice-Hall, 1971, p 127.
44. Scarce medical resources. Columbia Law Rev 69:690, April 1969.
45. Rescher N: "Introduction to Value Theory." Englewood Cliffs, New Jersey: Prentice-Hall, 1969, pp 41–45.
46. Davis J, Murray RF, Twiss SB: Panel discussion. Ann N Y Acad Sci 265:162–167, January 1976.
47. Steiner KC, Smith HA: Application of cost-benefit analysis to a PKU screening program. Inquiry 10:34–40, 1973.
48. Tsukahara T, Kadota RL: Economic considerations in genetic screening programs for Tay-Sachs disease. Claremont Economic Papers 150:12–13, November 1975.
49. Rawls J: "A Theory of Justice." op cit pp 284 ff.

17. Public Policy Issues in Genetic Counseling

James F. Childress, PhD and Kenneth Casebeer, JD

This chapter offers a framework for discussing issues in public policy relating to genetic counseling by considering the interaction of public policy and genetic counseling and the tensions between procreational freedom and other interests. It tries to identify and sort out some of the central arguments about whether and how genetic counseling should be made a matter of public policy, and to show that arguments that counseling should be a subject of public policy are not separate from arguments that a particular policy should be enacted. Our framework is also normative, for we hold that our society recognizes a rebuttable presumption in favor of procreational freedom.

PUBLIC POLICY AND GENETIC COUNSELING

"Public policy is whatever governments choose to do or not to do" [1]. An adequate definition would also stress that public policy is purposive action and, indeed, a course or pattern of action or inaction by government officials [2]. As such, public policies typically involve one or more of the following actions: allocation and distribution of benefits (eg services and goods) and burdens (eg taxation); regulation (eg prohibition or control of an activity); expression (eg affirmation of values). By no means exhaustive, these categories are designed to suggest some of the main types of public policies. Other essays in this volume treat directly some of these factors in relation to genetic counseling. For example, Twiss considers allocation, while Reilly and Capron discuss some issues in regulation such as licensing and confidentiality.

In defining "public policy" on a particular subject at a given time, our scrutiny must take in more than officially promulgated rules and regulations. Since a formal governmental policy may be one of inaction or laissez faire, various other forces, such as public opinion, may develop an informal or de facto policy. While de facto policies are sometimes only recognized in retrospect, they

Birth Defects: Original Article Series, Volume XV, Number 2, pages 279–290

often decisively influence the direction of technological developments, such as genetic intervention. Indeed, informal policies may be so strong that the scope of eventual formal licensing or regulation becomes a foregone conclusion.

It is not appropriate to view public policy as merely a dependent variable. We cannot assume that the subject matter — genetic counseling — is clear and determined so that public policy only responds to an independent technological reality. As other essays in this volume indicate, genetic counseling is not monolithic. Despite certain major trends, there are significant disagreements about the goals of counseling (eg whether it is primarily to facilitate individual decisions about risk-taking or to prevent risk-taking), about its loyalities (eg to the family or to the society), about the counselor's virtues (eg directive or nondirective), and about standards of effectiveness (eg understanding by the counselees or changes in reproductive patterns). The content of public policies toward genetic counseling will (or should) depend on an interpretation of trends within the activity and a judgment about its proper direction.

The current state of genetic counseling is in part the result of past public policies as well as private choices, many of which did not directly concern counseling or even genetics. First, the gene pool and the risks of defects have been influenced, even if only to a small degree, by mutagenic agents, social intercourse and mobility, consanguinity laws, and so forth. Second, public programs in other areas of genetic intervention (such as screening) place demands upon, sometimes complement, and sometimes compete with genetic counseling. Third, the tools (such as amniocentesis and abortion) available to a counselor depend on previous public policies and court decisions [3]. The policies which guide counseling in part reflect deliberate choices about genetics and in part are simply by-products of public or mixed public/private choices regarding genetics, reproduction, and numerous other matters.

It is possible to evaluate public policies from many different standpoints and by many different standards. Green, for instance, insists that the "correctness or ethical acceptability" of public policies in genetics is not "a really important element in the political framework" [4]. Yet we believe that an evaluation of policies must take account of principles which are moral, legal and constitutional as well as political but which are at a base implicitly ethical in nature. Our discussion focuses on the content of public policy rather than the many processes (such as legislation) through which governmental decisions are made; a complete analysis would include both the content and the processes.

PROCREATIONAL FREEDOM AS A RIGHT, VALUE, AND INTEREST

It would be unfortunate to conceive public policy debates about genetic counseling solely in terms of individual rights or interests against societal interest, for there is a collective interest in protecting individuals' freedom. Moreover, the view that society balances individual and collective interests may be misleading since it implies that society puts various and often incommensurable values and rights on a scale to determine the best policy. Such language does not recognize procreational freedom as a presumptive or prima facie right that society is willing to override only under certain circumstances. The specially protected nature of procreational freedom can be discerned in many laws, court decisions, and social practices. By now the Supreme Court cases that affirm a constitutional right to privacy in the area of procreational choice — Roe v Wade, Griswold v Connecticut, and Eisenstadt v Baird — are well known [5]. The First, Fourth, Ninth, and Fourteenth Amendments have been read to prohibit state control of or intervention into private reproductive relationships and medical advice or response in regard to them.

The Social Value of Free Choice

The interrelation of societal and individual interests can take a number of forms. First, the public policy of a society may display a commitment to the value of free procreational choice and not merely a recognition of the individual's right to be free of interference. Thus, the government might fund programs to increase freedom in procreational decisions. Freedom, according to this line of thought, is more than an arbitrary, capricious gamble. Real freedom to decide about reproduction requires sound information about the risks (both probability and severity) of genetic defects and about the options for avoiding and reducing these risks or for coping with untoward results. Policies to maximize freedom could stress formal rather than substantive rationality: the rationality of choices of means to ends regardless of the rationality of the ends. They could aim to remove barriers to free decisions, not to ensure that the counselees make the "right" decisions. From this perspective, society could insist that counseling be noncoercive and nondirective, that its goal be full communication, and that its efficacy be judged in terms of the counselees' level of understanding (not the "correctness" of their attitudes or behavior).

While freedom in reproduction has a high value in our society, there is little evidence that public policies primarily designed to enhance that freedom by facilitating informed choices have been given high priority in allocation of resources. Although the National Genetic Diseases Act [6] stresses "voluntary" choices, its paramount interest is not the increase of autonomy but the promotion of public health. It restricts its programs to voluntary counseling, but voluntariness is a "side constraint" not a goal [7]. Freedom is a limit on the pursuit of other ends, not an end in itself.

Freedom in the Positive Sense

A second type of interaction appears if we inquire about the obligations placed on the collectivity by the individual's rights regarding procreation. The focus here is on freedom in the positive sense, that is, the enhancement of choice rather than nonintervention by the state. If procreational freedom is a right of this type, there arises a positive duty on the part of the society not only to refrain from interference but to facilitate the full exercise of choice as well. It is apparent that past public choices in a complex social system markedly affect people's ability or options to implement procreational choice. Consequently, real liberty might depend on socially recognized responsibility toward individuals facing procreational choices. For example, the incidence and degree of genetic risk as well as the potential to respond to risk depend on the social process, especially when publicly funded advances in medical technology increase the likelihood that genetically defective newborns will survive, when rising medical costs restrict access of some segments of society to treatment for defective offspring, and when past public allocations of research funds place certain defective genotypes at risk of less attention than those thoroughly studied at public expense.

Freedom in the Negative Sense

The final area of concern includes those cases in which policy options that limit freedom of choice confront an individual's asserted right to be free from state interference. While procreational rights are recognized as fundamental, they have not been held to be absolute, and a compelling state interest can justify public intervention to restrict personal conduct that would otherwise be protected.

Any limits placed on the use of genetic counseling depend on its having markedly adverse social consequences. Such consequences may not only be attributed to the activity of counseling itself but to various techniques, procedures, and means of realizing the counselor's and counselee's goals. For example, screening and amniocentesis are important diagnostic procedures for identifying potentially "defective" offspring. Depending on what stage in reproduction that the counselees seek advice, a variety of options — nonmarriage, contraception, artifical insemination, abortion, allowing defective newborns to die, treatment, and so forth — may all be means of avoiding or coping with genetically defective offspring. Several adverse social consequences could follow from permitting some of these available means. For example, allowing defective newborns to die when they need medical intervention [8] appears to violate numerous laws; continuation of such practices may necessitate several legal changes for consistency and coherence or could lead to a policy of enforcing relevant laws because of prosecutors' view on the immorality of the practice and the danger of its creating a "slippery slope" [9].

Given the various court decisions and policies that recognize the legitimacy of abortion, it is difficult to argue for a restrictive policy regarding amniocentesis simply because it may lead to abortion. Yet many counselors are reluctant to offer amniocentesis to parents who merely want to determine the sex of the fetus. So long as amniocentesis is a limited resource it seems justifiable to give low priority to counselees who have only this interest. But if scarcity is not now or ceases to be a problem, a policy of withholding amniocentesis from families who only want to identify the sex of the fetus may lack compelling justification. In some cases, parents are merely curious, and there is no legitimate reason for the state to foreclose harmless curiosity. In other cases, the health of the family or particular members could be adversely affected by the birth of either a male or a female, consequences which society may have no reason to compel. Finally, in the remaining cases, parents may have personal reasons for wishing to abort a fetus of one sex or the other. Since no reasons are required for abortion at certain stages of fetal development, it would be awkward and inconsistent for the state to rule out abortion based on fetal sex. Unless there is a change in public policy toward abortion generally, the possibility of abortion on grounds of sex cannot appropriately be used to deny access to amniocentesis once scarcity ceases to be a problem. Nevertheless, such a practice may have other adverse social consequences (eg altering the ratio of males to females) that might justify state-imposed restrictions.

The fundamental right of free procreational choice not only limits societal interference with genetic counseling in the absence of adverse social consequences, but it also stands as a "side constraint" on governmental attempts to realize other ends through various mandatory and coercive programs. As C. Fried has remarked, a right that does not stick in the spokes of someone's wheels is no right at all. The National Genetic Diseases Act allocates funds to achieve several ends, including public health, but it adheres to the "side constraint" of free procreational choice. Observing that twelve million Americans are affected by genetic diseases that often are "severely handicapping and debilitating and result in tragic physical, emotional, and financial burden on the individuals, their families, and society," this bill holds that "reducing the burden of genetic diseases deserves a high priority in Federal health legislation and will be cost beneficial to the American public." Its rationale is "to preserve and protect the health and welfare of all citizens. . . ." Yet is supports only "voluntary genetic testing and counseling programs," holding that any individual's participation in the programs shall be "wholly voluntary and shall not be a prerequisite to eligibility for or receipt of any other service or assistance from, or to participation in, any other program."

Even when compelling public interests justify overriding fundamental rights, such as free procreational choice, those rights usually do not disappear without leaving some traces. Suppose for purposes of argument that public health considerations (such as protection of the gene pool) justify some form of mandatory genetic counseling. The state must first try to realize its compelling interest by the "least restrictive alternative" since a fundamental right is involved [10].

For instance, since only a few genetic defects can be detected and even fewer can be prevented or treated, the improvement in the overall quality of the gene pool may be problematic. Furthermore, we could possibly get the same improvement by identifying and reducing the mutagenic agents in the environment that cause the same defects. Although it is difficult to determine the causes of genetic change, such an approach would not necessarily be less effective than compulsory counseling programs especially if we assume that religious and moral convictions as well as simple resentment will result in significant noncooperation or noncompliance. Thus, the courts might require that policy-makers show that less restrictive alternatives including voluntary programs and attempts to control mutagenic agents or the environment are not available before allowing mandatory counseling. Yet ironically for public policy, while the constitutionality of a proposed compulsory program depends only on presently feasible technological alternatives, the need for such drastic means of compulson may be determined in part by wholly independent past public choices. Policy decisions to fund research and development to determine and alter the causes of genetic defects decided on their own merits thus set the future feasibility of alternatives to compulsion, illustrating the dynamic and continuous nature of public decision-making.

State regulations which restrict liberty (as, for example, mandatory amniocentesis) must also provide "procedural due process" in Constitutional terms. "Procedural due process" usually means that the person must be granted a hearing after notice of the proposed course of action, perhaps provided with counsel and given an opportunity to present and interrogate witnesses. Furthermore, compulsory counseling programs that aim only at specific genetic defects may also run afoul of the guarantee of equal protection of the laws. Laws that categorize compulsion by identifiable but inherent traits, whether ethnic, racial, national origin, or perhaps sex, are inherently suspect and demand strict scrutiny for a compelling interest in utilizing the suspect classification. Even if, for example, a sickle cell program does not use racial identification, but focuses on those "at risk of the disease," the classification may still be suspect if only one racial group is found to be "at risk." Indeed, genetic makeup itself (which after all determines race) may come to be recognized as an immutable characteristic that demands strict justification [11]. Thus, the means of classification as well as the state end must be justified, and a very heavy burden would be required for compelling a particular group to undergo compulsory genetic intervention. The dangers of manipulation aimed at subjugation of a particular group and the unavoidable danger of public stigma would make such a program extremely problematic.

Regulation of genetic counseling need not be limited to civil or constitutional remedies for violations of publicly sanctioned duties. Bad results can be prevented and counseling itself channeled and shaped by legislation under the traditional police powers of the states to protect the public health and welfare. The states may act indirectly through incentive or funding schemes or more directly by detailing the manner and form all counseling must take. All the standards incorporated into bases for liability could be reworked into direct regulations. Violations, rather than leading to private damage actions, could be policed by revocations of licenses or even criminal penalties.

Regulations that set limits and impose duties in counseling will form a significant part of public policy. By taking into account public desires as well as present practices, they may aim at remedying harms, preventing incompetence, or facilitating development and use, and each aim reinforces the others. The extent of regulation will depend upon the type and importance of the state interests involved.

STATE INTERESTS AS JUSTIFICATIONS FOR COERCION

Now, what are some of the state interests that might justify one or more coercive policies? One argument for coercive policies — and even for directive counseling — is paternalism, which can be seen as the collective interest in restricting a person's liberty for his or her own benefit. Examples of paternalistic legislation are laws that require motorcyclists to wear helmets, make attempting a suicide a criminal offense, or prohibit drugs that can harm their users. Since genetic counselors typically have a better understanding of the effects of particular genetic diseases and their probability than counselees, the argument runs, they should take necessary steps to ensure certain results, particularly since counselees may be swayed by numerous irrational factors such as religious beliefs that stress the positive effects of suffering or that restrict the means to be used to prevent the harm that will come to families from genetic defects.

Paternalism is in fact rarely offered as a sufficient justification. Stronger reasons for coercive interventions center around the prevention of harm to persons other than those whose freedom is restricted. (Sometimes paternalistic reasons may also be cited, to avoid the charge of unfairly imposing burdens on a person or group for society's benefit. Thus, it might be argued that a restriction on a one's procreational choice benefits one's family as much as it does society.) The list of "others" includes the genetically defective offspring, society and future generations.

Offspring

Some commentators have claimed that there is a tort of "wrongful life" and that every child has a right to a minimum quality of genetic inheritance [12]. Glass, for instance, maintains that "in a not-distant future time, owing to the advances of human genetics, the right of individuals to procreate must give place to a new paramount right: the right of every child to enter life with an adequate physical and mental endowment." [13] An argument such as Glass' might well point in the direction of a legal enforcement of genetic responsibility, although Glass, himself, was proposing only a moral, not a legal right. While the probable quality of life of potential offspring is relevant to parental decisions about risk-taking, it does not provide a solid foundation for coercive public policies, especially mandatory amniocentesis and abortion. Rarely does it appear by itself in discourse about public policies; and it seems to be limited to an exhortation to parents to base their decisions on what will be in their offspring's best interests.

Society

The public health, which appears in the National Genetics Diseases Act to justify funding voluntary programs, has also been invoked to justify coercive interventions in procreative decisions. For instance, in Buck v Bell in 1927, Justice Holmes appealed to the public health, along with other considerations including paternalism and fairness, to uphold a Virginia statute authorizing compulsory sterilization of the institutionalized mentally retarded: "The principle that sustains compulsory vaccination is broad enough to cover cutting the Fallopian tubes. . ."[14]. Much of our moral and legal reasoning is analogical. This is to be expected, since one fundamental principle of morality in general and justice in particular is that similar cases be treated in a similar way. Although analogical reasoning is necessary, particular analogies may be problematic. For Holmes, since the public health rationale is sufficient to sustain compulsory vaccination which invades privacy and bodily integrity, it is sufficient to uphold compulsory sterilization. Holmes overlooked the point that sterilization irreversibly prevents procreation and that it depends on uncertain theories of mental retardation and heredity. It is not at all clear that the holding in Buck v Bell would now be upheld, but regardless of the Supreme Court's decision, policy-makers can draw different and narrower boundaries on interference with procreation. While the strongest case for compulsory programs invokes the public health [15], even it depends on establishing clear connections between the classification of persons and the end that is sought; and those connections obviously hinge on well-founded theories of causation and prevention of genetic defects.

Many arguments about effects on society include the economic costs of trying to treat or care for defective offspring. The National Genetic Diseases Act refers to the "financial burden on the individuals, their families, and society," and insists that reducing genetic diseases will be "cost beneficial to the American public." Justice Holmes in Buck v Bell held that "three generations of imbeciles are enough" in part because they "sap the strength of the state. . . ." The drain on society's resources is a legitimate concern, but "there have also been intimations that a statute which compelled sterilization because of the potential financial drain on society posed by impecunious wards violates the Equal Protection Clause. . ."[16].

While economic costs cannot be ignored from the standpoint of public policy, a cost-benefit analysis that incorporates only such considerations is hardly adequate even if it is more quantifiable and manageable because it excludes other values. Furthermore, it is difficult to determine at what point economic values should override liberty.

Future Generations

Society has an interest in the quality of the gene pool particularly as it will affect the well-being of future generations. Interventions could be aimed at preventing further deterioriation of the gene pool and even at reducing the frequency of deleterious genes. Nevertheless, evidence on the effects of altered reproduction patterns on the gene pool is quite mixed. As long as the effects remain speculative, procreational freedom should be undisturbed.

Although these three rationales for state interest in "genetic decisions" do not appear to justify coercion, even this brief review has pointed in the direction of a "minimal ethic of genetic responsibility," [Twiss, in this volume, p 255] in which harm to others, including society, is a relevant moral consideration for families who are trying to decide what to do with genetic information. But while we may present these considerations to ourselves and others (even occasionally in our roles as counselors), they seldom justify forcibly overriding autonomy. Some fear that voluntary programs, such as the ones encompassed in the National Genetic Diseases Act, may evolve into coercive programs, mandating counseling and even dictating certain procreative decisions. Whether such an evolution could be morally justified depends on the weight of scientific and other evidence about the magnitude of harm of genetic defects to various individuals and groups and the available means of preventing such harm. Whether particular moral considerations should be legally enforced is a moral and political question since conflicting values are at stake. To avoid harm or certain costs to others and to society is surely a reason for considering whether to override liberty, but we start from a presumption in favor of liberty in procreative decisions and it is difficult to determine when avoiding harm or costs is a sufficient, decisive, or conclusive reason.

THE MORALITY INHERENT IN PUBLIC POLICIES

So far we have emphasized the choice of public policies in instrumental terms: which policies will enable us to realize or at least to respect certain values and rights including the reduction of genetic defects and the preservation of autonomy? But rarely are public policies merely instrumental. They also express certain values and convictions, and often have effects, sometimes unanticipated, on other values and convictions. We need to ask what policies toward genetic counseling express and what they may affect.

First, increased interest in genetic counseling and related procedures and techniques may well alter attitudes toward procreative decisions in far-reaching ways. While we have long been interested in healthy babies, evidence suggests that we are rapidly coming to think about optimal or perfect babies. We even seem to phrase the options in terms of optimal baby or no baby. As Kass has suggested, such attitudes bespeak a transformation in the process of procreation, away from the family and into the laboratory. What began as a procedure to increase voluntary decision-making cannot now easily exclude the demand for optimal babies [17]. The costs of such a shift should enter into the formulation of public policy even if these costs cannot be quantified as readily as the tangible costs of birth defects.

Second, with an emphasis on prevention of birth defects in conjunction with procedures and techniques to realize that aim, what will happen to efforts to treat such defects and to care for those who suffer from them? A shift from curative medicine to preventive medicine may be marked by a different attitude toward those who need cure and care, those who have slipped through the net of prevention. Such attitudinal shifts can be expected to be more pronounced where prevention is unsuccessful because the parents have religious or moral scruples against a method (such as abortion) and where the costs of care are exceedingly large. What will be the effects of such changes in attitude?

Third, faced with limited resources for health care, including both prevention and therapy, a society could decide to exclude whole classes of disease from treatment. As Outka has stressed, such a strategy need not violate the principle of formal justice (treat similar cases in a similar way). It might take the form of refusing to support particular diseases that are rare and noncommunicable, have little prospect for rehabilitation, and require extended and very expensive care [18]. If such a strategy were adopted, one would expect pressure to add another criterion: could the disease have been prevented or avoided? While this criterion seems to add retributive factors to distributive ones, few would deny the relevance of effort to distributive justice even if they dispute its weight and significance. At any rate, society might decide to exclude treatment of a genetic disease that could have been avoided through a different choice about marriage, conception and abortion if that disease requires expensive care without any prospect for rehabilitation. However formally just and rational such a policy may appear, it has its own symbolic and cultural costs. Justice does not exhaust our vision of society, and a society that is merely just may lack many elements of humane caring. That cost should not be overlooked or downplayed.

Finally, public policies reflect social notions of health and disease which may direct or limit genetic counseling. Appearing to encompass firm "harm" and "welfare" judgments, they may actually rest on other hidden moral principles and values. What is or should be a moral or political problem may be converted into a medical one. Thus, the putatively objective labels of health and disease may serve to legitimate restrictions of liberty when other justifications would fall short. The rather severe measures taken in the name of treating "mental disease" supply a harrowing catalogue of the potentially pernicious effects when the supposed neutral observations of medical science are translated into law. We should constantly probe assertions of harm and welfare, disease and health, to discover the unarticulated moral and political values on which the asserted justifications actually rest so as to determine whether they are strong enough to override other values and principles such as liberty and equality.

REFERENCES

1. Dye TR: Understanding Public Policy. Second edition. Englewood Cliffs, NJ: Prentice-Hall, Inc, 1975, p 1.
2. Anderson JE: Public Policy-Making. New York: Praeger Publishers, 1975, p 3.
3. For example, the increasing use of amniocentesis is controversial precisely because it may be utilized during the stage of fetal development when abortion is legally permissible, ie, prior to fetal viability. See Roe vs Wade, 410 US 113 (1973). Suppose that technological advances result in fetal viability at an earlier stage of development than amniocentesis can be effectively used. If the legal prohibitions of abortion remain wedded to viability, rather than genetic counseling techniques, we can expect a drop in the use of amniocentesis. Or at least the justification for its use would be limited to information — to identify sex or to alert parents to what defects they can expect their child to have. Similar effects on the use of amniocentesis might occur as de facto public policy following a shift in moral attitudes critical of abortion. Waltz JR and Thigpen CR: Genetic Screening and Counseling: The Legal and Ethical Issues. Northwestern University Law Review 68:738, note 215, 1974.
4. Green HP: Law and Genetic Control: Public-Policy Questions. Ann NY Acad Sci 265: 170–177, 1976.
5. Roe vs Wade 410 US 113 (1973); Griswold vs Connecticut 381 US 479 (1965); Eisenstadt vs Baird 405 US 438 (1972).
6. National Genetic Diseases Act, S 7801, 94th Congress, 2nd, 1975.
7. Nozick R: Anarchy, State, and Utopia. New York: Basic Books, 1974.
8. For a defense of the practice, see Duff RS and Campbell AGM: "Moral and Ethical Dilemmas in the Special-Care Nursey." N Engl J Med 289:890–894, 1973; and On Deciding the Care of Severely Handicapped or Dying Persons: With Particular Reference to Infants. Pediatrics 57:487–493, 1976.
9. See Robertson JA: "Involuntary Euthanasia of Defective Newborns: A Legal Analysis." Stanford Law Review 27:213–269, 1975.
10. Cf, eg Skinner vs Oklahoma, 316 US 535 (1942); Shapiro vs Thompson, 394 US 618 (1969).
11. See eg McLauflin vs Florida, 379 US 184 (1964). In McLauflin, a statute making interracial marriages a crime was struck down because of the per se use of race to distinguish the legal from the illegal. Similarly, the per se use of a particular genotype for a compulsory health treatment raises questions of definitional circularity in the rationale for using this means of classification.

12. For a legal analysis, see generally, Capron AM: Informed Decisionmaking in Genetic Counseling: A Dissent to the Wrongful Life Debate. Indiana Law Journal 48:581–604, Summer 1973.

13. Birch C, Abrecht P (eds): "Genetics and the Quality of Life." Elmsford, NY: Pergamon, 1975, pp 56–57. Glass' conception is a positive right to have a minimum level of genetic quality. This is an odd right since if the conditions are not present for its realization, the child is presumed to want no life at all. Furthermore, it is a right to something that we cannot guarantee. It might be better to avoid the language of rights in this context.

14. Buck vs Bell 274 US 200 (1927). But see also Skinner vs Oklahoma 316 US 535 (1942).

15. For example, the public health interest in compulsory vaccinations upheld in Jacobsen vs Massachusetts 197 US 11 (1905).

16. Price ME, Burt RA: Sterilization, State Action, and the Concept of Consent. Law and Psychology Review (Spring 1975): 62. They refer to Cook vs State, 9 Ore App 224, 495 P 2d 768 (1972).

17. See Kass L: Comments. "Early Diagnosis of Human Genetic Defects." Edited by Harris M. Fogarty International Center Proceedings No. 6 HEW Publication No. (NIH) 72–75, p 202. See also Kass L: Implications of Prenatal Diagnosis for the Human Right to Life. Ethical Issues in Human Genetics. Edited by Hilton B, et al. New York: Plenum, 1973, p 185.

18. Outka G: Social Justice and Equal Access to Health Care. Journal of Religious Ethics. 2:24, 1974.

18. Professional Identification: Issues in Licensing and Certification*

Philip Reilly, JD

GENETIC COUNSELING — A NEW PROFESSION?

Today most genetic counseling services are provided by clinics operating within large research hospitals. Because the patient load is not yet burdensome, the physician (a medical geneticist) who has made the diagnosis is often able to join counseling specialists (such as medical social workers) in at least some of the follow-up sessions with counselees. But this milieu is starting to change. Major advances, particularly in antenatal diagnosis, have been widely publicized by the lay press [1, 2]. Community-based genetic screening programs designed to detect carriers of Tay-Sachs disease or sickle cell anemia have created sudden, dramatic (albeit short-lived) demands for genetic counseling services [3, 4]. Although only rudimentary analysis of their impact is available [3], it is almost certain that such programs have elevated public awareness of hereditary disease.

It is safe to assume that the frequency with which patients ask private physicians for genetic advice will continue to rise. This should in turn lead to more clinic referrals and, consequently, a diminution of contact between the physician-geneticist and each patient after the initial, diagnostic counseling has been completed. On more and more occasions the counseling follow-up will be conducted by people with neither an MD degree nor doctoral training in human genetics. Persons trained in medical social work and pediatric nurse practitioners are among those most likely to provide such services. Graduates of the several "genetic associates" programs† constitute another important personnel source [5]. This essay is mainly concerned with the regulation of counseling by these

*Supported in part by the Commonwealth Fund.

†A master's degree in genetic counseling is offered by at least five schools in the United States: Sarah Lawrence, Rutgers, the University of Colorado, the University of California at Irvine and at Berkeley.

Birth Defects: Original Article Series, Volume XV, Number 2, pages 291–305

nonphysicians. In general, I shall use the term counselor to apply to any person (regardless of training) who helps persons to understand and cope with genetic problems. When it is necessary, I shall further refine the term.

Naturally, as they have acquired more experience, counselors have become more sensitive to the task of helping people comprehend the risks and burdens (medical, psychologic, and economic) of genetic disorders. This new sensitivity generated the first studies of the genetic counseling process [6] and caused a major shift in the meaning attributed to that term. Two counselors anticipated this trend in 1969 when they argued that although "genetic counseling in the past often stressed diagnosis and genetic risks . . . future definitions are likely to include more considerations about effective modes of communication between physician and families" [7]. By 1974 the "official" definition of counseling had fulfilled this prophecy [8]:

> Genetic counseling is a communication process which deals with the human problems associated with the occurrence, or risk of occurrence, of a genetic disorder in a family. This process involves an attempt by one or more appropriately trained persons to help the individual or family to (1) comprehend the medical facts, including the diagnosis, probable course of the disorder, and the available management; (2) appreciate the way heredity contributes to the disorder, and the risk of recurrence in specified relatives; (3) understand the alternatives for dealing with the risk of recurrence; (4) choose the course of action which seems to them appropriate in view of their risk, their family goals, and their ethical and religious standards, and to act in accordance with that decision; and (5) to make the best possible adjustment to the disorder in an affected family member and/or to the risk of recurrence of that disorder.

An inevitable consequence of the new emphasis on the communication's problem was the demise of the notion that physicians or persons with doctorates in human genetics should perform the bulk of the counseling. For example, in an editorial in the *New England Journal of Medicine* [9] two physician-counselors asked: "Does the neurologist, pediatrician or obstetrician have sufficient training to provide genetic counseling? Does the psychiatrist? Is the family physician adequately trained for this?" Three concerns motivated these questions: 1) most physicians were unfamiliar with the genetics of human disease, 2) effective counseling requires a set of skills not provided as part of a medical or scientific education, and 3) counseling can be a very time-consuming process. During the past five years, medical geneticists have reified these concerns to argue that genetic counseling should be viewed as a subspecialty over which they should have hegemony. In this view, a medical degree is necessary, but not sufficient, preparation for a person to operate a genetics clinic. Persons engaged to deliver the bulk of the follow-up (postdiagnostic) counseling need only minimal competence in medical genetics, but they should be trained in communications skills.

By 1974 a consensus seemed to be emerging about how genetic counseling services should be delivered and how the profession should be organized. The majority view was that counseling clinics should remain connected with the major medical institutions in which they had been spawned because the arcane problems often encountered in human genetics require a "team" approach for their solution. Only a medical center has sufficient bench strength. As Dr. Clarke Fraser, a leading medical geneticist, has stated [10], "No individual could set himself up as a counselor and provide satisfactory service without the support of a cytogenetics laboratory, a biochemistry department geared to do screening for a variety of genetic diseases, the diagnostic facilities of a modern hospital, and the clinical expertise of a variety of specialists." Despite general agreement among geneticists today that counseling should occur against this background of expertise, there are strong pressures to permit hospitals with maternity services to include diagnostic laboratories capable of performing antenatal chromosome studies. It remains to be seen whether health planners will insist that routine antenatal diagnosis be carried out solely at major medical centers simply because the maternity hospitals are not able to conduct other more esoteric tests.

The prevailing view on the operation of a genetics clinic is that the physician-geneticist must take responsibility for diagnosis and that other geneticists should be available to assist. Backing them up is a second tier composed, as Dr. Fraser writes [10], of "a variety of auxiliary personnel such as public health nurses, social workers or genetic associates (people with masters degrees in counseling) (who) can provide invaluable service in interviewing, searching files and literature sources, collating information, and following up families." Although Dr. Fraser failed to emphasize the important role that genetic associates can play in patient counseling, that fact is usually recognized. For example, in 1975 a committee of the American Society of Human Genetics advocated that genetic associates should be closely involved with the patient population and recognized that in some situations associates could assume a major role in counseling. Associates could "[enhance] the processes of communication and [assist] patients and families in dealing with their problems" [8]. The committee encouraged each counseling team to define for itself the extent to which associates should assume responsibilities for patients.

Arguments favoring an expanded role for nondoctoral counselors reflect the growing efforts to soften the hierarchic structure in medicine generally [11]. Although gradual, this important development is slowly being embodied as public policy. For example, a recent California law, written to increase access to medical care, declared that pediatric nurse practitioners would work in "consultation with" doctors. This is quite different from an earlier California statute on physician assistants which states that they must work "under the supervision of" doctors [12].

Although it is difficult to predict such matters with precision, it is likely that by 1985 at least 1,200 medical geneticists will be needed in the United States [10]. Assuming that each of these persons would require the aid of four follow-up counselors, several thousand such persons should be trained during this decade. Because existing "genetic associate" graduate programs could not possibly satisfy this demand, a large number of these positions will continue to be filled by people without formal education in genetic counseling who have received their training on the job. This is beginning to raise a number of questions for those already functioning as counselors, whether they have doctoral, masters-level, or no formal training in genetics. While perhaps originating in hierarchial and self-protective impulses, these questions are far-reaching: What makes a good counselor? And how, if at all, ought genetic counseling be regulated?

Incipient, but growing, interest in the regulation of genetic counselors can be detected in three different quarters. First, senior medical geneticists, concerned about the sudden demand for counseling services and the concomitant, rapid entry of new nonphysician counselors into the field, have expressed a desire for some kind of "quality control" [13]. No doubt this desire has been partly provoked by the malpractice crisis, since under common law principles, the negligent acts of counselors (and other employees) would be the responsibility of the physician and of the hospital's genetics clinic of which the physician is the director [14].

Naturally, the major concern of medical geneticists is that their patients be protected from incompetent counseling. This has reinforced the argument that medical genetics should be elevated to the status of a subspecialty. In a regulatory vacuum, notes Fraser [10], "it is possible for unqualified and ill-informed persons to set themselves up as genetic counselors." Because there is no evidence as to how often this has happened, it must be an uncommon event. Interestingly, despite occasional calls from physicians, the Ad Hoc Committee on Genetic Counseling of the American Society of Human Genetics has not yet taken a public stand on the issue of regulation, but in Canada a group of leading geneticists have already agreed to develop standards of performance for counselors. In Saskatchewan it has been decided that medical genetics should be made a board certifiable specialty.

Second, the advent of state-supported mass genetic screening programs (particularly the controversial efforts to identify carriers of sickle cell trait) have alerted public health officials to the need to provide high quality genetic counseling to screenees [15]. The injuries suffered by black persons who participated in poorly operated sickle cell screening programs have sensitized law makers to some of the more subtle aspects of mass genetic testing. First in 1972 when the "National Sickle Cell Anemia Control Act" became law and again in 1976 when an omnibus "Genetic Diseases Act" replaced it, Congress offered substantial funds to states which demonstrated that their screening programs complied with certain ethical principles. Among these is a guarantee that screenees be assured of "adequate genetic counseling" [16, 17].

The federal statutes have had a major impact on state legislation. Many states have adopted federal guidelines almost verbatim. The North Carolina sickle cell statute requires that "Counseling shall be done only by persons adequately trained and certified according to criteria established by recognized authorities in the field of human genetics" [18]. Kentucky law commands doctors who diagnose sickle cell anemia to refer affected persons to "an agency approved by the department (of public health)" for genetic counseling [19]. In Massachusetts a new omnibus genetic screening law permits public health officials to "promulgate rules . . . for the counseling of all susceptible persons" [20]. The Maryland Commission on Hereditary Disorders, created in 1973, provides "that counseling services for hereditary disorders be available to all persons involved in screening programs, that such counseling be non-directive; and that such counseling emphasize informing the client and not require restriction of childbearing" [21]. Thus far, with the exception of Maryland, no state seems to be actively applying principles embraced by its genetic screening law. Nevertheless, concerns about the quality of screening programs have elicited language in both state and federal laws which could be used to develop regulatory schemes for genetic counseling offered under state auspices. This could be a first step toward a system in which admission to the counseling profession was subjected to legal controls.

The third, and probably most important, source of pressures favoring the development of a formal scheme to control entry into the profession may be those persons who are coming to undertake the bulk of postdiagnostic counseling. Nurses, medical social workers, genetic associates, and other nonphysician counselors have identified several benefits that would accompany regulation*: 1) Formal recognition will enhance the frequency with which physicians refer patients to counseling units. This will be especially true if clinicians perceive nonphysician counselors to be noncompetitive health care personnel with professional status. 2) Institutional use of genetic counselors will expand since licensure will spur hospitals to list counseling as a job category and insurance companies to cover the cost of such services. 3) By forcing the debate over train-

*In July 1975, I attended a Conference on Genetic Counseling, sponsored by the University of California at Berkeley. The issue of regulation was among the major topics. I have abstracted these four benefits from discussions with nonphysician counselors far too numerous to list here.

ing and credentials to be resolved, licensure would help to coalesce the profession and facilitate its development. 4) Regulation is likely to enhance public awareness of genetic counseling services and normalize their use.

It is difficult to imagine a group for which the issue of regulation could have more importance than genetic associates and those persons directly involved in their training [22]. In 1976 I wrote to the faculties of the five schools that offer graduate degrees in genetic counseling asking: Do you favor licensing of genetic associates? Only one of the five professors who responded favored licensing without reservation; he thought it would greatly aid public use of counseling services. Other persons expressed serious doubt that licensing would ever be warranted. The majority view was that licensing could benefit both counselors and the public, that regulation was inevitable, but that it was premature to deploy such a scheme.

In her reply (letter to author dated 2/11/76), Dr. Patricia St. Lawrence of the University of California at Berkeley nicely summarized opinions that had been expressed by several respondents:

It is premature to consider licensure of genetic associates for several interconnected reasons. First, the extent and type of responsibilities which should properly be included in a position with such a title (or some other title such as genetic counselor) are not yet clearly enough defined to be described in legislation or administrative codes. Second, the appropriate training for such a specialty can only be specified when the position is clarified. Third, it is not clear whether the organized health care system, the public, and elected officials wish to expend resources on this type of service. I see little point in licensing unless there is a demonstrated need for the services to be provided. Fourth, it is not clear whether these persons will function as independent professionals or only in positions subordinate to physicians. The former would seem to necessitate some mechanism for certifying competence — to protect both the professional and the public — whereas the latter might not.

It thus appears that there are strong pressures to have genetic counseling recognized as a new profession in one fashion or another — either as medical and nursing subspecialties or as a distinct field for others with formal or on-the-job education in genetics and counseling techniques, or as both. Although such recognition is possible without formal steps being taken, it might be facilitated if laws were adopted requiring licensure. In order to evaluate them it will be useful first to review the history of licensure of the health professions in this country and to consider the arguments which are raised concerning licensing generally. Finally, we will return to the specific considerations that attach to the various alternatives now facing society concerning the regulation of genetic counseling.

MEDICAL LICENSING LAWS — AN OVERVIEW

The Development of Occupational Licensure in the Health Professions

A licensing system is a restraint on competition imposed by the state to achieve one or more benefits. The earliest, most important rationale offered in support of occupational licensing was to protect the public from incompetent persons who claimed expertise in matters about which the average person was uninformed. Since the first such law was enacted in Virginia in 1639, medical licensure has evolved away from a single-minded concern with quackery, and at least three other rationales have been developed: 1) to raise revenues through the imposition of licensing fees, 2) to legitimize new occupations, and 3) to provide an established occupation with a method to control its population and the direction in which it will develop [23].

Until recently most efforts to regulate the conduct of health care practitioners were generated by professionals, not consumers. Ordinances designed to control the practice of medicine began to acquire force in the middle of the 18th century. In 1767, 30 doctors from Litchfield County persuaded the Connecticut Assembly to authorize the review of the credentials of newcomers. This decision provoked one of the early debates over the advantages of consumer protection versus the disadvantages of monopolies. By 1800 fledgling medical groups existed in most states, and by 1820 some kind of prior approval was required of physicians in all but three states [24].

The following half century saw the erosion of the licensing system. Rapid population growth and westward expansion led to a shortage of physicians. On the frontier unlicensed healers were often the only ones available. Early licensing systems, aimed primarily at the apprenticeship system, had conferred automatic recognition on graduates of medical school. But in the early 19th century there were many medical schools which offered education of dubious quality. Moreover, licensing was incompatible with popular notions of laissez-faire economics and with the democratic, antiaristocratic tenor of the times. For these and other reasons, quality control of medical practice entered a state of desuetude that lasted until about the 1880s. By that time the various national medical associations which had been formed in midcentury began to acquire political clout. Reform movements in European medical schools and the new interest in public health also contributed to the renaissance. New licensing laws, often solicited by medical groups, began to reappear [24].

The new laws were, of course, resisted by many doctors, especially those whose training did not meet standards proposed by the American Medical Association (founded in 1847) and other reform groups. But the licensing movement overcame both political and legal challenges. West Virginia, for example, had enacted a law requiring doctors to meet one of three standards: 1) to have graduated from an approved medical college, 2) to have practiced medicine within the state for ten years, or 3) to pass an examination prepared by the new licensing board. Dr. Charles Dent refused to sit for the examination; instead, he sued the state for depriving him of his "right to work" in violation of the due process clause. The case eventually came before the Supreme Court of the United States, which in 1888 ruled that it was reasonable for the state to require that a doctor demonstrate that he had acquired "necessary learning and skill" [25]. During the subsequent decade, state courts routinely rejected challenges brought by irate physicians [26].

As the number of specialized occupations proliferated, state licensing schemes grew apace. The heyday of expansion came at the height of the progressive era (1890—1910) as part of the trend toward a more organized economy. Physician licensing laws were rapidly extended to cover allied health personnel. Virginia first licensed nurses in 1903; by 1920 nursing licenses were required in 47 states with most states adopting a uniform law written by the American Nursing Association [27].

A major change in the use of licensing became apparent between 1910 and 1930. Both inside and outside the health care occupations, groups of professionals, representing the majority, but certainly not all members, gained firm control of state licensure boards. In some cases these groups imposed rules which brought about fundamental changes in the organization of the professions. For example, after the requirement that doctors graduate from "approved"medical schools was widely adopted, the number of schools shrank rapidly from the 154 that had existed in 1904, so that by 1932 there were only 66 in operation [24]. The elimination of marginal schools elevated the general quality of medical education and reduced the problem of incompetent physicians. Of course, it also served to protect the competitive position of existing physicians.

The concentration of power spawned a shift in the use of licensing laws. As the state license became a symbol of competence and as it became more obvious that government would delegate control of the licensing process to members of the occupation, regulatory legislation was actively sought. Chiropractors, osteopaths, and podiatrists, threatened by the medical profession, lobbied arduously for separate laws. There was little resistance within government circles to such requests. At the behest of various professions, more than 130 state laws were written to regulate conduct in 14 separate health care occupations between 1910 and 1920 [27]. Today, there seems to be an endless number of special licensing statutes. In California alone more than 25 separate health care licenses are now recognized [18]. Few of these occupations involve conduct that places the patient-consumer at any significant risk. Clearly, the regulatory system has evolved far beyond the goal of protecting the public from physical harm at the hands of quacks.

The Case Against Licensing

The incredible web of occupational licensing laws has been subjected to searching, severe criticism since the late 1950s. Professor Walter Gellhorn first argued that the licensing boards had not only proliferated unnecessarily but that the top-heavy, moribund bureaucracy had been co-opted to serve as a bottleneck on entry into the professions while doing little to monitor the performance of licensees. He advocated a single, well-financed health occupation licensing board that would be composed of professionals and laymen [29].

During the 1960s conservative economists sharply criticized state licensing schemes. Milton Friedman, who offered the most vigorous attack, characterized licensure as a return to the medieval guild system in which economic power was concentrated in the hands of few. He felt that the "paternalistic" arguments offered to justify licensing could not make up for the erosion of the right of the individual to enter into voluntary contracts which such a system caused. Medical licensure especially troubled him [30]:

> I am myself persuaded that licensure has reduced both the quantity and quality of medical practice; that it has reduced the opportunities available to people who would like to be physicians, forcing them to pursue occupations they regard as less attractive; that it has forced the public to pay more for less satisfactory medical service; and that it has retarded technological development both in medicine itself and in the organization of medical practice. I conclude that licensure should be eliminated as a requirement of the practice of medicine.

Recently, less conservative economists have also begun to criticize occupational licensing. Alex Maurizi, of the United States Department of Labor, surveyed the admission statistics of selected licensing boards between 1940 and 1950. Asking whether rising consumer demand for certain services could be correlated with changes in the rate of entry into occupations, he found that as demand increased, admission frequencies declined. To Maurizi, this meant "the power of licensing boards is often used to prolong the period of higher incomes resulting from increases in excess demand for the services of the occupation in question and that the instrument then used to accomplish this purpose is alteration of the pass rate in the licensing examination [31].

The American Medical Association (AMA) began making sporadic criticism of state licensing boards as early as 1960. Agreeing in part with Professor Gellhorn, the AMA found that boards were not adequately monitoring the conduct of physicians. But more fundamentally, the AMA objected to the ever larger involvement of the state in medical practice that is inherent in licensing, particularly when it is vigorously pursued. An editorial in the *Journal of the American Medical Association* in 1969 warned that "increased governmental regulation of health occupations related to physician services would tend to freeze existing classes of personnel into current standards and lead to unnecessary multiplication of officially recognized classes of workers" [32] .

Today, a vast majority of those who have studied the question favor a moratorium on licensure of new health occupations. Among those groups that have called for a halt are the AMA Council on Health Manpower, the American Hospital Association, and the National Advisory Commission on Health Manpower [33] . Most legal writers agree with health professionals that licensing schemes, as they are currently operated, retard innovations in manpower usage (especially delegation of tasks) and the overall dissemination of medical care [34] .

Modern Variations on Licensure

Despite cogent arguments against licensing, new laws continue to be enacted. For example, during the early 1970s many states decided to recognize and license "physician assistants." The idea of the physician assistant was developed more than a decade ago as a proposed solution to the doctor shortage. Proponents hoped that platoons of assistants could be trained to perform the more mechanical aspects of medical care. An assistant would work under the supervision of a doctor, although not necessarily in his presence. It was thought that the great number of corpsmen returning from Vietnam and the large number of persons rejected by medical schools would provide a ready pool of assistants.

The evolution of the physician assistant laws illustrates the inertial force of the licensing system [35] . At first a few states passed "delegation amendments." These were intended to clarify the right of doctors to delegate the performance of certain tasks to persons not specifically trained in medicine or nursing (in fact physicians have always had this option, as well as the corresponding responsibility for the errors of their employees). Although the new laws did not diminish the scope of the physician's liability, they seemed to make doctors more willing to delegate. The "delegation amendments" had two important effects: first, they diminished the already small risk that an assistant might be prosecuted for practicing medicine without a license [36] . Second, the laws offered a new channel of entry into auxiliary health care occupations. More formal legislation soon followed. The term "physician assistant" first appeared in an Oklahoma law in 1967. By 1971 the term had been locked into statutory solutions to the health manpower problem. In that year laws recognizing and licensing "physician assistants" were enacted in 12 states. A doctor could still delegate duties, but obvious pressures demanded that the delegation be to licensed assistants.

Fortunately, advocates of reform had some influence on the development of licensing laws for physician assistants. Most of the 37 states which adopted such laws chose to require that the physician assistant complete an "approved training program." Since training programs have a vested interest in a large student population, licensure of schools is less likely to permit special interest groups from holding down the number of persons joining the occupation each year. Moreover, most states retained a broad definition of the scope of activity delegable to a physician assistant.

Of course such statutes and their corresponding regulations are constantly subject to attack by professional groups that perceive them to pose an economic threat. For example in 1977 organizations representing physicians and nurses led a major drive to revise the New York rules to rescind the right of physician assistants to prescribe medication [37] . Similarly, for the past few years a battle has raged in Wisconsin over whether third party payments for psychotherapy should be limited to counseling provided by psychiatrists or should continue to include psychologists and other nonphysicians [38] . Such events suggest that advocates of reform in the licensing of health professionals have had little impact on the traditional use of such laws to protect the economic power of the entrenched groups.

HOW SHOULD GENETIC COUNSELORS BE REGULATED?

The major argument against the use of state licensure laws to regulate genetic counselors is the obvious failure of similar laws to control the quality of practice in other health care occupations. Political scientists [39] , lawyers [34] , health care administrators [40] , and physicians [32] who have studied the question agree that licensure does not guarantee meaningful quality control. Yet, even if one posits a reformed, efficient, and equitable licensing system, other factors argue against the choice of this regulatory route.

Although the number of people who are employed as genetic counselors will probably increase greatly during the next decade, it will eventually reach a plateau that is not very high. The advent of a system of nationalized health care may stimulate the propagation of genetic counseling services since it is reasonable to expect that widespread counseling would help to reduce the number of children born with incurable genetic disease. Nevertheless, it is difficult to imagine that in a society of 230,000,000 people with a static birthrate there will be a demand for more than 5,000 full-time "follow-up" (nonphysician) counselors. Assuming that trained counselors practice their profession for at least a decade, once the plateau is reached the annual replacement demand should rarely exceed a few hundred persons. Thus, the problem of monitoring the quality of persons wishing to enter the profession in no sense compares to the difficulties involved in regulating the entry of 15,000 physicians into the medical profession each year. The number of genetic counselors whose knowledge and abilities must be tested in advance is sufficiently small to dilute the classic argument in favor of licensure. I see little value in writing special laws and setting up special administrative units in states where as few as ten persons may apply for genetic counseling licenses each year. There is a less complicated way to protect the public which is already in effect.

The bulk of formal genetic counseling will continue to be offered by "groups" operating out of genetic clinics. Most persons burdened with genetic disease will in fact receive diagnostic information and make therapeutic decisions in consultation with physicians. It is possible that follow-up counselors could occasionally mislead persons about therapeutic alternatives, but such events should be rare. The traditional practice of periodic review of difficult cases by the entire counseling team provides the best insurance against injury to the counselee.

Eventually certain functions performed by the human genetics clinic will be subject to federal regulation. Since 1967 when the "Clinical Laboratories Improvement Act" became law [41], the federal agency charged with its implementation (the Center for Disease Control) has gradually extended the scope of its monitoring. In 1973 officials from CDC, working in cooperation with representatives of the American Society of Human Genetics, began to develop standards for some of the diagnostic activities of human cytogenetics laboratories. Although the federal government is notorious for its failure to provide funds for adequate inspection teams, the publication of regulations for cytogenetics laboratories will no doubt influence practices in some laboratories. The development of rules for certain technical aspects of genetic diagnosis such as the number of amniocentesis cell cultures permitted per volume of incubator space is easily managed. Similar rules cannot be written to guide the subjective nature of genetic counseling.

Further, there are few real benefits to be gained by nonphysician counselors from a licensing law. Their occupational ceiling will remain substantially below that of the medical geneticists with whom they work. Although licensure creates the possibility that the nonphysician counselor could practice independently, such an enterprising person would probably have little chance of success. The layman with a health problem wishes to visit a physician. The independent counselor would depend greatly on referrals and it is unlikely that many physicians would send patients to such an individual rather than to a genetics clinic operating out of a large hospital in a nearby city. Finally, it is highly unlikely that counselors could use licensure to prohibit physicians from providing primary counseling services to their patients. The licensed physician has traditionally been permitted to stray into all health care fields.

There is one major alternative to the licensing route. Experienced genetic counselors (medical geneticists, persons with a doctoral degree in genetics, and other counselors) could attempt to control the development of the profession by a system of certification and accreditation. A policy of hiring only diplomates of accredited schools (that is, institutions with programs approved by the

American Society of Human Genetics or some similar group) would greatly influence the development of the genetic counseling profession.

I see little chance that such a policy will be formally adopted. The job prospects of graduates of genetic counseling programs are too uncertain and the demand too small to stimulate a significant number of universities to develop master's degrees in this field. In reality local demand for follow-up counselors is unpredictable and ad hoc. It is as much a function of good fortune with a grant application or a strong interest on the part of a medical school dean as anything else.

But even if a system of certification does evolve I doubt that it can promise graduates of special competence. First, it is against the best interests of colleges to flunk students. Second, the requirement of advanced training reduces the number of potential counselors. Further, it is contrary to the experience of many medical geneticists who know that with minimal training, health professionals without previous knowledge of genetics can readily learn to offer counseling services.

So long as the bulk of counseling is offered by highly trained "genetic groups" in medical research facilities, a regulatory scheme ought not be imposed. The members of the counseling team are in the best position to judge the kind of person whom they wish to join the group. There is no evidence that unlicensed counselors are offering their services to the public in a manner that raises a specter of serious harm to laymen. It is possible that the failure to secure licensing laws could injure the development of graduate training programs for "genetic associates." It is more likely that the associate's degree would continue to provide an important advantage in the search for employment. Should evidence emerge that indicates that the public would benefit from a formal system of regulation, I would advocate the development of a system of certification with two separate tracks. Persons should be given the alternatives of completing an academic program or getting training on the job. Formal degree requirements should not be made absolute.

REFERENCES

1. Galton L: Prenatal tests help cure defects and save babies. Parade, Apr 11, 1974, pp 10–12.
2. Bylinsky G: What science can do about hereditary diseases. Fortune, Sept, 1974, pp 148–160.
3. Childs B, Gordis L, Kaback MM, Kazazian HH: Tay-Sachs screening: Social and psychological impact. Am J Hum Genet 28:550–558, 1976.
4. Chamberlain N: A workable approach to testing. In Sinnette CH, Smith JA (eds): "Legislative and Socio-Economic Aspects of Sickle Cell Disease." New York: Harlem Hospital Center — Columbia University, 1973, pp 45–53.

5. Marks JH, Richter ML: The genetic associate: A new health professional. Am J Public Health 66:388–390, 1976.
6. Shaw MW: Review of published studies of genetic counseling: A critique. In de la Cruz F, Lubs HA (eds): "Genetic Counseling." New York: Raven Press, 1977, pp 35–49.
7. Reismann LE, Matheny AP: "Genetics and Counseling in Medical Practice." St. Louis: C V Mosby, 1969, pp 26–38.
8. Ad Hoc Committee on Genetic Counseling: Genetic counseling. Am J Hum Genet 27: 240, 1975.
9. Hecht F, Holmes LB: What we don't know about genetic counseling. N Engl J Med 287:464, 1972.
10. Fraser FC: Genetic counseling. Am J Hum Genet 26:636–659, 1974.
11. Bullough B: The law and the expanding nursing role. Am J Public Health 66:249–254, 1976.
12. California Business and Professions Code Section 2510 et seq. (West, 1973).
13. Epstein CJ: Who should do genetic counseling, and under what circumstances? In Bergsma D (ed): "Contemporary Genetic Counseling." White Plains: The National Foundation, BD:OAS IX(4):39–48, 1973.
14. Leff A: Medical devices and paramedical personnel: A preliminary context for emerging problems. Washington U.L. Quarterly 1967:332–399, 1967.
15. Reilly PR: State supported mass genetic screening. In Milunsky A, Annas G (eds): "Genetics and the Law." New York: Plenum Press, 1976, pp 359–376.
16. "National Sickle Cell Anemia Control Act." Pub. L. No. 92–294, 86 Stat 136.
17. "National Sickle Cell Anemia, Cooley's Anemia, Tay-Sachs and Genetic Diseases Act." Pub. L. No. 94–278, 90 Stat 407 et seq.
18. General Statutes of North Carolina 143B-196 (1973 Supp).
19. Kentucky Revised Statutes 402.330 (1972).
20. Annotated Laws of Massachusetts Ch. 76, Section 15B (1974 Supp).
21. Annotated Code of Maryland Art 43, Section 814 et seq (1973 Cum Supp).
22. Lustig L, Poskanzer L: Genetic associates. N Engl J Med 295:1436, 1976.
23. Moore JE: The purpose of licensing. J of Law and Economics 4:93–117, 1961.
24. Shryock RH: "Medical Licensing in America: 1650–1965." Baltimore: Johns Hopkins Press, 1967.
25. Dent v. West Virginia 129 U.S. 114 (1889).
26. See, for example, Iowa Eclectic Medical College Ass'n. v. Schrader, 87 Iowa 659, 55 N.W. 24 (1893).
27. Pennell MY, Stewart PA: State licensing of health occupations. Monograph published by the National Center for Health Statistics, Washington, D.C. Public Health Service (No. 1758), 1968.
28. See generally California Business and Professions Code, Section 500 et seq. (West, 1974).
29. Gellhorn W: "Individual Freedom and Governmental Restraints." Baton Rouge: Louisiana State University Press, 1956.
30. Freidman M: Occupational licensure. In "Capitalism and Freedom." Chicago: University of Chicago Press, 1962, p 158. See also: A pitch for 'caveat emptor' medicine. Medical World News, Mar 8, 1976, p 32.
31. Maurizi A: Occupational licensing and the public interest. J Pol Econ 82:399–413, 1974.
32. Editorial: Licensure of health occupations. JAMA 208:640, 1969.
33. Forgotson E, Cook J: Innovations and experiments in uses of health manpower – The effect of licensure laws. Law and Contemporary Problems 32:731–750, 1967.

34. Gellhorn W: The abuse of occupational licensing. The Univ of Chicago L Rev 44:6–27, 1976.
35. Kissam PC: Physician assistant and nurse practitioner laws: A study of health law reform. Kansas Law Review 24:1–65, 1975.
36. Magit v. Board of Medical Examiners 57 Cal. 2d. 74, 366 P. 2d. 816 (1961).
37. Meislin RJ: Physicians' assistants face loss of right to prescribe medication. New York Times, Feb 20, 1977, p 17.
38. McDonald MC: The medical psychotherapy dispute. Psychiatric News, May 7, 1976, p 1.
39. Holmer R: The role and functioning of state licensing agencies. State Gov't 40:34–45, 1967.
40. Shimberg B, Esser B, Kruger D: "Occupational Licensing: Practices and Policies." Washington: Public Affairs Press, 1973.
41. "Clinical Laboratories Improvement Act Of 1967." Pub. L. No. 90-174, 58 Stat 702.

19. Autonomy, Confidentiality, and Quality Care in Genetic Counseling

Alexander M. Capron, LLB

Like any new area, genetic counseling has raised a host of problems, many of which are addressed in this volume. Some of these present difficult ethical dilemmas, others pose novel points for public policy debate, and still others raise questions of technique and biomedical knowledge for practitioners in the new field. It is therefore not surprising that genetic counseling is thought to require special attention from the law — that there might be, in other words, a "law of genetic counseling" which addresses many "serious if not altogether unique, legal problems" [1]. Yet on closer inspection the legal issues involved in genetic counseling are fairly straightforward. Some novel issues may be raised, and some points may remain unresolved. For the most part, however, the issues of legal liability for genetic counselors will reflect the main body of the law of professional practice and malpractice.

I. FRAMING THE ISSUES

The general concern of the law in the area of genetic counseling as elsewhere will be to minimize the harm the activity causes while maximizing the benefits it confers. Society accomplishes this in a number of ways. First, it attempts through the subsidization and accreditation of educational programs for future health professionals to reduce the dangers of incompetent or uninformed practitioners. Similarly, professionals must pass certain tests and become licensed before engaging in practice, and the movement toward continuing education (particularly important in new fields like genetics) and relicensure is growing. Human genetics is receiving increasing attention in medical school research and teaching, and proposals for specialized licensing have been made. Philip Reilly's chapter treats these concerns.

Birth Defects: Original Article Series, Volume XV, Number 2, pages 307–340
© 1979 The National Foundation

Further prospective steps to diminish risks include governmental regulation of facilities providing health care services, such as the inspection and certification of hospitals and laboratories. The provision of safe, effective care is also encouraged by the support which the legal system gives to peer review by holding practitioners to standards determined by the professional community itself and by upholding professional censure.

After an injury has occurred, the legal system is primarily concerned with redressing the damage through the law of malpractice, the branch of tort law involving civil remedies for the wrongful acts of persons practicing a profession. The avoidance of future injuries is also encouraged by the suspension or revocation of the licenses of those shown to have deviated in a gross fashion from professional standards and by the deterrent effect an adverse judgment is expected to have, specifically on the conduct of the defendant and generally on the conduct of his or her peers. (The effectiveness of tort law in achieving its wider objectives is much debated; one would not expect genetic counseling to be unusual in this regard, one way or the other.)

All of these standard prospective and retrospective concerns of the law can be expected to manifest themselves in the practice of genetic counseling. Indeed, one of the most interesting questions for a lawyer examining genetic counseling is whether a distinct field exists. The assumption in this article will be that genetic counseling is comparable to the practice of medicine; that is, as a general matter, the legal issues raised will be framed in terms of the law of medical malpractice, including the principles of contract and battery as well as of negligence. Nonetheless, the first point which must be addressed here concerns the problems raised by that assumption. These problems are of two sorts: First, whether the relationship of physician to patient accurately characterizes the field of genetic counseling, and second, whether a single such "field" exists, as part of medicine or otherwise. The conclusions reached lead to the use in this chapter primarily of the terms "counselee" and "counselor"; the occasional use of such terms as "patient" and "physician" to reflect clinical realities, particularly in circumstances requiring physical diagnosis and treatment, is not intended to convey any substantive legal difference. Further, while our initial exploration of the "practice" of genetic counseling reveals practical as well as legal problems in regarding it as a unified field, strong reasons favoring such a view exist and seem also to point to the conclusion that medical jurisprudence will be the major reference point for the resolution of the problems which arise.

Despite the alleged "crisis" in medical malpractice litigation, the law in this field is not greatly disputed. Of course, some matters of medicolegal concern are unlikely to arise in the genetic counseling context, for example, abandonment of the patient, unauthorized autopsies, failure to report child abuse, or determination of the time of a patient's death. Most standard medicolegal concerns will nevertheless be pertinent to genetic counseling. Furthermore, certain unusal aspects of genetics and the involvement of persons not trained in medicine enlarge the confines of the field and present legal issues beyond those applicable to medical practice.

II. DEFINITION OF THE FIELD

The suggested analogy of genetic counseling to the practice of medicine rests on several factors, most importantly that the knowledge base on which counseling proceeds has largely (though far from exclusively) been developed by physicians and that most counseling takes place at genetics centers within medical institutions. This ought not, however, lead automatically to the conclusion that those receiving counseling are "patients" nor that those dispensing it are "physicians."

A. The Status of Counselees

The term "client" is sometimes used to describe a counselee [2], apparently with the intent to differentiate such a person from one denominated a "patient." The latter term may carry rich and diverse connotations, but as a part of the legally defined relationship of doctor *and patient,* it is merely a particular way of saying "client," that is, one who employs the services of a professional. Using the word "patient" does not justify *in law* treating a person as an infantile nondecision-maker, just as using the word "client" does not assure *in reality* that a person will be free from feelings of dependence (as psychotherapists have discovered from their efforts to substitute "client" for "patient" terminology).

As is developed more fully in what follows, the operative legal principle is that the professional owes the person relying on his or her services duties of fidelity, of full disclosure, and of such care as is exercised by a prudent person possessing the expert skill and knowledge relevant to the field. To the extent that physicians (or others) employ a concept of "patient" that would replace these duties with a notion of professional dominance [3] in the relationship between those supplying and those receiving genetic counseling, they expose themselves to liability. It is interesting, moreover, to note that such a counseling posture transgresses not only the law's expectations about the professional-client relationship but also the norms articulated by many of the leading professionals in the field. Sheldon Reed's pioneering description of the geneticist's role emphasized information-giving rather than active intervention in decisionmaking [4].

In recent years that position has faced dissent. The psychological aspects of genetic counseling, initially little considered or assumed to be within the competence of any practitioner, have been increasingly emphasized. The encouragement of an active interventionist stance for counselors may carry with it impetus to be "directive," whether they are unaware of this tendency or even state their conscious opposition to it [5]. Still other geneticists believe that the counselor's role includes helping counselees to make a "responsible adjustment" to their genetic status [6].

While it is possible to detect similar normative drives in the guidance of those, like Reed, who emphasize the educative function of genetic counseling, it is apparent that in a number of ways a single dominant professional norm has yet to emerge. This leads us, then, to the second problem of "defining" this field, especially as that definition begins from the assumption that genetic counseling is comparable, for purposes of the law, to the practice of medicine.

B. Professional Standards

Genetic counseling is still a relatively young field. In the absence of any form of licensure or certification, people with a wide variety of backgrounds and orientations toward treatment can legitimately hold themselves out as genetic counselors. This diversity is inevitable in a new discipline and moreover is probably something to be applauded rather than criticized. But diversity can create difficulties for people involved in the legal process, because of the confusion it creates concerning the professional standards governing counselors' conduct.

Suppose that a couple sues a genetic counselor for malpractice alleging negligent counseling. Assuming for the moment that there is no difficulty in showing that the defendant's conduct caused the plaintiffs measurable harm, the primary issue will be whether the defendant deviated from the due care that can be expected from genetic counselors. Since the standard of care in genetic counseling is not something which is familiar to the average layperson, the plaintiffs will be required to establish the standard through expert testimony [7]. Any expert called to testify for either side must have such skill and knowledge in the field that his or her opinion would rest on a substantial foundation and would tend to aid the trier of fact in its search for truth [8]. A witness' expertise may, nonetheless, be acquired solely by practical experience rather than professional education; this aspect of the rule is especially important in a new field, such as human genetics [9].

The actual application of these rules to the field of genetics is complicated by the very question of whether one is speaking of a single, identifiable field. Does a single standard apply to all who practice genetic counseling regardless of their professional training? Generally, each professional group or subgroup is held to its own standards: physicians are not judged by nursing standards nor vice versa because differences in training and skills would make cross-professional judgments unreliable. Since a nurse is not taught to behave like a doctor, it would be unfair to penalize her when she did not do what a doctor is expected to do. Consequently, if nurses, social workers, physicians from different specialities (pediatrics, obstetrics, psychiatry, and internal medicine), and others engaged in genetics counseling in fact perform different functions according to different types of training, then each would be governed by the expectations of his or her subgroup of genetic counselors: nurse-counselors, obstetrician-counselors, and so forth. Although in a negligence suit a person from another subgroup might be qualified as an expert to testify on the proper standard of conduct for a person in the defendant's subgroup, the trial judge would have to be satisfied that the expert is knowledgeable about the norms of the *defendant's* subgroup and the expert would have to confine his or her testimony to that subgroup [10] . Conversely, if genetic counselors from differing professional backgrounds perform interchangeable functions, then there would be no basis — at least as to those functions — to treat them as belonging to separate subgroups. Anyone who attempted to perform those functions may be expected to know the proper means of doing so and will be held responsible for harm caused by lapses from the norms of genetic counseling.

The application of a single standard to everyone in the field seems sensible for a number of reasons. First, it probably best reflects reality. A person with a master's degree from a specialized graduate program in genetic counseling can be expected to counsel a couple with a Down syndrome baby in the same fashion as a person with training in pediatrics. If the service offered the counselee requires skills or knowledge that either type of counselor does not possess, such a counselor should not attempt to offer the counseling alone without the inclusion of other persons having the necessary skills.

Second, one usual reason for applying separate standards — meaning, in effect, a lower standard for a defendant than a plaintiff would like to see applied — is frequently missing here. Someone who has chosen to be treated by a nonspecialist or a nonphysician cannot reasonably complain of injury because the person providing the care did not meet the higher standards of physicians or specialists or so forth [11] . (It may, of course, be that some things once expected only of the specialist are now expected of the competent nonspecialist or nonphysician, but that does not amount to the ad hoc application of a standard higher than that expected of the defendant's peers.) In most instances the recipient of genetic counseling will have contacted the genetics clinic at a medical center, either through self- or physician-referral. The clinic staff member or members who provide counseling will be determined by the people running the clinic. Since it would be highly inefficient if each person has to be seen and counseled by the most highly trained physician on the staff, someone who accepts counseling from a nonphysician can expect that, whatever the applicable requirements for the type of counseling provided, the counselor meets them. Of course, someone who sought genetic counseling from a nonspecialist — for example, a general practitioner — cannot complain if that person did not measure up to the knowledge and skills of a genetic counseling specialist, provided, of course, that the nonspecialist was not negligent in failing to refer the patient to a specialist because the problem was one which he or she should have known was beyond his or her competence [12] .

Finally, a single standard for all genetic counselors providing the same category of services is appropriate because it will promote society's desire, as expressed in tort law, to see victims compensated. The reason to have separate standards is to go easy on those who are less proficient, but in doing so one deprives some injured people of compensation. Since the use of liability insurance funds allows the burden of compensation to be spread over the entire class of consumers of the service (rather than being borne solely by either plaintiff or defendant), there is no unfairness to the counselor in holding him or her to a standard which may occasionally be higher than he or she expected. Furthermore, as has already been mentioned, the choice of which staff member does the counseling will typically be determined by routine clinic policy or by the persons running the genetic service; since the insurance policy will cover all staff of the clinic, it is appropriate that the insurer bear the cost of an injury that resulted from the assigned counselor being unable to carry out the task properly.

The differences in genetic counseling are not limited to, or defined primarily by, differences in counselors' professional backgrounds, however. A variety of opinions exists, as chapters in this book demonstrate, on the true ends of counseling and hence on the means that may properly be adopted in pursuit of those ends. These differences concern matters that are not likely soon to be settled by scientific evidence (as was the need for sanitary precautions in surgery). Indeed, since the differences are largely reflective of divers philosophical presuppositions they are not subject to proof one way or the other.

The disagreements existing in the field could be of great significance to the defendant in our hypothetical malpractice action. Suppose that the claimed fault of the counselor was failure to take account of the counselees' anxiety, guilt, and ambivalent feelings, because the counselor follows the school of thought that genetic counseling is solely an information-giving process; and suppose that the counselees claim damage both from their emotional suffering and consequent marital discord and from the harm that arose from the decisions about reproduction, which they made because of their confused and anxious mental condition. The defendant counselor will then most certainly object if the counselees attempt to prove negligence through the expert testimony of a genetic counselor who believes that the primary function of counseling is to overcome the counselees' anxiety, assuage their guilty feelings, and resolve their ambivalent ones.

The objection of the defendant would be that the proposed line of testimony comes from a different "school" of genetic counseling than the one to which he adheres. Usually, a physician (or other professional) who abides by one school of thought is judged by the standards of that school and the testimony of someone from another school is inadmissible, unless, of course, the proposed witness is expert in the standards of the defendant's school as well as his own and confines himself to the former standards [13] . In order to enjoy this testimonial protection, the defendant's school must have the support of a considerable body of competent medical opinion. The traditional concern of the law has been to prevent quackery from insulating itself from outside scrutiny; accordingly, a school must be grounded in sound scientific principles, attested to by professional expert witnesses

[14] . The precedents in this area are of only marginal relevance to genetic counseling. They involve, for example, whether Chinese herb doctors constitute a school of medicine (they do not, and hence the testimony of a conventional physician was admissible to establish the relevant standard of care) [15] . Genetic counselors are very likely to be operating generally within the bounds of the health care professions, although it is not unimaginable that someone lacking any biomedical credentials would claim to be a "genetic counselor."

Today the major question about "schools of thought" rules on testimony is whether two or more alleged schools really are separate. The recognition of separate schools depends upon there being an identity of practice by people within the school and a distinction between the behavior of those people and ones outside the school [16] . Furthermore, it is necessary for the defendant's distinctive procedures to be ones that more than just "some" practitioners follow; they must be supported by at least a "respectable minority" within the professional group, if the judge is going to direct a verdict for the defendant rather than leave the question in the hands of the jury based upon the conflicting testimony of the proponents of the two opinions [17] .

The potential for conflict among the principles that guide various groups of genetic counselors is thus almost certain to pose difficult issues as litigation arises. Moreover, the uncertainty about proper professional standards for this emerging field may itself have an interesting impact on the development of those standards. Although it is generally true that the legal system is a check on any activity, calling it to account for its "progress" (or lack thereof) and passing on the "standards" by which it is guided, the professions have traditionally been given special deference. To an unusual degree — explained though not fully justified by their esoteric subject matter, the inherent imperfections of their efforts, and a social desire to promote their development [18] — the professions have been allowed to set their own pace and judge their own performance. Formally, the law on this subject has changed little, but in actual practice the increased frequency with which professionals have been called to account for their actions amounts to a substantive change (even though the overwhelming majority of such lawsuits are decided in the professional's favor).

The increase in scrutiny is especially important for a somewhat inchoate field like genetic counseling. In effect, it must grow up in public. Its development of goals and norms will not result solely (or perhaps ever primarily) from a slow process in medical schools and other training programs or in professional associations. Instead, that process is certain to be shaped by the need, which will arise in the context of individual litigation, to define its contours as a professional discipline and to determine whether a variety of practices — which might well be tolerable for members of a vaguely defined "field" with diverse professional antecedents and traditions — is acceptable or constitute "malpractice." Moreover, to the extent that differences in practices follow preexisting disciplinary lines, there will probably be a tendency for the field as a whole to embrace the views of the professional constituencies with the greatest prestige (namely, physicians and secondarily, nurses) to lend legitimacy to the practices adopted.

The influence of the legal process on the formation of practices in genetic counseling is likely to be further increased by the nature of the questions that are likely to divide differing "schools" of thought. The techniques at issue are not likely to be the biologically sophisticated ones (eg whether a particular method for staining chromosomes is proper for the type of karyotype analysis desired). Rather, the issues are likely to revolve around matters of information conveyance (eg whether the defendant used the proper technique to inform the plaintiff about the risks of having a child with Tay-Sachs disease). Such matters might be seen as involving expert judgment but they are just as likely to be seen by many courts as issues which laypersons can legitimately decide. Thus, the effect of outside scrutiny on the development of standards for genetic counseling will probably be more pronounced than would be the case were surgery now in its infancy.

Our examination of professional standards points to two conclusions. First, genetic counseling will probably come to be regarded as a field with defined standards comparable to those that prevail under the law of medical malpractice, without its practice being limited to physicians. Within the field, everyone legitimately undertaking a particular function will be judged by the same standard of due care. Second, to the extent that different philosophies divide genetic counselors, the law is unlikely to give such divisions decisive weight. Instead, the process of judicial scrutiny will accelerate the development of standards of practice and may even shape aspects (particularly nonbiologic ones) of those standards.

III. STAGES OF COUNSELING

A. Diagnosis

Before genetic counseling can take place — and usually before the need for such counseling will be perceived — an accurate diagnosis of the condition in question is necessary. This will typically arise in the context of either treatment of affected individuals or reproductive counseling. In the former, the initial diagnosis is likely to be made by someone other than a geneticist, although the medical geneticist may, in the exercise of due care, be obliged to perform further clinical or laboratory tests to confirm or refine the initial diagnosis. On the other hand, a geneticist not trained in medicine could offer counseling based upon a diagnosis given by a physician who had previously examined the patient, but it would violate both ordinary expectations of due care and customary state statutes for a person not licensed as a physician to diagnose the patient's medical status.

The steps involved in diagnosis create many opportunities for legal concern. First the physician must understand enough about the patient's apparent condition to obtain proper clinical and laboratory tests and to gather relevant facts through a medical, and perhaps a family, history. This involves as much as the need to discern the correct tests as to perform them properly. Moreover, small differences in diagnostic results may be crucial in determining what condition is involved and in recognizing whether it is classified as a "genetic disorder." If harm occurs because a practitioner reasonably relies on tests negligently conducted by an independent laboratory, he or she would not be liable [19]. Suit should be brought against the laboratory itself, unless, of course, the practitioner was negligent in the choice of laboratory or in failing to detect the error.

For the nonspecialist the question may be one of clinical acumen to recognize the need for any tests whatsoever. In this regard the physician will be held to the standards of due care defined by his own professional group, and not by the subspecialty of genetic counseling. For example, a pediatrician confronted with a child with progressive mental retardation may be expected to consider diagnostic tests for phenylketonuria (PKU), a disease with a genetic pattern of causation. The diagnosis of PKU depends upon the expertise of pediatricians in recognizing symptoms and employing the appropriate metabolic tests, which are not in themselves genetic [20]. Once a condition has been recognized its treatment may similarly not involve anything that specifically requires the knowledge of a genetic counselor, as for example the dietary therapy for PKU, although there may be certain types of treatment, as well as specialized diagnoses, which do presume such expert knowledge. In the latter cases the duty of the nonspecialist is limited to recognizing the need for the patient to consult with a geneticist.

The second context in which a diagnosis will lead to genetic counseling is the medical care of people contemplating reproduction. Counseling about genetic risks in reproduction has traditionally occurred largely as a result of the birth to couples of children with genetic disorders. The issues here are the ones already surveyed — completion of necessary tests and histories, accuracy in the acquisition and analysis of data, and reasonable use of the information obtained. But reproductive genetic counseling now increasingly involves diagnosis of a different type, namely predictive "diagnosis" based upon risk factors rather than upon the appearance of a proband in the family. The development of more sophisticated biochemical and cytogenetic tests constantly increases the importance of this aspect of medical genetics for physicians generally. For example, the availability of a carrier detection test for Tay-Sachs disease and of prenatal diagnosis makes it possible to offer advance counseling and accurate diagnosis of fetal status to couples of Ashkenazic Jewish extraction to whom previously only statistical risks could be conveyed. The failure of an obstetrician to perform a carrier test for Tay-Sachs has already been alleged as the basis for liability in at least one lawsuit [21]. The speed with which new diagnostic capabilities developed by genetic specialists are absorbed into physicians' routine practice is largely a matter within the hands of practitioners themselves. The existence of a group of knowledgeable specialists creates pressure for more rapid adoption, as does the increased awareness of medical consumers about genetics and available diagnostic procedures. For example, the lay press' coverage of amniocentesis for pregnancies at risk for chromosomal aberrations because of advanced maternal age has generated more use of the technique than would have occurred had it remained a matter of esoteric medical knowledge.

Reproductive counseling, whether by a genetic counselor, an obstetrician, or a general medical practitioner, raises some difficult issues of potential damages and their measurement. Those issues that depend upon the birth of a defective child because of a failure to warn of the risks of the defect are treated more fully below [22]. Harm of the opposite sort may also occur if inaccurate advice is given, leading to unnecessary protective steps, such as abortion or sterlization; liability may also be imposed if the couple is counseled into unnecessary contraception, artificial insemination, or adoption, although these steps would be less likely to give rise to substantial irreversible harm. Moreover, in addition to its inappropriate use, a procedure might be carried out negligently or without sufficient warnings and consent. Judgment for the plantiff in such a case would depend upon proof that the revelant standard of care had been breached and had given rise to measurable damages, including the emotional trauma of an unnecessary procedure.

B. Treatment

As in other health fields, genetic counseling diagnosis may be followed by treatment. In some instances, treatment involves conventional medical or surgical procedures, such as a special diet for a patient with an autosomal recessive condition like galactosemia, or the removal of a tumor for a patient with retinoblastoma, a dominant disorder. But more commonly the "treatment" associated with genetic counseling will consist of advice about the expected course of the disorder and about methods for preventing its recurrence in future offspring.

The quality of the communication between the treaters and the treated doubtless plays an important, if largely undocumented, part in all health care. What passes, for instance, between a surgeon and a patient may well influence the outcome of surgery in some unknown fashion or provide the basis for informed or uninformed consent. But the efficacy of surgery is never measured in such terms. By contrast, the nature and purpose of the communication is a vital aspect of genetic counseling. Although opinion is not unanimous on the propriety of measuring counseling efficacy by the quality of the communication involved, it is widely held that this provides a better measure than the alternatives, such as measuring counselees' compliance with counselors' recommendations or deciding whether the choices made by counselees were "correct" (since in both cases it is difficult to know whether any particular choice of either counselor or counselee is the "right" one to make or to be followed).

Some aspects of the counselor—counselee communication are not difficult to evaluate, namely the information presented by the counselor. A medical counselor will be expected to supply an accurate diagnosis (or, when necessary, a tentative one, with whatever qualifiers are needed to explain the uncertainty), an explanation of the hereditary basis, if any is known for the condition in question, and the range of available therapeutic options, preventive measures, and further diagnostic procedures. A genetic counselor would not be expected, any more than other medical practitioners, to supply error-free explanations. The field is too new and the knowledge involved is far too incomplete and esoteric for a mistake to bespeak negligence in and of itself. Consequently, a counselee suing a genetic counselor must produce expert testimony that the counselor's information fell below that which would have been supplied by a prudent and knowledgeable practitioner in the field [23]. The doctrine of res ipsa loquitor allows a plaintiff to prove negligence from the occurrence of an event which does not usually happen absent negligence [24]. But the rule is not available in situations that require one to possess special expertise to know whether a bad result bespeaks negligence. Therefore, a plaintiff—counselee's case would be dismissed if testimony on the counselor's malpractice was not given by the counselor's peers, because the field is not one with which ordinary people are sufficiently familiar.

In areas outside of the medical profession, courts have established the minimum standards of due care so as not to permit an industry to set its standards too low [25]. This rule has been applied to medical practice in only one case, Helling vs Carey [26], a 1970 Washington Supreme Court case. This case may have particular relevance for genetics if and when certain tests become so safe, inexpensive, and routine that failure of a practitioner to employ them would be inexcusable, even if the practitioner's professional peers rarely used such tests.

As important as the accuracy of the information may be, it is only part of the counseling function and not the most difficult from a legal vantage point. Two other important aspects are: a) The extent that good counseling depends on the manner in which the information is conveyed to the counselees; and b) the obligations, if any, of the counselor beyond the obligation to convey accurate information.

A correct statement of "the facts" about a genetic condition may mean nothing to a layperson, although a fellow counselor would find it pellucid. At a minimum, the function of genetic counseling is to inform patients about genetically based conditions and risks, so counseling that fails to be informative would seem to be inadequate counseling.

There are two legal approaches to this inadequacy. First, the manner in which information is conveyed could be judged by the standards established by genetic counselors themselves. This would represent an application of the traditional malpractice formula to a novel area. It assumes that the profession has developed procedures and criteria for adequate counseling such that counselors will have some way of knowing whether they are measuring up to their peers' expectations or are behaving negligently or incompetently. Two questions arise from these assumptions: Is there a professional consensus — rather than diverse schools of thought — on the right way to counsel, and do genetic counselors have tools to evaluate whether they are counseling properly and achieving the results that should be expected? At the moment, the answer to both questions appears to be "no." This does not invalidate following usual malpractice rules but it at the least suggests that they should be applied with great caution.

The second way to approach the question of adequacy of genetic counseling methods would be through the developing law of informed consent. This doctrine is usually invoked in a suit against a physician when a patient alleges that surgical or medical procedures caused injuries to which the patient was not properly alerted and the risks of which the patient did not accept. Although no further physical manipulation of the counselee may occur after the genetic diagnosis is conveyed, the basic notion of the informed consent cases — to render the patient an informed decisionmaker able to participate in his or her own care [27] — would still apply. Moreover, even in a narrower sense informed consent may be deemed pertinent, since in most instances some physical intervention by the physician will follow counseling — for example, obstetrical care and examinations after the commencement of pregnancy. If the initial counseling was deficient, then all subsequent interventions by the counselor may be said to be based on invalid consent. And if the subject matter of the counseling was the reproductive decision to be made by a couple, then the man has as much of an interest in being adequately informed as does the woman, even if any subsequent physical interventions involve solely her person. The determination whether counseling provided sufficient information in a comprehensible fashion can be made by reference either to the traditional malpractice reference point — "what other physicians typically do" — or to a lay standard — "what a patient would want to know under the circumstances."

The latter standard has been gaining increasing recognition, spurred especially by three important legal decisions in 1972 [28]. The lay standard is particularly appropriate for genetic counseling. There appears to be no fixed professional standard to turn to as an alternative, and the conduct in question — the comprehensible conveying of information from one person to another — is not a matter of medical expertise but comes within common understanding and experience. Furthermore, the adequacy of the informing process will involve value questions that are more within the province of community standards of reasonableness than within the expertise of a clinical subspecialty [29]. Of course, the constraints of present genetic knowledge and available procedures place practical limits on the information that counselors can impart, but within such confines it seems proper for the counselor to aim at informing the counselees about everything the latter would find material for the decisions they have to make.

Beyond information-giving, some counselors (including R. Antley and S. Kessler in this volume) suggest that genetic counselors have larger responsibilities. The very term "counselor" and its usual context, which is one of reproduction and marriage, suggests concern for the psychological adjustment of the counselees to the information they have been told. If this is indeed the case, perhaps genetic counselors should be judged by the professional standards of psychiatrists, psychologists, and marriage counselors. This adds further significance to the legal rules concerning different professional schools of thought.

Suppose, for example, that a couple who have had a stillborn child come for genetic counseling. If the counselor knows that the woman is Rh-negative and has had previous spontaneous abortions early in pregnancy and that, in the absence of an autopsy, the records on the stillbirth note edema, he many conclude hydrops (based on heart failure secondary to severe anemia) and be prepared to advise the couple about the recurrence risk and preventive measures for fetal hemolytic disease. If questioning of the couple reveals that the father was shown the dead fetus which manifested other rare anomalies, the counselor must be prepared to rechart his course. Should the counselor's primary mission be to establish the condition responsible for the stillbirth? Or to reassure the couple if their own pediatrician has told them never to attempt to have children again? Or to confront the anxieties of the woman, who never was shown the dead fetus (a fact which she reiterates during the counseling session at various appropriate and inappropriate moments)? Should he let them known in advance that, even after further testing, there may be wide variations in the risk to which they are exposed — from near zero (if the condition was a mutation) to twenty-five percent (if the condition was recessive) to fifty percent (if the correct diagnosis is of a dominant disorder) — with no way to know for sure which risk figure is correct? Or, alternatively, should the counselor construct a "rough average" risk figure, in a fashion more appropriate to lay then to statistical reasoning, based on an educated guess about the probability that one diagnosis rather than another is correct, even though such an average figure makes no sense intellectually?

The initial resolution of such questions lies with genetics, not the law. That resolution will depend upon such underlying aspects of professional orientation as whether counselors take their task to be the treatment of a case of "X genetic disease" or a case of "parental anxiety following the birth of an affected child." But eventually, in cases in which harm is claimed to have arisen because of "mistakes" made by genetic counselors in just such situations, judges and juries will be called upon to resolve the propriety of the professional conduct. In most American jurisdictions today, the issue would probably be treated as one of professional expertise. But, as suggested previously, a good case can be made that a lay, rather than a professional, standard of information disclosure and conveyance is preferable, and this is likely to be the direction in which the law will move. Adopti a lay standard does not render the genetic counselor's professional judgment irrelevant, but it avoids dismissal of counselees' cases merely because they lack expert testimony. In effect, the lay standard compels the counselor at least to explain the reasons why information was or was not disclosed, why certain means of communication were used, and what, if anything, was done to ascertain whether the counselees understood and had some means of remembering (such as a follow-up letter) what the counselor had tried to tell them. Moreover, the explanation given the counselees must be rooted in professional understanding of the field and in the proper way to practice it and not merely in the personal preferences of the counselor, divorced of any scientific basis or peer verification.

In much genetic counseling, diagnosis followed by the "treatment" of counseling will not end the relationship, since it can lead to the need for further diagnosis and treatment if, for example, a pregnancy is at risk for a condition discoverable through antenatal techniques. These techniques themselves raise no major legal issues. Until recently, the major technique — amniocentesis and examination of the harvested cells — was experimental, but with the completion in 1975 of a collaborative study sponsored by the National Institute of Child Health and Human Development, it has come to be regarded as of proven efficacy and safety. The judgment that the status of the procedure had changed was made by the profession, which is appropriate; the characterization of the procedure as experimental or accepted has no direct legal consequences, although it will affect such issues as the relative risks and benefits, the degree of specialized skill needed to undertake the procedure, and the formality of institutional review. The informed consent of patients must be obtain for all procedures, whether experimental or not; the fact that a procedure is still under study must, of course, be disclosed and will also effect the precision with which its risks and benefits can be described.

If the medically and prudentially necessary steps are carefully followed and proper consent obtained, no liability should arise from the performance of antenatal diagnosis as a follow-up to counseling. For example, Reilly has noted that proper consent in amniocentesis procedures may well include informing the patient of the possibility of cell culture failure [30]. Antenatal diagnostic techniques are neither absolutely safe nor perfectly accurate, but harm alone is not a basis for liability. If the risks and uncertainties of the procedure and the resulting diagnosis, if any, are correctly communicated to the patient, the counselors are not responsible for the perfection of the result or the wisdom of the choices made by counselees. Potential liability would result, however, if the genetic counselors misrepresented the data — for example, the counselors, thinking the risk is small even though the test results are ambiguous, tell the parents not to worry in a misguided effort to reassure them.

IV. THREE LEGAL PROBLEMS

While most of the legal issues raised by genetic counseling are straightforward matters of professional responsibility and liability, there are several special legal problems that arise. Among them are issues of confidentiality, damages, and duty and allegiance.

A. Confidentiality

People frequently expect others to keep information in confidence, but there are few settings in which the law actually secures this expectation. The doctor–patient relationship is one in which confidentiality is not only a professional norm — going back to the Hippocratic Oath's admonition not to divulge that "which ought not to be spoken of abroad" and reiterated in modern ethical codes — but a rule that may have legal consequences if breached. Among these are penalties applied by state licensing and disciplinary bodies and a judgment for damages in a suit brought by a patient who is harmed by an unauthorized disclosure. Further, the law protects some confidential disclosures by granting testimonial immunity to those involved, privileging them to remain silent in court. The common law did this for the client–attorney relationship, while statute law has created the same for doctor–patient communications in approximately thirty American jurisdictions [31]. The privilege belongs to the patient and only he or she can waive it.

Confidentiality poses unusual legal issues for genetic counseling on three points: The application of the legal rule to nonphysician counselors, the permissibility of unauthorized disclosures to benefit other persons, and the availability of data about family relationships in confidential judicial records.

The origin of civil liability for breaches of confidentiality lies primarily in state licensing statutes [32], which typically provide for license revocation for unauthorized betrayal of patients' confidences, and secondarily in the doctor–patient privilege statutes, which have been read to protect against unconsented disclosures out of court as well as in [33]. Moreover, the expectations of patients that medical care is a private matter will make the revelation of even nondefamatory information actionable if it offends the community's standard of ordinary decency [34] or an explicit privacy statute [35]. Only the latter two bases (which are the weakest ones) would reach beyond counselors who are physicians and nurses [36], so long as there are no licensing or testimonial privilege statutes for nonphysician geneticists from which a duty of confidentiality could be derived.

It does not necessarily follow that these counselors are free to violate their counselees' privacy, however. First, if they operate in a medical setting, particularly in a genetics clinic headed by a physician, they may be bound by the rules governing physicians' conduct. Not only could their activities be seen as being under the direction of, and an adjunct to, the activities of the physician–geneticist, but the nature of the facility may create a reasonable expectation in the minds of counselees that all communications would be governed by the usual norms of medical confidentiality. Consequently, medical geneticists who may be held liable, under the doctrine of respondeat superior, for the actions of their subordinates would be well advised to assure that the subordinates are familiar with and adhere to the norms of medical confidentiality. Second, liability could arise for contractual as well as tortuous lapses, or duties assumed contractually could give rise to tort liability if breached [37]. The counselees' expectations, or an explicit statement assuring confidentiality, would be regarded as part of the counselor—counselee "contract" for service.

Thus, it is likely that all members of the genetic counseling team, whether physicians or not, are bound by a duty to keep private the information they gather, whether directly from the counselees' lips or through their clinical and laboratory studies. However, it is permissible (or in some instances even professionally obligatory) to discuss the case with colleagues within and without the genetics clinic; this does not breach confidentiality but merely expands the circle of those with a professional interest in the counselee. As that circle is further expanded through conferences, meetings, and even publication, it becomes advisable, indeed, essential to remove unnecessary identifying data about the counselee.

Another problem for genetic counselors is that the discovery of one affected person may indicate to them a need to alert other members of that person's family about a possibly urgent genetic risk. In many situations, an accurate determination of the patient's condition will depend upon examination of relatives; the geneticists may also have a research interest in studying the family, particularly when, for example, the discovery of undetected cases elsewhere in the pedigree may indicate that a disease thought to arise largely from spontaneous mutations is actually frequently dominant but unexpressed or only mildly manifested. (Setting the foregoing concerns aside, the following discussion will be limited to the issues posed by a proposed disclosure to relatives solely for their benefit, rather than benefit to either the original counselee or the counselor.)

Once a diagnosis has been arrived at, the typical response of counselees may well be to supply the necessary information concerning the existence and location of their at-risk relatives or to contact these relatives directly and suggest that they come in for necessary tests and counseling. Yet this is not always the case, for there are various reasons why a person may not wish to reveal a medical condition to some or all members of his or her immediate, much less extended, family or simply may not wish to warn them about their risk. Two issues are thus presented for a genetic counselor with a counselee who will not consent to the contacting of relatives: Would communication by the counselor fall outside the bounds of normal medical confidentiality, and if so, would it nevertheless be permissible as an exception to the norms?

Although the rule of confidentiality forbids unconsented disclosure of medical information to family members as well as to strangers, it is often assumed by both medical [38] and legal writers [39] that information may, or even should, be disclosed in some circumstances. In many cases, the patient will have given express or implied consent to the sharing of the information. When this is not the case, the usual justification is that the information is too distressing for the patient, especially one who is already ill or who is facing a serious operation, and yet some one or more members of the immediate family (spouse, children) ought to be informed of the diagnosis and proposed treatment, in lieu of informing the patient.

While the paternalism inherent in this course of conduct may be questionable, at least it is clear that the sharing of confidential information is based upon an intent to benefit the patient directly. When this intent is absent, a sharing with family members has been held to give rise to liability [40], even when the defendant is physician both to the plaintiff and to other family members [41]. In the context of an impending legal action, where the medical testimony would have been available to the adverse party, a different result has been reached [42]. Thus, the bounds of normal confidentiality, while broadened for consensual or therapeutic reasons, are too narrow to encompass a genetic counselor's unconsented disclosure to relatives solely for the latter's benefit rather than the counselee's.

There are, however, some exceptions to a physician's confidentiality obligations, both in the common law and under public welfare statutes. The latter are of little relevance to the present topic, except as they indicate the authority of the state to compel the disclosure of otherwise private information which is of potential significance to the health and welfare of other individuals or of the community at large [43]. Until a "genetic risks family disclosure act" is adopted, the breaches of confidentiality that result from vital statistics (including abortion), child abuse, and venereal disease reporting laws provide no analogical support for a breach of confidence by a genetic counselor.

The common law has recognized that under certain circumstances a physician may betray a confidence to protect the public or other particular individuals. Simonsen vs Swenson [44], a leading case decided by the Nebraska Supreme Court in 1920, illustrates the type of situation in which disclosure has been held to be justified. Mr. Simonsen, a traveling telephone company employee, registered at a small hotel and then went to see the town doctor about some sores. The doctor informed him of the probable diagnosis (veneral disease) and told him that he should move out of the hotel because he was contagious. When Simonsen refused, Dr. Swenson informed the landlady to be careful to avoid spread of the infection. She fumigated the room and forced Simonsen to leave; he sued the doctor. The court upheld a directed verdict for the defendant, holding that the disclosure of confidential information is permissible, if there is no other way to prevent the spread of a highly contagious disease.

Cases of this sort provide some foundation for a genetic counselor's decision to warn his patient's relatives of a risk that he has discovered based on diagnosis of his patient's condition and analysis of the pedigree according to the known rules of inheritance for the disease in question. But some distinctions are worth noting. Prime among these is the difference between the threat posed by a patient with an infectious disease and that of a patient with a genetic disorder. If warning is not given in the former case people who are free of disease may become infected, while in the latter the relatives of the patient either are or are not affected by the genetic condition regardless of the patient's conduct. The law has traditionally held that people have a duty to avoid intentionally hurting others or exposing them to an unreasonable risk of harm, but there is no duty to act when the harm arises from forces outside their control. Nevertheless, while a patient may be under no legal obligation to inform his or her relatives and hence the counselor would not be justified in remedying this dereliction of duty, the fact that the relatives may in ignorance miss an opportunity to prevent the manifestation of a harmful genetic condition suggests the existence of a strong moral obligation to inform.

The view taken of the danger of syphilis in Simonsen points to another limiting factor in the application of its reasoning to genetic counseling. It may well be justifiable to breach confidence when a prompt and accurate diagnosis will lead to early or presymptomatic treatment of a serious, progressive disease and thereby greatly improve chances of survival and cure (as, for example, with multiple polyposis of the colon). Such life-threatening but undetectable conditions are rare, however. Even in the case of warnings about reproductive risks, Simonsen may not justify disclosure. Certainly, in some instances — such as dominant disorders (particularly with late onset), X-linked conditions, and chromosome translocations — the risk and burden are very grave. Yet frequently, either the diseases involved will be mild and not life-threatening or the probability of an unborn or as yet unconceived niece, nephew, or cousin being affected will be small. Moreover, if an autosomal recessive carrier is turned up in a routine screen (for Tay-Sachs disease or sickle cell anemia, for example) it would not be unreasonable to assume that the carrier's relatives will get the same test, if they desire it, before having children. In any event, the 50% chance that brothers and sisters of the patient are also carriers becomes a relevant factor only if their spouses are carriers, which is only as probable as the general population risk. At least one court has held, however, that a physician's revealing information is justified to protect "well-being or other important interests" as well as life [45], which might sweep in a wider range of genetic disorders.

It would appear, therefore, that a genetic counselor acting in good faith and without malice may, over a patient's objections, reveal to persons at great risk (or to their physicians) such information as is necessary to alert the relatives to a preventable hazard that may arise from their genetic make-up. The privilege of disclosure is conditional and not absolute; a revelation that is false, is not made with due care, is made to unnecessary parties or conveys superfluous data would subject a counselor to liability. Refuge to this legal option ought seldom to be sought, since it suggests some breakdown in the counseling process. The diagnosis transmitted in the reported cases — veneral disease, psychopathy, and the like — typically had pejorative social connotations; counselees should be helped to understand that having a genetic disorder need carry no social onus. Of course, in some cases the feelings of shame and guilt — baseless as they may be — will remain too great and the counselees will remain adamant for nondisclosure. Perhaps, then, the nondefamatory nature of the information can still serve to help justify its necessary revelation, since whatever embarrassment may subjectively be felt by the counselee, he or she will not usually be scorned or ridiculed by relatives if the diagnosis is known.

Finally, a further prudential strategy emerges from the cases on disclosure. The Court's holding in Simonsen vs Swenson was actually that the disclosure of the contagious disease there was "not . . . a betrayal of the confidence of the patient," [46] since he must have known that such information would have to be revealed. Given the present understanding of genetic counseling in the general population, a patient entering genetic counseling would probably not contemplate that his or her condition would have to be revealed to anyone. Consequently, the counselor could avoid the need for an after-the-fact overriding of the counselee's wishes by informing him or her (at the outset or as soon as the possibility becomes revelant because testing is contemplated) of the clinic's policy on contacting relatives at risk. It is unlikely that any counselees would for that reason decline to go further with the diagnostic procedure except those for whom the thought of any revelation would be extremely distasteful. For this group, the risk of revelation would have to be weighed against the harm of not getting a needed diagnosis from this counselor. Perhaps the counselor can be persudaded to alter the usual policy, or the reluctant counselee can seek help from someone else. In any event, an advance statement of policy can serve to make any ultimate decision seem less arbitrary and ad hoc and to place it for the counselee into a larger picture of social expectations about familial obligations.

A third unusual facet to confidentiality arises in the context of genetic counseling when a diagnosis of genetic disorder is made concerning a family that has been involved in an adoption. If a person found to have a genetic condition gave up a child for adoption at some earlier time, he or she may wish to contact the child to alert it to its genetic risk, or the adopted person (or, if he or she is still young or otherwise ignorant of the adoption, the adoptive parents) may wish to contact the biological parents and collateral relatives to seek confirmation of the diagnosis or to warn them about their genetic risk.

Adoptions are handled through the courts. By law such proceedings are usually held in private and the records are sealed after the decree has been finalized. The rule of secrecy may be statute, regulation, or common law apply also to the records of the state and private agencies involved in the adoption process or charged with keeping health and birth records and other vital statistics.

There are several ways to resolve the conflict between the policy of confidentiality, which is usually appropriate to protect all parties to the adoption, and the equally important goal of aiding in the diagnosis of disease or risks in reproduction. First, the problem could be handled on a case-by-case basis, requiring an individualized application by the counselee (and/or adoptive parents), supported by information from the genetic counseling staff, to the court having jurisdiction over the records for an order unsealing them. The danger in such an approach is that "genetic risks" might become a pretext for adoptees to discover information about their natural parents. Alternatively, but still on the basis of an individual petition, the counselor could seek to learn the relevant information in order that the counselor could contact the persons at risk, without informing the counselee who such persons may be or telling the persons contacted the identity of the proband who led to their being contacted.

The second alternative has much to recommend it. Rather than destroying confidentiality it would merely take the counselor, a person who should be used to confidential relationships, into the circle of secrecy. By placing the initial contact with the persons identified in the hands of the counselor, the risk of an adverse impact from the disclosure of the unsolicited and probably unwelcome information about the genetic risk is minimized. The judicial or other governmental official who possesses the secret data is unlikely to be qualified to convey the information accurately or otherwise properly. But a case-by-case approach leaves much to be desired. It would seem preferable, either through statutory amendment or judicial interpretation, to authorize the statewide keeper of birth (and adoption) records to release the relevant data to genetic counselors who provide reasonable grounds for believing the information is necessary for the diagnosis, treatment, or prevention of a genetic disorder.

B. Damages

Damages may not be difficult to determine in many cases in medical genetics— for example, were a sterilization procedure to be done negligently, giving rise to medical complications and further surgery, or were it to have been undertaken because of an erroneous diagnosis. But more often than not, when counseling is being sought because of a concern for reproductive risks, the measurement of damages is a difficult issue when the risk materializes, allegedly due to the counselor's negligent error.

The difficulties are of three sorts. First, can there, as a matter of law, ever be a cognizable injury in the birth of a child, however afflicted with genetic burdens? Second, if the only means of preventing the injury would have been to prevent the child's birth, is the child barred for reasons of policy or logic from recovering damages from a counselor? And third, if the physical injury is suffered solely by the child, have the parents any basis for recovery for their nonpecuniary loss?

In one leading case, Gleitman vs Cosgrave [47], the New Jersey Supreme Court denied damages to the parents of a child born with severe malformations after the defendant doctors had assured the mother that the rubella which she contracted early in her pregnancy posed no risk to her child. The court held that it was impossible to strike a balance between the benefits of parenthood and the anguish of having a deformed child. Gleitman is consistent with several other cases from the 1960s and more recently, but a majority rule in this country seems to be taking shape to the contrary [48].

The Texas Supreme Court recently held in Jacobs vs Theimer [49] that the parents of a child with rubella-related injuries could recover the cost of care and treatment necessitated by the child's impairment, although not for their own emotional suffering.

> Perhaps the court felt that if courts began allowing such damages there would be an overwhelming burden on physicians, which could lead to physicians protecting themselves by revealing all the horrendous possible outcomes of all pregnancies a result which would surely be detrimental to prospective parents as a class. This concern is a real one and deserves notice; however, the court did not actually state it [50].

Moreover, physicians do not escape malpractice by engaging in professionally inexcusable "overkill." If risks are realistic ones for a counselee, he or she *should* be properly (not inflammatorily) informed of those risks.

The Wisconsin Supreme Court in 1975 recognized a cause of action for the extra medical expenses caused by the birth of a child deformed by undiagnosed rubella [51], although it had earlier concluded that no damages arose from a physician's failure to detect pregnancy in time for an abortion [52], apparently on the rationale that it would be unseemly for parents to complain of the birth of a healthy child and the law must always treat a birth as worth more than its opposite. Some courts have given damages even in the latter situation. The plaintiffs in Custodio vs Bauer [53] were permitted to recover for any measurable changes in the family's status resulting from the mother's having to spread herself more thinly after the birth of a child consequent to failed tubal ligation. Courts allowing damages apply the "benefits rule," under which the trier of fact sets off the benefit of parenthood against the costs imposed by the child's existence in calculating net damages [54]. One New York appellate court has extended the measurement of damages for the birth of an unwanted but healthy child to all the detriment proximately caused thereby, whether it could have been anticipated or not [55]. The burdens imposed on the parents of a child with a serious genetic defect that would have been prevented, but for the defendant's negligent or wrongful act, should be subject to proof and counterproof by defendant, rather than ruled out by a matter of law.

Although recovery by the parents seems patently justified, more understandable doubts have been raised about recovery by a child of a damage award against the physicians who negligently or wrongfully failed to take steps necessary to prevent its birth with deformities. The Jacobs court, in dictum, indicated that had the child sought to recover, its claim would have been dismissed as too speculative "as to the quality of life" [56]. The holding of the New Jersey court in Gleitman is a landmark on this issue as well. That opinion states that it is logically impossible to weigh the value of life with impairments against the child's nonexistence [57]. The "logical impossibility" has two meanings, neither persuasive. The court is first suggesting that since there is no known way for the trier of fact to comprehend nonexistence, it is not possible to calculate the difference in value between that state and the pain the child plaintiff experiences in life. It would be unfair to the defendant were the fact finder not to offset the damages experienced by some substantial amount; otherwise, it would be as though the child would have been healthy had it not been for the defendant's act, which is clearly not the case for a child with an irremediable genetic disorder. Yet it is equally unfair to the child plaintiff to rule out any recovery because the damages require both great care and an imaginative leap for their calculation. There may be some situations in which common understanding would lead to the conclusion that it would be better to be dead (or never to have existed) — and it is for the trier of fact (typically a jury) to determine just how much better it would be [58]. Similar subjective calculations about the "value" of lives cut short, of pain and suffering, and other intangibles, are made every day.

The second reading of the "logical impossibility" presents a difficulty more of philosophy than of policy. The Gleitman court would not allow the child to recover because it could find no logic in permitting a party to complain of its "wrongful life," when that very life was the precondition for the party's ability to appear in court to assert his or her claim. Although attractive at first blush, this conclusion is nothing more than a restatement of the idea that any life must be better than nonlife. There is nothing illogical in a plaintiff saying "I'd rather not be here suffering as I am, but since your wrongful conduct preserved my life I am going to take advantage of my regrettable existence to sue you." To say, as courts [59] and commentators have [60], that such plaintiffs are suing for their "wrongful lives," mistakes the real basis of such complaints. The wrong actually being complained of is the failure to give accurate advice on which the child's parents, acting in his or her behalf, can make a decision whether not being born would be preferable to being born deformed [61].

> If one objects to awarding damages for the violation of this right, it would seem that the objection is directed either at the policy of allowing abortions . . . or at giving parents who may have conflicting motivations the authority to make this decision. The fact remains that the Gleitman court departed from the rule that the choice in this matter lies with the patient, not the physician.

The rejection of the child's right to recover, based upon the ground that he or she would be nonexistent if his or her claimed preference had been followed in the first place, seems almost metaphysical. As a legal matter, it resembles the common judicial interpretation of the wrongful death statutes which precludes maintenance of an action on behalf of a fetus that died prior to being delivered [62]. Assuming this construction of the statutes to be correct (ie that legislators did not intend to include that nonperson or not-yet-person, the fetus, within the coverage of a statute permitting recovery for the wrongful *death* of "a person") a child born with a genetic disorder does not cast him- or herself into the same legal limbo merely by asserting that, *if* the defendant physician had done the proper thing, the plaintiff would never have been born. For in fact the plaintiff child *was* born to suffer with the burdens which nonception or abortion would have prevented ever being manifested.

In most of the "wrongful life" cases, the courts assumed arguendo that the pregnant woman could legally have obtained the abortion she claimed she would have wanted had she possessed the information that the physician negligently or intentionally failed to disclose or discover. Nevertheless, it is difficult (given the language of the opinions and the highly charged nature of the abortion issue in our society) not to suppose that the need for an abortion to prevent the harm of which the plaintiffs complained contributed to the courts' reluctance to allow damages. Conversely, it is not surprising that in Park vs Chessin [63], the first reported case to base a claim for damages on the failure to give proper *preconception* genetic counseling, the plaintiffs' claim on behalf of their deceased child was held to be legally enforceable. Although a warning to the parents about the recurrence risk for congenital polycystic kidney disease would apparently have meant that the child would never have been conceived, much less born, the court was able to escape from the logical fallacy of the Gleitman line of cases [64].

The third damage issue — the ability of parents to collect for emotional injuries although they are not the ones suffering the physical injury — has recently been considered in the decision of the New York Court of Appeals in Howard vs Lecher [65]. In that case, the first appellate case to involve a failure to warn a pregnant woman of a genetic risk, the plaintiffs alleged that Mrs. Howard's obstetrician–gynecologist knew that the couple was of Ashkenazic Jewish background and hence was at special risk for Tay-Sachs disease. Plaintiffs further alleged that Dr. Lecher neglected to employ the tests available for carrier detection, to construct a proper genealogical history, or to advise them of the risks and the means of avoiding these risks. Their daughter, born in August 1972, died nearly two years later of Tay-Sachs disease. Had they known that she was affected, the Howards stated that they would have terminated the pregnancy.

The Howards sought damages for, among other things, their "mental distress and emotional disturbances" consequent to their daughter's condition. The defendant argued that this cause of action should be dismissed because damages could not be awarded for their distress in seeing someone else's illness. The trial court denied the defendant's motion, but in a split decision the Appellate Division reversed; its judgment was subsequently affirmed by the Court of Appeals, four to three.

The reasoning of the Court of Appeals was that the parents are in the same position as if they had witnessed their child being injured in an accident. New York, like most American jurisdictions, has abandoned the old "impact" rule which required physical contact resulting directly from defendant's conduct before mental or psychological injuries could be recompensed. It follows the "zone of physical danger" rule, which permits recovery for injuries resulting from fear for a member of one's family if the plaintiff was also in physical peril. But "no cause of action lies for unintended harm sustained by one, solely as a result of injuries inflicted directly upon another, regardless of the relationship and whether the one was an eyewitness to the incident which resulted in the injuries," as the Court of Appeals had held in Tobin vs Grossman [66]. The court concluded that no reasonable limits could be drawn on the emotional injuries to bystanders which a tort-feasor might cause. Morever, the court stated that "the risks of indirect harm from the loss or injuries of loved ones is pervasive and inevitably realized at one time or another" [67]. In effect, the court held that everyone assumes the risk of such injuries just by living in society. Since not every wrong can have a remedy — and since most of the risk of emotional injury is not associated with the culpable acts of third parties — the court decided that it was better to let such indirect injuries go uncompensated than to expand liability beyond directly or intentionally inflicted harm.

The Tobin decision thus rejected the conclusion of the California Supreme Court in Dillon vs Legg [68] that "recovery should be had in such a case if defendant should foresee fright or shock enough to cause substantial injury to a person normally constituted." The California court left the elaboration of its rule to case-by-case adjudication based on the plaintiff's proximity in distance and time to the accident and the closeness of the relationship between plaintiff and victim.

Some courts have gone further than the California Supreme Court in extending liability for injuries to bystanders. The Supreme Court of Hawaii went so far as to permit recovery for the emotional suffering of people who viewed the flooding of their homes caused by the defendant's negligence in the construction of a road [69]. The Hawaii court has seemed willing to impose liability whenever the defendant could reasonably foresee some harm to another and the nature of the harm actually suffered was reasonably foreseeable [70]. In a subsequent case [71], however, the court denied recovery where the plaintiff was too physically remote from the accident — although the *existence* of the plaintiff (whose daughter and granddaughter were killed by the defendant) and the type of injury the plaintiff suffered were perfectly foreseeable.

It is apparent, however, that even the broadest rules for bystander recovery for emotional suffering fit the genetic counseling cases very poorly. Negligent counseling, resulting in the birth of a child affected with a genetic disorder, exposes the parents to their child's course of suffering, perhaps drawn out over a long period of time, but not to a sudden, traumatic injury. It is not surprising to discover that in nongenetics cases of injuries arising from alleged malpractice, parents were denied recovery when the illness was drawn out [72] but were able to recover when, for example, a child choked to death in their arms [73]. Even when the parents are present, it has been held that they must have an "understanding observation" of what they see. Thus, fathers who had been present in the delivery room when their sons were stillborn were denied recovery because of their shock did not arise from "sensory and contemporaneous observation" but only later when they were informed that the sons had been born dead [74].

C. Duties and Allegiances

The difficulty in fitting the facts of Howard vs Lecher to the Procrustean bed of bystander law could be avoided if the court accepted the parents' characterization of their injury rather than the physicians'. The Howards claimed that their distress resulted from the defendant's failure to test for, ascertain, and advise plaintiffs of a serious genetic condition of which they were the carriers. In effect, they alleged that the obstetrician's primary duty was to them — in their own right and not merely as representatives of the unborn fetus [75]. The failure to conduct the tests that would have uncovered the disease of the fetus would in this view be a breach of the due care owed to the parents (assuming that a nonnegligent obstetrician in New York in the spring of 1972 would have known of the risk of Tay-Sachs disease in such patients and of the availability of the tests). The primary injury would be depriving them of their role as "informed decisionmakers" concerning their reproductive choices; the measurement of the damages here would be the costs (not of the benefits of parenthood) of raising and caring for the child.

Such a "duty" analysis has been followed by intermediate appellate courts in New York in two recent cases. In Karlsons vs Guerinot [76], a mother complained of her physicians' failure to advise her of the special risk she ran of bearing a monogoloid child. The appellate court reversed the dismissal of plaintiffs' action and held that they should be permitted to prove, if they could, that the defendants had breached their "duty to plaintiff wife to provide her with proper medical care during her pregnancy . . . by not properly diagnosing the condition of the child, thus precluding a decision to abort" [77]. If the defendants breached a duty owed the plaintiffs (rather than one owed only to their child), under accepted tort theory they would be liable for those injuries flowing to the plaintiffs *directly* from the breach, including mental anguish and other emotional injuries [78]. The Karlsons' judges simply chose not to follow the contrary views of their appellate brethren in Howard vs Lecher [79].

This course was not open to the Appellate Division panel which decided Park vs Chessin [80], however, since in the interim the state's highest court had affirmed the Howard holding that no cause of action existed for the parents' emotional injuries. Instead, the Park court limited Howard to cases in which plaintiffs seek to compel an obstetrician "to take lengthy genealogical histories of both parents, whether the patient affirmatively requested it or not, [and] whether the medical circumstances indicated cause for alarm or not." The Howards, the Park court wrote, had "sought to impose an unwarranted and clearly intolerable burden upon the physician" which would make the physician "a virtual insurer of the genetic health of newborns" [81]. It is understandable that the majority in Park would wish to distinguish Howard, which lends itself to this absurd reading. If others follow the Park view of Howard's holding, the latter will have only a brief life, for no plaintiff (including the Howards themselves) would seriously contend that the law should require that obstetricians and other physicians become "forced genetic counselors" who must always take genealogical histories of their female patients — and of "the nonpatient father" — when the "medical circumstances" do not suggest any need for concern [82]. Rather, a plaintiff in a malpractice case would merely be contending that the physician had breached the standard of care, including knowledge of genetic and other risks in reproduction, established by and for members of his or her own professional group. Whether that would include any particular means of ascertaining the risk of a genetic disorder in the prospective mother and, if appropriate, in her partner would depend upon all the circumstances of the individual case under the practices established in the profession [83].

In any event, Judge Damiani and his colleagues [84] were satisfied that Mrs. Park, in alleging that she had been erroneously advised in response to her specific request for information about the risk of bearing a second child with polycystic kidney disease, had stated a cause of action which she should be allowed to prove. Curiously, the Park majority apparently shrank from the logical conclusion of its holding, that if the plaintiffs show a breach of duties *owed to them* they may recover for *all* injuries directly caused thereby, including psychic and emotional harm. Such damages are "specifically excluded from recovery under the parents' cause of action" [85]. This statement may be purely descriptive — that is, as the parents had not appealed the trial court's dismissal of the counts dealing with recovery for mental anguish such damages were "excluded from" — indeed, were beyond the scope of — the court's judgment. It is likely, however, that the court did intend to reach out to express its obiter dictum on the matter, for it gives reasons for the exclusion: "the inability to calculate damages, and the absence of duty" [86], citing Howard and Tobin vs Grossman [87], which established the no-recovery-for-bystanders rule discussed above. The calculation difficulty is hard to take seriously, since the Park court would allow recovery by the affected child, whose net damages (life with suffering versus no life) are plainly much harder to calculate than the parents' emotional anguish would be.

The second objection, that no duty exists, is puzzling in light of the reliance (later in the paragraph) on Karlsons, which recognized a right to recover for emotional anguish, and in light of the Park opinion's own careful exposition that a duty of due care *to the parents* does indeed exist, at least so long as the physician has been alerted to the need to give advice on reproductive risks. Any suggestion that the duty is limited to avoiding financial but not emotional injuries is so unrealistic as to be nonsensical. Surely, in seeking medical advice, prospective parents like the Parks desire to avoid not only the medical expenses of having a child with a severe disease which will prove fatal within a few years, but also — indeed very likely, primarily — to avoid the terrible anguish of producing such a child (especially when the birth could have been avoided), caring for the child and then waiting and watching (helplessly) as the child dies. Since, in Judge Cardozo's classic statement, "the risk reasonably to be perceived defines the duty to be obeyed" [88], the duty of physicians in such circumstances must include the giving of professionally competent advice such as would permit the parents to avoid the grave risk of psychological and emotional harm.

A breach of this duty occurs when the advice given is not professionally competent or does not cover points which would be material for decisionmaking by persons in the position in which the physician (or genetic counselor) knows or should know his or her clients to be. The customary tort standard of "reasonableness" should apply to the professional's conduct but not to the highly personal and subjective decisionmaking of the clients [89]. Causation is made out if it is established that the clients (again, not the "reasonable person" but the actual individuals, with the personal values on which the trier of fact determines they would have acted) would by contraception, abortion, artificial insemination, or other means have avoided the injury (manifested in the birth of the affected child) had the counselor or physician not breached his or her duty [90]. Damages for the net harm (the additional economic and emotional burden of the child with a genetic disorder less the benefits to the parents of the child's existence) are then appropriate.

The conclusion that a person providing genetic counsel — or a physician who ought to recognize the need for such counseling — is liable for a breach of disclosure comports with the emerging constitutional jurisprudence on the zone of privacy that surrounds decisions about reproduction. Since the consequences of such decisions will rest on the parents and not in any significant degree on health care personnel, justice and good public policy are also best served by legal rules which encourage the exercise of due care by visiting the costs of breaches of this duty on the personnel responsible [91]. This is especially true when the failure to disclose is based on a "therapeutic privilege" rationale. This "privilege," often mentioned but rarely actually relied upon in the decision of a case, excuses a physician's withholding of information necessary for informed consent when the physician believes that the information would be too distressing or otherwise harmful to the patient. The usurpation of a counselee's decision by a counselor not only deprives the former of the freedom that the law is supposed to guarantee but is likely to lead to unhappy results since there is little reason to predict congruence between the value judgments of counselees and counselors [92].

Counselors may find themselves pulled, moreover, by an allegiance to the unborn child — whose well-being is, after all, the ultimate object of their concern as well as the motivating interest of the parents. As understandable as this concern may be, in the end it must give way to the duty owed to the counselee—parents. The policy adopted, for example, by some genetics clinics not to disclose certain diagnoses from amniocentesis appears to be based in part on a concern that parents learning of certain facts may decide to abort fetuses that the genetic counselors believe will not be seriously burdened. This problem may be finessed if an advance understanding is reached with counselees on the limits of disclosure that the counselors plan to observe [93]. Where an unexpected or ambiguous result occurs in the absence of such an understanding, the withholding of information cannot be justified out of a duty to protect the unborn child from its parents, although the competent counselor will make every effort to convey the information in a fashion which will cause the least unnecessary shock (there being no way to make it completely innocuous) and will maximize the parents' understanding of the facts (as well as the unavoidable uncertainities). In this fashion, counselors fulfill their primary obligation — which is to the parents — while also reducing the suffering of both parents and fetus to the extent possible consistent with parental exercise of their rights and responsibilities in reproduction.

It is not possible to predict how soon the problems some courts have had in measuring damages will cease being a barrier to recovery against those who negligently or otherwise give inaccurate or improper genetic counseling. But the trend in the law is clear. As we have seen, the courts have begun first with the cost to the parents of care and treatment. They will probably next recognize the emotional injuries consequent to preclusion of the parental choice to avoid the birth, and finally the net harm to the child (the amount by which his or her pain, suffering and other burdens exceeds the detriment of not having been born at all). Indeed, the judicial acceptance in Park vs Chessin [94] of a right of recovery for the child's suffering (instituted by her parents after her death from hereditary polycystic kidney disease) shows that the courts are capable of overcoming the confusion created by the "wrongful life" framework.

The distinction between the failure in Park to provide advice *pre*conception rather than *post*conception, as in all the prior cases, cannot withstand analysis.

The cause of action rests on the same theory in both situations: That the defendant physician negligently failed to provide information and technical skills which would have permitted the child's parents to prevent its being born and suffering the illness for which it was at risk. And the metaphysical or logical difficulty of asserting that nonexistence would be preferable to existence with the defect is, if anything, more pronounced in the case of nonconception (where the plaintiff would never have existed as a genetic being at all) than of nonbirth (where the plaintiff existed as a fetus — entitled to legal protection from harm that manifests itself after birth — but would have been aborted prior to birth).

Once the damage hurdle is overcome, the substantive legal rules — about the establishment and enforcement of reasonable care — will be felt more clearly by those participating in the new field of genetic counseling. Basic control over the field's development will remain with its practitioners, but they will in the years ahead need to be prepared to justify their practices — particularly those with roots in philosophical stances rather than biomedical science — in public fora. It seems likely that the process of legal review will influence the development of genetic counseling in subtle and not entirely predictable yet nonetheless important ways.

ACKNOWLEDGMENTS

This research was supported in part by a grant from the National Institutes of Health (GM-20138) to the University of Pennsylvania Human Genetics Center.

REFERENCES

1. Milunsky A, Reilly P: The "new" genetics: Emerging medicolegal issues in the prenatal diagnosis of hereditary disorders. Am J Law Med 1:71–72, 1975.
2. See eg Reed SC: "Counseling in Medical Genetics." 2d Ed. Philadelphia: WB Saunders, 1963.
3. Freidson E: "Professional Dominance: The Social Structure of Medical Care." Chicago: Aldine Publishing, 1970.
4. Reed SC: History of genetic counseling. Soc Biol 21:332, 1974.
5. Reilly P: "Genetics, Law, and Social Policy." Cambridge, Massachusetts: Harvard University Press, 1977, pp 152–155.
6. Thompson JS, Thompson MW: "Genetics in Medicine." 2d Ed. Philadelphia: WB Saunders, 1973, p 337.
7. See eg Price v Neyland, 320 F.2d 674, (D.C.Cir. 1963); Brown v United States, 419 F.2d 337 (8th Cir. 1969); Fear v Rundle, 506 F.2d 331 (3rd Cir. 1974), cert. denied sub. nom. Anderson v Fear, 421 U.S. 1012 (1975); Edwards v United States, 519 F.2d 1137 (5th Cir. 1975).
8. Eg Gardner v General Motors Corp., 507 F.2d 525 (10th Cir. 1974); Southern Cement Co. v Sproul, 378 F.2d 48 (5th Cir. 1967).

9. Faircloth v Lamb-Grays Harbor Co., Inc., 467 F.2d 685 (5th Cir. 1972) (plant engineer with 20 years experience qualified as expert).

10. Arnold v Loose, 352 F.2d 959 (3d Cir. 1965) (expert is competent only if possesses "reasonable pretension" to specialized field.

11. Firman G, Goldstein M: The future of chiropractics: A psychosocial view. New Engl J Med 293:639–642, 1975.

12. King v Flamm, 442 S.W.2d 679 (Tex. 1969) (physician has duty to seek consultation with specialist if, in the exercise of reasonable care, the physician knew or should have known that a specialist's services were necessary); Manion v Tweedy, 257 Minn. 59, 100 N.W.2 124 (1960) (for failure to consult to be negligence, must be shown that defendant should have discovered that patient's condition was beyond the defendant's knowledge or ability to treat with likelihood of reasonable success). Cf Larsen v Yelle, 246 N.W.2d 841 (Minn. 1976) (if general practitioner breaches duty to consult with a specialist, he will be held to the specialist's standard of care).

13. Siirila v Barrios, 398 Mich. 576, 248 N.W.2d 171 (1976) (pediatrician not allowed to testify as to requisite standard of care required of defendant general practitioner as ̩pediatrician was unaware of the applicable standards of defendant's school); Fraizer v Hurd, 380 Mich. 291, 157 N.W.2d 249 (1968) (testimony of medical doctor, unaware of the procedures and standards of osteopathic medicine, defendant's school, was inadmissible).

14. Kelly v Carroll, 219 P.2d 79 (Wash. 1950) (drugless healer held to standards of accepted medical treatment).

15. Hansen v Pock, 57 Mont. 51, 187 p. 282 (1920).

16. Nelson v Harrington, 72 Wisc. 591, 40 N.W. 228 (1888) (defendant-clairvoyant not permitted to defend on grounds that his action was consistent with usual procedures of spiritualists).

17. Hamilton v Hardy, 549 P.2d 1099 (Colo. App. 1976).

18. Ewing v Goode, 78 F. 442, 443, (C.C.S.D. Ohio 1897) (Taft, J.).

19. Reilly P: Genetic Counseling and the Law. Houston L Rev 12:640, 656, 1975.

20. Naccarato v Grob, 12 Mich. App. 130, 162 N.W.2d 305 (1968).

21. Howard v Lecher, 42 N.Y.2d 109, 397 N.Y.S.2d 363, 366 N.E.2d 64 (1977).

22. See section IV B infra.

23. See note 7, supra, and accompanying text.

24. See Prosser WL: Handbook of the Law of Torts, 4th Ed. St. Paul: West Publishing, 1970, pp 211–228.

25. The T.J. Hooper, 60 F.2d 737 (2nd Cir. 1932).

26. 83 Wash.2d 514, 519 P.2d 981 (1974). The court held that failure by defendant opthamologist to employ simple, harmless pressure test for glaucoma to woman under 40 years old, who manifested some symptoms of the disease, was negligence as a matter of law despite professional testimony attesting that use of the test in such a case was not the norm and despite the fact that risk of disease in under-40 population is only 1 in 25,000. Cf Morgan v Sheppard, 188 N.E.2d 808, 816–817 (Ohio App. 1963) (in determining whether defendant used due care, jury may consider "usual and customary methods," but no matter how long or how generally such methods have been used they do not establish a standard of safe conduct if they "are in fact negligent").

27. Capron AM: Informed Consent in Catastrophic Disease Research and Treatment. Univ Pa L Rev 123:340, 364–376, 1974.

28. Cobbs v Grant, 8 Cal.3d 229, 502 P.2d 1, 104 Cal. Rptr. 505 (1972); Canterbury v Spence, 464 F.2d 772 (D.C.Cir.), cert. denied, 409 US 1064 (1972); Wilkinson v Vesey,

110 R.I. 606, 295 A.2d 676 (1972). But see NY Public Health Law 2805-d(1) (McKinney Supp. 1976) (expert testimony necessary in informed consent cases arising after July 1, 1975).

29. Capron AM: Informed Decisionmaking in Genetic Counseling: A Dissent to the "Wrongful Life" Debate. Ind L J 48: 581, 589–593, 1973.
30. Reilly P: Genetic Counseling and the Law. Houston L Rev 12:640, 655, 1975.
31. Waltz JR, Inbau FE: Medical Jurisprudence. New York: Macmillan, 1971, pp 235–236.
32. Clark v Geraci, 29 Misc.2d 791, 208 N.Y.S.2d 564 (1960) (physician's disclosure to Air Force of plaintiff's alcoholism was unprofessional and would be actionable except that in this set of circumstances, plaintiff had waived his confidentiality rights by requesting that physician send some information to Air Force); Simonsen v Swenson, 177 N.W. 831 (Neb. 1920) (propriety of physician's disclosure, which was upheld, judged by whether it violated professional standards).
33. Schaffer v Spicer, 215 N.W.2d 134 (S.D. 1974) (plaintiff held to have cause of action against her psychiatrist for disclosing to plaintiff's husband's attorney information for use in custody action).
34. Hammonds v Aetna Casualty & Surety Co., 243 F.Supp. 793 (N.D. Ohio 1965) (plaintiff has cause of action against insurance company for allegedly inducing physician's divulgence of confidential information by intimidating physician with non-existent malpractice claim); Bazemore v Savannah Hosp., 155 S.E. 194 (Ga. 1930) (parents' claim against hospital, photographer and newspaper for damages after publication of picture of malformed child stated a cause of action).
35. Griffin v Medical Society of New York, 11 N.Y.S.2d 109 (Sup. Ct. 1939) (plaintiff has cause of action against physician and magazine for publishing pictures of patient entitled "saddle hose" without permission). Cf Horne v Patton, 287 So.2d 824 (Ala. 1974) (physician's disclosure to plaintiff's employer of information acquired during treatment of patient held to be an invasion of privacy).
36. Lynch v Lewis County, 68 Misc. 2d 78, 326 N.Y.S.2d 243 (1971); In re Schermerhorn, 98 N.Y.S.2d 361, reversed on other grounds, 277 A.D. 845, 98 N.Y.S.2d 367, aff'd, 302 N.Y. 660, 98 N.E.2d 475 (1950); Williams v State, 65 Okla. Crim. 366, 86 P.2d 1015 (1939).
37. Horne v Patton, 287 S.2d 824 (Ala. 1974); Hammonds v Aetna Casualty & Surety Co, 243 F.Supp. 793 (N.D. Ohio 1965); Quarles v Sutherland, 389 S.W.2d 249 (Tenn. 1965).
38. Leake CO (ed): "Percival's Medical Ethics." Baltimore: William & Wilkins, 1927.
39. Nishi v Hartwell, 52 Haw. 188, 473 P.2d 116 (1970) (in an action against physicians for nondisclosure to patient and wife of risks attendant to aortography, court said that although the law does not require such disclosure, relaying the information would be a considerate act, good public relations and may benefit both patient and physician); see also Patrick v Sedwick, 391 P.2d 453 (Alaska 1964) (dictum) (physician may withhold information from patient which would cause unnecessary anxiety and may inform family instead).
40. Kitson v Playfair, 1 Br Med J 815, 882 (1896) (plaintiff able to collect against physician who, after examining plaintiff, determined she had miscarried and, since her husband had been away for months, surmised that she had committed adultery. He informed his wife and relatives of plantiff of his suspicions.)
41. Furniss v Fitchett, N.Z.L.R. 396 (Sup. Ct. 1958) (upholds recovery against doctor for disclosure of diagnosis to husband).

42. Pennison v Provident Life & Accident Insurance Co., 154 So.2d 617, writ refused, 244 La. 1019, 156 So.2d 226 (1963) (disclosure to husband of wife's medical records which were pertinent to divorce proceeding does not constitute violation of privacy).
43. Whalen v Roe, 45 U.S.L.W. 4166 (1977) (N.Y. dangerous drug reporting statute upheld as within state's broad police powers); State v Jacobs, 75 Misc.2d 840, 348 N.Y.S.2d 907 (Sup. Ct. 1973) (NY statute requiring filing of patient's name and address post-abortion on fetal death certificate upheld); but, cf, Schulman v New York City Health and Hospitals Corp., 75 Misc.2d 150, 346 N.Y.S.2d 920 (Sup. Ct. 1973) (same reporting statute held to be invasion of privacy and contrary to public policy).
44. 177 N.W. 831 (Neb. 1920).
45. Berry v Moench, 331 P.2d 814, 817–818 (Utah 1958) (physician is bound by duty of confidentiality but that may be outweighed by a higher duty to disclose for the protection of a sufficiently important interest, here the informing of the future wife's family of the plaintiff husband's psychiatric history).
46. 177 N.W. at 832 (Neb. 1920).
47. 49 N.J. 22, 227 A.2d 689 (1967).
48. Reilly P: "Genetics, Law, and Social Policy." Cambridge, Massachusetts: Harvard University Press, 1977, pp 172–175.
49. 519 S.W.2d 846 (Tex. 1975).
50. Kass M, Shaw MW: The Risks of Birth Defects: Jacobs v Theimer and the Parent's Right to Know. Am J Law & Med 2:213, 240, 1976–77. Accord Park v Chessin, 60 App. Div. 2d 80, 400 N.Y.S.2d 110 (1977) (reversing refusal to dismiss claim for emotional injuries).
51. Dumer v St. Michael's Hosp., 69 Wis.2d 766, 233 N.W.2d 372 (1975).
52. Rieck v Medical Protective Co., 64 Wis.2d 514, 219 N.W.2d 242 (1974).
53. 251 Cal. App. 2d 303, 59 Cal. Rptr. 463 (1967).
54. Stills v Gratton, 55 Cal. App. 3d 698, 127 Cal. Rptr. 652 (1976) (unwed mother has cause of action for failed abortion and subsequent misprescription of contraceptives; normal tort damages apply with benefits offset); Troppi v Scarf, 31 Mich. App. 240, 187 N.W.2d 511 (1971) (benefits of having child may be offset against elements of damage claimed by plaintiffs whose unwanted child resulted from defendant pharmacist's negligence in supplying tranquilizers rather than birth control pills).
55. Ziemba v Sternberg, 45 App. Div. 2d 230, 357 N.Y.S.2d 265 (1974) (parents have cause of action against physician for failure to diagnose woman's pregnancy in time for her lawfully to terminate it). See also Karlsons v Guerinot, 57 App. Div. 2d 73, 394 N.Y.S.2d 933 (1977) (parents have stated cause of action for pain, suffering and mental distress from birth of deformed child which they would have aborted if properly diagnosed and disclosed by defendant physicians).
56. 519 S.W.2d at 849.
57. 49 N.J. at 28, 227 A.2d at 693.
58. See Story Parchment Co. v Paterson Paper Co., 282 U.S. 555, 562–566 (1931) (jury using "good sense" may determine "probable" amount of damages on all circumstances of the case without needing "positive proof," and the risk of uncertainty in determining damages should be upon wrongdoer whose action was responsible for difficulty of measurement not upon the injured party).
59. Williams v New York, 18 N.Y.2d 481, 276 N.Y.S.2d 885, 223 N.E.2d 343 (1966) (infant, born to unwed mentally deficient mother subsequent to sexual assault on mother while confined in state mental institution, has no right to recover damages from state which negligently failed to prevent assault); Zepeda v Zepeda, 41 Ill. App.2d 240, 190 N.E.2d 849 (1963) (action dismissed against father for admitted damages

resulting from plaintiff's being born adulterine bastard, because of sweeping public policy ramifications of permitting children to complain legally about circumstances of their birth).

60. Tedeschi G: "On Tort Liability for Wrongful Life." Israel Law Rev 1:513, 1966.
61. Capron AM: Informed decisionmaking in genetic counseling: A dissent to the "wrongful life" debate. Indiana Law J 48:581, Summer 1973.
62. See eg, Endresz v Friedburg, 24 N.Y.2d 478, 248 N.E.2d 901, (1969).
63. 88 Misc. 2d 222, 387 N.Y.S.2d 204, (Sup. Ct. 1976), aff'd in part & rev'd in part, 60 App. Div.2d 80, 400 N.Y.S.2d 110, (1977), modified, No. 560 (Ct. App., Dec. 27, 1978).
64. Note: A cause of action for "wrongful life:" A suggested analysis. Minn L Rev 55:58, 1970. See also Becker v Schwartz, 60 App. Div. 400 N.Y.S.2d 119, 1977.
65. 42 N.Y.2d 109, 397 N.Y.S.2d 363, 366 N.E.2d 64, (1977).
66. 24 N.Y.2d 609, 611, 301 N.Y.S.2d 554, 555, (1969).
67. 24 N.Y.2d at 619, 301 N.Y.S.2d at 561–62.
68. 68 Cal.2d 728, 740, 69 Cal. Rptr. 72, 80, 441 P.2d 912, 920, (1968).
69. Rodrigues v State, 52 Haw. 156, 472 P.2d 509, (1970).
70. Leong v Takasaki, 55 Haw. 398, 520 P.2d 758 (1974) (held that minor plaintiff had a cause of action to recover damages for nervous shock and psychic trauma suffered without physical impact when he saw his stepgrandmother struck and killed by automobile driven by defendant).
71. Kelley v Kokua Sales & Supply, Ltd., 56 Haw. 204, 532 P.2d 673, (1975).
72. Hair v County of Monterey, 45 Cal. App.3d 538, 119 Cal. Rptr. 640 (1975) (no recovery for parents mental distress from witnessing their child's serious and permanent injuries after oral surgery); Jansen v Children's Hosp. Medical Center, 31 Cal. App.3d 23, 106 Cal. Rptr. 884 (1973) (visibility to mother of progressive decline and death of five-year-old daughter, allegedly caused by hospital's malpractice, not sufficient for recovery for emotional shock absent physical proximity to accident).
73. Mobaldi v Bd. of Regents of University of California, 55 Cal. App.3d 573, 127 Cal. Rptr. 720 (1976) (foster mother had cause of action for alleged emotional trauma occurring when foster child, after receiving incorrect dosage in glucose injection before pyelogram, became spastic, convulsant and comatose in her arms); Huber v Aengst, 28 Citation 88 (1974), (Cal. Super. Ct., Los Angeles Co., Docket No. NEC 12214, May 17, 1973) (mother allowed to recover for her emotional distress caused when son choked to death in her arms).
74. Justus v Atchinson, 139 Cal. Rptr. 97 (1977).
75. See Howard v Lecher, 53 App. Div.2d 420, 425–431, 436–437, 386 N.Y.S.2d 460, 463–467, 470–471 (1976) (Margett, J., dissenting). Cf. Howard v Lecher, 42 N.Y.2d 109, 116, 397 N.Y.S.2d 363, 368, 366 N.E.2d 64, 68 (1977) (Cooke, J., dissenting) (would limit cause of action to mother, since physician owed no direct duty of care to father).
76. 57 App. Div.2d 73, 394 N.Y.S.2d 933 (1977).
77. Id at 77, 394 N.Y.S.2d at 936.
78. See eg Johnson v New York, 37 N.Y.2d 378, 372 N.Y.S.2d 638, 334 N.E.2d 590 (1975).
79. 53 App. Div.2d 420, 386 N.Y.S.2d 460 (1976).
80. 60 App. Div.2d 80, 400 N.Y.S.2d 110 (1977).
81. Id at 84, 400 N.Y.S.2d at 112.
82. Id at 84–85, 400 N.Y.S.2d at 112.
83. See eg, Johnson v Yeshiva University, 42 N.Y.2d 818, 364 N.F.2d 1340, 396 N.Y.S.2d 647 (1977) (sustaining judgment for defendants on ground that plaintiffs had not established negligence in failure to perform amniocentesis in 1969 to detect cri-du-chat syndrome).

84. Judges Rabin and Margett (the latter having authored the dissent in Howard v Lecher, in which Judge Damiani joined) concurred in the opinion; Judge Cohalan concurred in upholding the child's claim for "wrongful life" but he would have dismissed the parents' claims for their own damages; and Judge Titone, who had written for the Appellate Division in Howard, dissented on all counts.

85. 60 App. Div.2d at 86, 400 N.Y.S.2d at 113.

86. Id.

87. 24 N.Y.2d 609, 301 N.Y.S.2d 554, N.E.2d 419 (1969).

88. Palsgraf v Long Island Railroad Co., 248 N.Y.339, 162 N.E. 99 (1928).

89. See Capron A: Informed Consent in Catastrophic Disease Research and Treatment. Univ Pa L Rev 123:340, 407–414, 1974, which argues that the position adopted in a number of informed consent cases that materiality is determined by what a reasonable patient would want to know undercuts the very logic of these cases and robs the patient of "the undisputed right . . . to receive information which will enable him to make a choice." Wilkinson v Vesey, 110 R.I. 606, 625, 295 A.2d 676, 688 (1972).

90. See Capron, supra note 89; Riskin L: Informed Consent — Looking for the Action. Univ Ill L Forum 1975; 580, 600–606, 1975.

91. Birnbaum SL, Rheingold PD: 1976 Survey of New York Law — Torts. Syracuse L Rev 28:525, 559–566, 1977; Katz LG: Howard v Lecher: An Unreasonable Limitation on Physician's Liability in a Wrongful Life Suit. New Engl L Rev 12:819, 833–840, 1977; Case Note, Albany L Rev 41:162, 170–172, 1977 (all reviewing Appellate Division opinion in Howard).

92. Capron AM: Informed Decisionmaking in Genetic Counseling: A Dissent to the "Wrongful Life" Debate. Indiana L J 48:581, 589–593, 1973. See also note 39 supra.

93. Committee for the Study of Inborn Errors of Metabolism: Genetic Screening — Programs, Principles and Research. Washington: National Academy of Sciences, 1975, pp 185–186.

94. 60 App. Div.2d 80, 400 N.Y.S.2d 110 (1977).

Index